Hidden and Lesser-known Disordered Eating Behaviors in Medical and Psychiatric Conditions

Emilia Manzato • Massimo Cuzzolaro
Lorenzo Maria Donini
Editors

Hidden and Lesser-known Disordered Eating Behaviors in Medical and Psychiatric Conditions

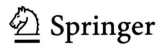

Editors
Emilia Manzato
Private Hospital "Salus" of Ferrara
University of Ferrara
Ferrara, Italy

Massimo Cuzzolaro
Formerly Sapienza University of Rome
Founding Editor of Eating and Weight Disorders
Campiglia Marittima, Livorno, Italy

Lorenzo Maria Donini
Experimental Medicine Department
Sapienza University of Rome, Editor-in-Chief of Eating and Weight Disorders
Roma, Roma, Italy

ISBN 978-3-030-81173-0   ISBN 978-3-030-81174-7   (eBook)
https://doi.org/10.1007/978-3-030-81174-7

© Springer Nature Switzerland AG 2022

This work is subject to copyright. All rights are reserved by the Publisher, whether the whole or part of the material is concerned, specifically the rights of translation, reprinting, reuse of illustrations, recitation, broadcasting, reproduction on microfilms or in any other physical way, and transmission or information storage and retrieval, electronic adaptation, computer software, or by similar or dissimilar methodology now known or hereafter developed.

The use of general descriptive names, registered names, trademarks, service marks, etc. in this publication does not imply, even in the absence of a specific statement, that such names are exempt from the relevant protective laws and regulations and therefore free for general use.

The publisher, the authors, and the editors are safe to assume that the advice and information in this book are believed to be true and accurate at the date of publication. Neither the publisher nor the authors or the editors give a warranty, express or implied, with respect to the material contained herein or for any errors or omissions that may have been made. The publisher remains neutral with regard to jurisdictional claims in published maps and institutional affiliations.

This Springer imprint is published by the registered company Springer Nature Switzerland AG
The registered company address is: Gewerbestrasse 11, 6330 Cham, Switzerland

Preface

At the beginning of the third decade of the twenty-first century, the two major psychiatric classifications—DSM-5 [1] and Chapter VI of ICD-11 [2]—include in the field of feeding or eating disorders (FEDs) six main diagnostic categories (anorexia nervosa, bulimia nervosa, binge eating disorder, avoidant-restrictive food intake disorder, pica, rumination-regurgitation disorder) and two residual categories (other specified feeding or eating disorders, and feeding or eating disorders, unspecified).

In this group (FEDs), both taxonomies gather abnormal and harmful eating behaviors that are not explained by other pathological conditions, are not typical of a specific developmental stage, and do not depend on religious or cultural rules.

The 37 chapters of this book describe several hidden and lesser-known disordered eating behaviors that pose the clinicians with problems of recognition and assessment and require specific interventions for treatment and prevention. The authors attempted to offer a synthesis of knowledge useful to physicians, nutritionists, psychiatrists, and psychologists.

Abnormalities in eating and weight control behaviors can occur in the course of many medical and psychiatric conditions. In some cases, they meet the diagnostic criteria given for the six major FEDs, but in other cases, they do not. Always, however, they affect the course and outcome of associated diseases and disorders and contribute to impairment of personal and family quality of life. Twenty-five chapters address these issues:

- addictive disorders (Chap. 6)
- post-traumatic disorders (Chap. 7)
- psychotropic drug-induced disordered eating behaviors (Chap. 8)
- disordered eating behaviors in other psychiatric disorders (Chap. 9)
- drunkorexia (Chap. 11)
- post-bariatric disordered eating behaviors (Chap. 12)
- achalasia (Chap. 18)
- cancer (Chap. 19)
- celiac disease (Chap. 20)
- craniopharyngioma (Chap. 21)
- cyclic vomiting syndrome (Chap. 22)
- cystic fibrosis (Chap. 23)
- type 2 diabetes (Chap. 24)

- type 1 diabetes (Chap. 25)
- food allergies (Chap. 26)
- Hirschsprung's disease (Chap. 27)
- hypermobility spectrum disorders. Ehlers–Danlos syndrome (Chap. 28)
- Kleine-Levin syndrome (Chap. 29)
- Klinefelter syndrome (Chap. 30)
- Parkinson's disease (Chap. 31)
- polycystic ovary syndrome (Chap. 32)
- Prader-Willi syndrome (Chap. 33)
- Turner syndrome (Chap. 34)
- non-HIV lipodystrophy (Chap. 35)
- androgen insensitivity syndrome (Chap. 37)

Age of life, sex at birth, gender identity, sexual desire orientation, physical activity, and sports are closely related to body image, body weight control, and eating behavior [3]. Here is a list of chapters that address these issues:

- muscle dysmorphia (Chap. 1)
- infants and toddlers (Chap. 2)
- males (Chap. 3)
- midlife and old age (Chap. 4)
- sexual and gender minorities (Chap. 5)
- avoidant/restrictive food intake disorder in adults (Chap. 10)
- adipositas athletica (Chap. 36)
- anorexia athletica (Chap. 36)

Finally, some chapters are devoted to disorders that generally receive less attention than anorexia nervosa, bulimia nervosa, and binge eating disorder, and to symptomatic pictures that DSM-5 and ICD-11 classify as other specified feeding or eating disorders:

- night-eating syndrome and nocturnal sleep-related eating disorder (Chap. 13)
- orthorexia nervosa (Chap. 14)
- pica (Chap. 15)
- purging disorder (Chap. 16)
- rumination disorder (Chap. 17)
- chewing and spitting (Chap. 36)
- eating disorders by proxy (Chap. 36)
- emetophobia (Chap. 36)
- picky eating (Chap. 36)

This volume is not intended to expand the number of FEDs.

DSM-5 and ICD-11 list an increasing number of psychiatric diagnostic categories and treat them as morbid entities separated by natural, time-stable boundaries. For years now, the critique of current psychiatric classifications and diagnostic crystallizations has led toward a transdiagnostic view, more focused on the evolution of pathological phenomena observed during the same individual's lifetime. It is a position proposed to both researchers and clinicians to redefine the concepts of diagnosis and comorbidity in psychopathology.

Moreover, longitudinal epidemiological studies suggest that the major psychiatric syndromes, including FEDs, appear in 75% of cases at a young age (before 24 years) and, over time, in the same individual, different symptoms tend to associate, transform, replace each other (fluid comorbidity) [4–8].

Some supporters of the transdiagnostic paradigm take their cue from the medical model of *clinical staging* [9]. It consists of following the clinical manifestations along the axes of the *progression* of symptoms (worsening, persistence, recurrence, partial, or total remission) and of the *extension* of the pathology with other psychic and somatic manifestations, which are associated or succeed each other, with new symptoms, complications, and consequences.

The purpose of this volume is to widen the angle of view on disturbed eating behaviors.

References

1. American Psychiatric Association DSM-5 Task Force. Diagnostic and statistical manual of mental disorders, DSM-5™, 5th ed. Arlington, VA: American Psychiatric Publishing, Inc.; 2013.
2. World Health Organization. ICD-11, International classification of diseases for mortality and morbidity statistics. Geneva: World Health Organization; 2019. https://icd.who.int/browse11/l-m/en. Accessed 11 Dec 2020.
3. Cuzzolaro M, Fassino S, editors. Body image, eating, and weight. Cham: Springer; 2018.
4. Kessler RC, Berglund P, Demler O, Jin R, Merikangas KR, Walters EE. Lifetime prevalence and age-of-onset distributions of DSM-IV disorders in the National comorbidity survey replication. Arch General Psychiatry. 2005;62(6):593–602.
5. Uhlhaas PJ, McGorry PD, Wood SJ. Toward a paradigm for youth mental health. JAMA Psychiatry. 2021;78(5):473–4.
6. Keski-Rahkonen A, Mustelin L. Epidemiology of eating disorders in Europe: prevalence, incidence, comorbidity, course, consequences, and risk factors. Curr Opin Psychiatry. 2016;29(6):340–5.
7. Caspi A, Houts RM, Ambler A, Danese A, Elliott ML, Hariri A, et al. Longitudinal assessment of mental health disorders and comorbidities across 4 decades among participants in the Dunedin birth cohort study. JAMA Netw Open. 2020;3(4):e203221.

8. Plana-Ripoll O, Pedersen C, Holtz Y, et al. Exploring comorbidity within mental disorders among a Danish national population. JAMA Psychiatry. 2019;76(3):259–70.
9. Shah JL, Scott J, McGorry PD, Cross SPM, Keshavan MS, Nelson B, et al. Transdiagnostic clinical staging in youth mental health: a first international consensus statement. World Psychiatry. 2020;19(2):233–42.

Ferrara, Italy Emilia Manzato
Campiglia Marittima, Italy Massimo Cuzzolaro
Rome, Italy Lorenzo Maria Donini

Contents

1 **Muscle Dysmorphia and Disordered Eating Behavior** 1
   Stuart B. Murray and Rachel F. Rodgers

2 **Eating Disorders in Infants and Toddlers**....................... 5
   Antonia Parmeggiani and Jacopo Pruccoli

3 **Eating Disorders in Males** 15
   Giovanni Gravina, Malvina Gualandi, and Emilia Manzato

4 **Eating Disorders in Midlife and in the Elderly** 23
   Emilia Manzato and Eleonora Roncarati

5 **Eating and Weight Disorders in Sexual and Gender Minorities** 33
   Massimo Cuzzolaro

6 **Food and Addictions**.. 49
   Umberto Nizzoli

7 **Post-Traumatic Eating Disorder** 63
   Romana Schumann, Valentina Fasoli, and Chiara Mazzoni

8 **Psychotropic Drug-Induced Disordered Eating Behaviors**.......... 77
   Enrica Marzola, Maria Musso, and Giovanni Abbate-Daga

9 **Disordered Eating Behaviors in Other Psychiatric Disorders** 87
   Anna Rita Atti, Maurizio Speciani, and Diana De Ronchi

10 **Avoidant/Restrictive Food Intake Disorder (ARFID) in Adults**...... 103
   Patrizia Todisco

11 **Drunkorexia**... 123
   Crystal D. Oberle

12 **Eating Disorders and Bariatric Surgery**........................ 129
   Donatella Ballardini, Livia Pozzi, Elena Dapporto, and Elena Tomba

13 **Night Eating Syndrome and Nocturnal Sleep-Related Eating Disorder**... 147
   Caterina Lombardo and Silvia Cerolini

14 When "Healthy" Is Taken Too Far: Orthorexia
    Nervosa—Current State, Controversies and Future Directions 159
    Valeria Galfano, Elena V. Syurina, Martina Valente,
    and Lorenzo M. Donini

15 Pica 177
    Alexandra Höger and Andrea Sabrina Hartmann

16 Purging Disorder 185
    Norbert Quadflieg

17 Rumination Disorder 193
    C. Laird Birmingham

18 Achalasia and Disordered Eating Behaviours 199
    Aurélie Letranchant

19 Cancer and Disordered Eating Behavior: The Issue of Anorexia 207
    Alessio Molfino, Maria Ida Amabile, Giovanni Imbimbo,
    Antonella Giorgi, and Maurizio Muscaritoli

20 Celiac Disease and Eating and Weight Disorders 217
    Patrizia Calella and Giuliana Valerio

21 Craniopharyngioma and Eating Disorders 223
    Marta Bondanelli, Emilia Manzato, Irene Gagliardi,
    and Maria Rosaria Ambrosio

22 Cyclic Vomiting Syndrome 233
    Toshiyuki Hikita

23 Current Knowledge on Eating Experiences and Behaviours
    in Cystic Fibrosis: Exploring the Challenges and Potential
    Opportunities for Interventions 239
    Helen Egan and Michail Mantzios

24 Type 2 Diabetes and Eating Disorders 247
    Walter Milano

25 Type 1 Diabetes and Disordered Eating Behavior 253
    Rita Francisco

26 Food Allergies 261
    Elaine Kathleen Tyndall and Fabrizio Jacoangeli

27 Hirschsprung Disease and Eating Disorders 273
    Anna I. Guerdjikova, Francisco Romo-Nava, and Susan L. McElroy

28	**Hypermobility Spectrum Disorders/Ehlers–Danlos Syndrome and Disordered Eating Behavior**................ 279 Carolina Baeza-Velasco, Paola Espinoza, Antonio Bulbena, Andrea Bulbena-Cabré, Maude Seneque, and Sebastien Guillaume	
29	**Kleine–Levin Syndrome and Eating and Weight Disorders**......... 287 Antonio F. Radicioni, Chiara Tarantino, and Matteo Spaziani	
30	**Klinefelter Syndrome and Eating and Weight Disorders**........... 293 Antonio F. Radicioni and Matteo Spaziani	
31	**Parkinson's Disease and Eating and Weight Disorders**............ 299 Massimo Cuzzolaro and Nazario Melchionda	
32	**Polycystic Ovary Syndrome and Eating and Weight Disorders**...... 313 Francesco Pallotti and Francesco Lombardo	
33	**Prader-Willi Syndrome and Eating and Weight Disorders**......... 319 Massimo Cuzzolaro	
34	**Turner's Syndrome and Eating and Weight Disorders**............ 333 Massimo Cuzzolaro	
35	**Eating Behavior and Psychopathology in Non-HIV Lipodystrophic Patients**...................................... 347 Federica Ferrari, Pasquale Fabio Calabrò, Giovanni Ceccarini, and Ferruccio Santini	
36	**Adipositas Athletica, Anorexia Athletica, Chewing and Spitting, Eating Disorders by Proxy, Emetophobia, Picky Eating ... Symptoms, Syndromes, or What?**............................. 357 Massimo Cuzzolaro	
37	**CAIS Syndrome and Eating and Weight Disorders**............... 379 Emilia Manzato and Malvina Gualandi	

Muscle Dysmorphia and Disordered Eating Behavior

Stuart B. Murray and Rachel F. Rodgers

1.1 Introduction

Muscle dysmorphia (MD) is a relatively recently identified psychiatric phenotype which encapsulates the pathological pursuit of muscularity and a pervasive belief that one is of insufficient muscularity [1]. Crucially, the belief around insufficient muscularity is not related to one's actual degree of muscularity, and MD has often observed in those with a range of physiological dimensions, even those with ostensibly large muscularity, suggesting a degree of body image distortion in MD. Behaviorally, the hallmark feature of MD relates to (i) excessive working out and muscle-building endeavors and (ii) muscularity-oriented disordered eating—pathological eating patterns which aim to optimize muscular development. Extreme anxiety is often reported if either gym-related or dietary regimens are disrupted, and case reports have reported men resigning from professional jobs that interfere with rigorous workout or dietary regimens, continuing intensive muscle-building regimens despite serious injury, and not attending important social events (e.g., best friend's wedding) if the food available did not support dietary ideals [2]. Importantly, MD is also associated with elicit androgenic anabolic steroid use [3] and elevated rates of suicidality [4].

S. B. Murray
Department of Psychiatry and Behavioral Sciences, University of Southern California, California, USA
e-mail: stuart.murray@ucsf.edu

R. F. Rodgers (✉)
Department of Applied Psychology, Northeastern University, Boston, USA

Department of Psychiatric Emergency & Acute Care, Lapeyronie Hospital, Montpellier, France
e-mail: r.rodgers@northeastern.edu

© Springer Nature Switzerland AG 2022
E. Manzato et al. (eds.), *Hidden and Lesser-known Disordered Eating Behaviors in Medical and Psychiatric Conditions*,
https://doi.org/10.1007/978-3-030-81174-7_1

1.2 Characteristics

Phenomenologically, MD was originally conceptualized as a reverse form of anorexia nervosa [5], owing to its similarity with anorexia nervosa, including rigid dietary and exercise-related practices in pursuit of opposing extremes of body ideals, body image distortion, high diagnostic crossover, and similar psychological profiles [2, 3]. However, MD was reconceptualized as a body dysmorphic disorder phenotype and re-termed muscle dysmorphia, in 1997, owing to the centrality of muscularity concerns. Specifically, it was thought that since muscularity cannot be developed without muscle-building exercises, exercise must therefore be the primary pathogen and eating practices were peripheral, meaning therefore that MD could not be considered an eating disorder phenotype. However, an abundance of research has now illustrated the centrality of disordered eating practices in MD [3, 6–8]. Notwithstanding, MD is currently conceptualized as a body dysmorphic disorder subtype in DSM-5 [9], a classification that has been supported through recent meta-analytic work [10].

1.3 Epidemiology and Prevalence

In the last few years, the number of studies examining the rates and prevalence of MD symptoms has multiplied. Due to substantial methodological limitations, previous estimates had ranged extremely widely, from 1% to over 50% [11]. Recent studies have reported more conservative rates with clear gender differences, with estimates of 5% (7.0% of men and 3.4% of women) of a mixed gender sample of Italian students [12] and 7% of male students from Buenos Aires [13]. In another study of US entry-level military personnel, MD was reported by 12.7% of males and 4.2% of females [14]. Large-scale population studies on MD are currently lacking, and additional epidemiological investigations are warranted.

1.4 Correlates

Perhaps the most robust correlate of muscle dysmorphia is eating psychopathology, as confirmed through meta-analysis [15]. In addition to this, robust associations have been found with obsessive-compulsive symptomatology [2].

Given the central role of body image concerns in muscle dysmorphia, it has been conceptualized within the growing emphasis on extreme muscularity as an important dimension of appearance ideals for men and growing pressures on men to pursue the lean-and-muscular ideal. Consistent with this, biopsychosociocultural theories have been used with some success to frame investigations of the correlates of muscle dysmorphia [16]. In this way, muscle dysmorphia has been found to be associated with sociocultural dimensions including the internalization of the lean-and-muscular ideal, as well as media and interpersonal appearance pressures and influences and appearance comparison [16–19]. Psychological dimensions such as low self-esteem, perfectionism, and negative affect have also been found to be associated with muscle dysmorphia symptoms [16]. Evidence for the role of body weight or pubertal development, frequently considered biological dimensions, has been more mixed. Nevertheless, overall a number of psychological and sociocultural dimensions have been supported as important correlates.

More recently, these theoretical frameworks have been expanded to include gendered aspects of muscle dysmorphia, building on the centrality of muscularity in masculinity. Such integrated approaches highlight, for example, the role of self-objectification, a construct initially developed to describe the process through which female bodies were reduced to objects in contemporary culture and the male gaze, but expanded to account for the increasing importance placed upon male appearance ideals. Among men, self-objectification, that is, the adoption of an external objectifying perspective, has been found to be associated with muscle dysmorphia [20]. Interestingly, and consistent with muscularity as a core element of masculinity, among women, muscle dysmorphia has been found to be associated with several dimensions of gender role stress, while these relationships were less evident among men [18].

1.5 Treatment

At present, the evidence base relating to the treatment of muscle dysmorphia remains sparse. Owing to the challenges around its diagnostic conceptualization, frequent misdiagnosis, and the notion that symptomatology is often socially endorsed and ego-syntonic, few controlled treatment studies exist. To date, the only treatment study of MD is a case study of one male adolescent patient, who was treated with a modified form of family-based treatment [21]. This treatment, as in family-based treatment for restrictive eating disorders [22], involved the central leveraging of parental support in directly intervening into the adolescent's behavioral symptom profile. In this case, however, parents were charged with the task of ensuring the adolescent did not compulsively screen the protein content of foods he consumed or compulsively engage in muscle-building exercise practices [23]. In concert with this clinical treatment study, prevention studies have successfully aimed to disrupt muscularity-oriented body dissatisfaction [24], and while this out not to be conflated with MD, these efforts may nevertheless form a critical component in the efforts to ameliorate MD psychopathology.

1.6 Conclusion

MD is a devastating illness which renders broad impairments to quality of life and functioning and has been linked to elevated suicidality. With this increasing awareness of the dangers associated with MD, alongside a steadily increasing prevalence, focused efforts must now go toward the development of evidence-based treatment approaches.

References

1. Pope HG Jr, et al. Muscle dysmorphia: an underrecognized form of body dysmorphic disorder. Psychosomatics. 1997;38(6):548–57.
2. Murray SB, et al. Muscle dysmorphia and the DSM-V conundrum: where does it belong? A review paper. Int J Eat Disord. 2010;43(6):483–91.
3. Murray SB, et al. A comparison of eating, exercise, shape, and weight related symptomatology in males with muscle dysmorphia and anorexia nervosa. Body Image. 2012;9(2):193–200.
4. Pope CG, et al. Clinical features of muscle dysmorphia among males with body dysmorphic disorder. Body Image. 2005;2(4):395–400.
5. Pope HG Jr, Katz DL, Hudson JI. Anorexia nervosa and "reverse anorexia" among 108 male bodybuilders. Compr Psychiatry. 1993;34(6):406–9.
6. Murray SB, Rieger E, Touyz SW. Muscle dysmorphia symptomatology during a period of religious fasting: a case report. Eur Eat Disord Rev. 2011;19(2):162–8.
7. Murray SB, Griffiths S, Mond JM. Evolving eating disorder psychopathology: conceptualising muscularity-oriented disordered eating. Br J Psychiatry. 2018;208(5):414–5.
8. Murray SB, et al. The emotional regulatory features of bulimic episodes and compulsive exercise in muscle dysmorphia: a case report. Eur Eat Disord Rev. 2012;20(1):68–73.
9. American Psychiatric Association. Diagnostic and statistical manual of mental disorders, 5th ed. Arlington: American Psychiatric Association, 2013.
10. Cooper M, et al. Muscle dysmorphia: a systematic and meta-analytic review of the literature to assess diagnostic validity. Int J Eat Disord. 2020;53(10):1583–604.
11. Tod D, Edwards C, Cranswick I. Muscle dysmorphia: current insights. Psychol Res Behav Manag. 2016;9:179.
12. Gorrasi ISR, et al. Traits of orthorexia nervosa and muscle dysmorphia in Italian university students: a multicentre study. Eat Weight Disord. 2020;25(5):1413–23.
13. Compte EJ, Sepulveda AR, Torrente F. A two-stage epidemiological study of eating disorders and muscle dysmorphia in male university students in Buenos Aires. Int J Eat Disord. 2015;48(8):1092–101.
14. Campagna JDA, Bowsher B. Prevalence of body dysmorphic disorder and muscle dysmorphia among entry-level military personnel. Mil Med. 2016;181(5):494–501.
15. Badenes-Ribera L, et al. The association between muscle dysmorphia and eating disorder symptomatology: a systematic review and meta-analysis. J Behav Addict. 2019;8(3):351–71.
16. Tod D, Lavallee D. Towards a conceptual understanding of muscle dysmorphia development and sustainment. Int Rev Sport Exerc Psychol. 2010;3(2):111–31.
17. Diehl BJ, Baghurst T. Biopsychosocial factors in drives for muscularity and muscle dysmorphia among personal trainers. Cogent Psychol. 2016;3(1):1243194.
18. Readdy T, Cardinal BJ, Watkins PL. Muscle dysmorphia, gender role stress, and sociocultural influences: an exploratory study. Res Q Exerc Sport. 2011;82(2):310–9.
19. Compte EJ, Sepúlveda AR, Torrente F. Approximations to an integrated model of eating disorders and muscle dysmorphia among university male students in Argentina. Men Masculin. 2018:1097184X17753039.
20. Heath B, et al. The relationship between objectification theory and muscle dysmorphia characteristics in men. Psychol Men Masculin. 2016;17(3):297.
21. Murray SB, Griffiths S. Adolescent muscle dysmorphia and family-based treatment: a case report. Clin Child Psychol Psychiatry. 2014;20(2):324–30.
22. Lock J, Le Grange D. Treatment manual for anorexia nervosa: a family-based approach. New York: Guilford Publications; 2015.
23. Murray S, Griffiths S. Muscle dysmorphia and family-based treatment: a preliminary case report. Clin Child Psychol Psychiatry. 2015;20(324):e30.
24. Brown TA, et al. A randomized controlled trial of The Body Project: more than muscles for men with body dissatisfaction. Int J Eat Disord. 2017;50(8):873–83.

Eating Disorders in Infants and Toddlers

Antonia Parmeggiani and Jacopo Pruccoli

2.1 Introduction

Parents frequently refer to medical attention reporting that their children eat poorly. Commonly this trouble does not represent a severe problem; however, in a small percentage of cases, children may present significant feeding difficulties. Paediatricians and child neuropsychiatrists should be informed about these disorders in order to support parents by offering appropriate guidance and treatments.

In this chapter, the authors will consider feeding disorders (FD) and eating disorders (ED) in infants and toddlers and describe their main features and variables. They will also describe the characteristics of ED in a neurodevelopmental disorder, namely, autism spectrum disorder [1].

2.2 Nutrition, Eating Behaviour and Feeding Difficulties/Disorders

Eating behaviour, together with sleep, represents an important function of regulation in infancy. The development of adequate feeding and eating functions relies on the proper integration of a range of physical and psychological competencies. Feeding represents a critical source of interaction between caregivers and their child in the first years of life, particularly for children with neuropsychiatric disabilities [2]. FD in infancy result from impairments in developmental milestones needed to

---

A. Parmeggiani (✉) · J. Pruccoli
IRCCS Istituto delle Scienze Neurologiche di Bologna, Centro Regionale per i Disturbi della Nutrizione e dell'Alimentazione in Età Evolutiva, Child Neurology and Psychiatry Unit, Bologna, Italy

Dipartimento di Scienze Mediche e Chirurgiche (DIMEC), Università di Bologna, Bologna, Italy
e-mail: antonia.parmeggiani@unibo.it; jacopo.pruccoli@studio.unibo.it

achieve proper eating skills [3]. FD might be the result of a lack of balance among parents' feeding style, organic causes, and child behaviour. FD present themselves on a clinical spectrum from mild to severe and are characterized by food refusal, lower amount of food intake or a more significant food selectivity than that appropriate for the age. FD have a prevalence among children in western countries around 20–30%, including cases misperceived by parents [4], and they represent a risk factor for severe long-lasting physical and psychosocial morbidity. Recurrence of severe FD/ED during lifetime is around 1–5% [5].

Problems of feeding in children encompass a broad range of conditions. Notably, paediatric patients display malnourishment more quickly than adults, causing negative effects of prolonged malnutrition on their growth and development. Physicians should consider that a FD in infancy could lead up to an ED in adolescence and in adulthood.

Nowadays, in developed countries, nutrient deficiencies may be a consequence of inflammatory bowel diseases, chronic diarrhoea, cystic fibrosis, congenital heart defects, prematurity, intestinal failure, liver diseases, chylothorax, cancer, poor wound healing, metabolic dysfunction, food allergies, gastroesophageal reflux disease, esophagitis, macroglossia, etc. [5, 6]. But they may also be a consequence of an inappropriate dietary intake in children without a balanced support of mineral/vitamins [7]. Feeding problems or dysphagia is seen in up to 25% of all children in developed countries. Prematurely born children present an increased prevalence of swallowing disorders, developmental disorders and cerebral palsy [8–10].

Literature reports a number of medical definitions for feeding difficulties, such as neophobia (food rejection), picky eating (fussy children) and avoidant/restrictive food intake disorder (ARFID), a newly introduced diagnosis in the DSM-5 [11].

An exhaustive medical approach to patients reporting FD should include a detailed anamnesis, physical and neurological examinations, dietary assessment and appropriate exams regarding possible organic failure. Dysphagia or swallowing in children with premature birth, cerebral palsy or metabolic diseases should always be considered. Once organic disorders have been ruled out, physicians should consider non-organic aetiologies: incorrect feeding behaviours as selective intake, fear of feeding, low food intake or even food refusal may be present. Behavioural problems may coexist. Clinicians should investigate early depressive mood or psychosocial deprivation, including maternal depression. Physicians should examine the interaction between child and caregivers during mealtimes, postpartum depression of the mother, selective food intake in parents and mood disorders. Whenever a patient is diagnosed with a FD, physicians should provide a thorough assessment by a multidisciplinary team, including paediatricians, child neuropsychiatrists, nutritionists, psychologists and speech pathologists.

2.3 Classification of FD and ED in Infants and Toddlers

Classifications of FD in infancy have formerly established a rigorous dichotomy between organic and nonorganic failure to thrive [12] by separating medically diagnosable causes from infant and maternal psychopathology. Later studies have raised concerns regarding this distinction as being misleading and rarely possible in practice [13, 14].

In 1994, the DSM-IV presented "Feeding Disorder of Infancy and Early Childhood" as a new diagnostic category, not modified in the DSM-IV-TR [15]. This disorder was defined by persistent failure to eat adequately, with significant failure to gain weight or significant loss of weight over at least 1 month. This disturbance was not caused either by an associated gastrointestinal or other medical condition or accounted another mental disorder or lack of available food. The onset was before the age of 6 [16]. In 2002, Chatoor expanded this diagnostic entity and identified six subgroups of "Feeding Behaviour Disorders" in the first 3 years of life [17]. This new classification was adopted by the Diagnostic Classification of Mental Health and Developmental Disorders of Infancy and Early Childhood (DC:0-3) [18], recently updated to a new version (DC:0-5). In DC:0-5, eating disorders are distinguished according to observed pathologic eating behaviours, rather than to hypothetic aetiologies, and eating disorders of infancy/early childhood are classified as overeating disorder, undereating disorder and atypical eating disorder (hoarding, pica and rumination) [19]. The target of this classification system is to evidence developmental differences in psychopathological descriptions and to separate pathological conditions from transient, age-related behaviours [20].

In 2013, the DSM-5 presented "Feeding and Eating Disorders" in one chapter, providing diagnostic criteria for pica, rumination disorder, ARFID, anorexia nervosa, bulimia nervosa, binge-eating disorder, other specified feeding or eating disorder and unspecified feeding or eating disorder [11]. In infancy and in childhood, these eight categories of FD/ED may all occur. In fact, cases in individuals younger than 13 years of age are reported in literature [21]. With regard to FD in infancy, the main innovation brought by DSM-5 consists in replacing the former DSM-IV-TR "Feeding Disorder of Infancy and Early Childhood" with ARFID as an entirely new diagnosis. The diagnosis of ARFID has no age restriction. Consistent with the DSM-5, the latest version of the International Classification of Diseases and Related Health Problems (ICD 11) includes ARFID as a new diagnosis, replacing the former ICD 10 "Feeding disorder of infancy and childhood" [22]. ARFID being a relatively newly defined diagnostic category, further research should provide deeper knowledge about the disorder and potential subtypes [21].

2.3.1 ARFID

The main diagnostic feature of ARFID is avoidant or restrictive eating behaviour, with persistent difficulty in meeting nutritional needs. Patients with ARFID manifest a series of clinical features as a result of their eating behaviour disturbance. Notably, ARFID is associated with significant weight loss, or infants may show failure to achieve weight or height as expected from their developmental trajectory. Clinical and laboratory assessments may reveal significant nutritional deficiencies causing anaemia, hypothermia, bradycardia and low bone mineral density [23]. Patients frequently develop dependence on enteral feeding or oral nutritional supplements, involving hospitalization. The DSM-5 criteria require that ARFID should not be explained with lack of available food or associated cultural practices. Different from anorexia nervosa, a diagnosis of ARFID requires physicians to rule out a significant disturbance in body weight or shape perception. Lastly, no medical or psychiatric condition should provide a better explanation of the eating disturbance [11, 22, 24].

Literature does not report data on population-based incidence and prevalence rates for ARFID in infants and toddlers. A review conducted in 19 paediatric gastroenterology clinics in the United States found 33 patients out of 2231 (1.5%) meeting diagnostic criteria for ARFID [25]. Further studies investigated prevalence of ARFID among clinical settings specific for ED. The introduction of ARFID as a new diagnosis dramatically reduced the former number of eating disorders not otherwise specified (EDNOS) as classified in DSM-IV [16]. A review of 177 patients treated for ED in Switzerland revealed that 22.5% subjects met DSM-5 criteria for ARFID; in line with other studies, all of these patients would have previously been diagnosed with EDNOS [26]. Literature consistently reports that patients diagnosed with ARFID are younger and male and present greater psychiatric and medical comorbidity compared to another ED [27, 28, 29]. Many studies report higher rates of generalized anxiety, obsessive-compulsive, autism and learning disorders [28, 30]. Congenital malformations, very low birth weight, cerebral palsy and diseases of the gastrointestinal tract may also be associated with a picture similar to ARFID. Consequences of any underlying medical or psychiatric condition may have triggered food aversion. Moreover, DSM-5 criteria neither presuppose nor exclude any aetiology previously and assume that ARFID may occur concurrently with medical or comorbid psychiatric diagnoses, if the feeding or disturbance implies clinical attention beyond that expected for the co-occurring illness [11, 25]. For this reason, to distinguish between medical conditions and ARFID is frequently challenging [31].

When food refusal dominates the clinical picture, a relevant differential diagnosis should be made between ARFID and pervasive refusal syndrome (PRS). Pervasive refusal syndrome is a rare, potentially life-threatening condition, characterized by the following: partial or complete refusal in eating, mobilization, speech and/or personal care; active resistance to help; social/school withdrawal; and clinical conditions requiring hospitalization, in the absence of co-occurring organic or psychiatric conditions. Pervasiveness of symptoms in different domains and rejection of any offer of help may distinguish this condition from ARFID [32].

2.3.2 Autism Spectrum Disorders and FD

Infants with autism spectrum disorders (ASD) experience a variety of developmental, cognitive, medical and behavioural problems. Among these difficulties, FD implicate significant social and biological distress. Ledford and Gast [33] presented the first literature review of FD in ASD, describing rates of prevalence of problematic feeding behaviours from 46% to 89%. The latest meta-analysis on this topic has been published by Sharp, Berry and colleagues [34]. Findings from their study show that children with ASD are five times more likely to manifest FD than their peers without ASD. Recently, possible links between ASD symptomatology and the clinical picture of eating and feeding disorders have been documented in literature. Autistic traits in infancy have been reported by parents of patients with anorexia nervosa (AN). This evidence may suggest that autistic features, documented in patients with AN, pre-exist to the occurrence of eating disorder symptomatology [35].

FD in children with ASD may include deficient motor skills (handling, chewing and swallowing), abnormal sensory processing, gastrointestinal disorders, behavioural problems (obsessive-compulsive or repetitive behaviours, imitation impairment and limited interests), maladaptive mealtime behaviours and food selectivity [1, 36]. FD as selective or scarce feeding may represent a warning early sign suggesting an ASD and are frequently associated with delay or stagnation of development [37]. Earliest alterations may be evident since the 6th month of life [38]. Food selectivity represents the most predominant feeding problem in ASD, affecting approximately 70% of patients; texture, taste, smell and temperature of foods may be involved. Carbohydrates, snack foods and processed foods are usually preferred over vegetables and fruit [39]. Abnormalities in sensory integration, as well as social and familial factors, could play a role in determining feeding difficulties; no definite causal relationship between feeding disorders and ASD, however, has been demonstrated so far [40]. Feeding difficulties among children with ASD have been positively related to parent-reported autism core symptoms, behavioural disorders, sleep difficulties and parental stress [41].

Clinical monitoring of FD among infants with ASD has prominently focused on growth impairment. Yet, literature reports no significant disparity between children with and without ASD concerning height, weight and BMI. Energy intake, as consumption of carbohydrates and fats, is not usually impaired, despite feeding difficulties. Exhaustive nutritional analysis, however, reveals significant distinctive deficits, e.g. lower calcium and protein intake, and suggests susceptibility to multiple long-term complications. Deficits of vitamins A, B12 and D have been documented as well. Thus, relying only on classic anthropometric measurements in children with ASD may reveal regular health status and cover underlying specific nutritional deficits [35].

Recent studies attest to a growing interest in dietary manipulation (e.g. gluten-free casein-free diet, GFCF) for children with ASD. Elimination diets, based on the removal of complex carbohydrates and processed foods, have been documented as well. These interventions have been reported to contribute to dietary insufficiencies and nutritional deficits in children with ASD [42].

Based on this evidence, clinicians should regularly assess nutritional conditions of patients with ASD. Feeding difficulties should be systematically investigated and considered together with the analysis of anthropometric parameters and nutritional deficits or excesses. Furthermore, physicians should inform parents about the potential risks involved in putting children with ASD on an elimination diet or diet modifications [43].

2.3.3 Treatment

FD/ED in infancy show heterogeneous clinical pictures, which encompass medical, behavioural and psychological factors and thus entail individualized and multidisciplinary treatment programmes. Since unaddressed FD frequently persist into adolescence and adulthood, causing multiple complications, early referral for diagnosis and treatment is mandatory.

Currently, literature confirms behavioural therapy as the main empirically supported treatment for FD in paediatrics. Comparative studies have revealed its markedly greater efficacy in improving oral intake, when compared to other non-behavioural interventions [44–46]. Non-behavioural treatments include sensory integration [47], oral-motor exercises and nutritional manipulation [48]. Literature concerning such interventions currently lacks empirical support [49]. A few recent studies have investigated the efficacy of pharmacologic interventions on FD in infancy; low-dose olanzapine [50], cyproheptadine [51] and D-cycloserine [52] have shown promising results. Nonetheless, research on this topic remains limited, and pharmacotherapies continue to be considered as adjunct treatments to behavioural interventions [50].

Concerning ARFID as a specific condition, the recent Canadian guidelines for the treatment of eating disorders indicate that day treatment may provide weight restoration. Cognitive behavioural therapy and atypical antipsychotics represent promising treatments, requiring further research [53]. Concerning PRS, literature lack official guidelines for treatment; a recent report has described the case of a patient successfully treated with cognitive behavioural strategies like prompting, fading, modelling and task analysis [54].

In conclusion, at present, behavioural interventions represent the mainstay of treatment for FD in infancy. Considering the high prevalence of these conditions among paediatric population, additional studies are needed to provide stronger empirical evidence for existing interventions.

2.3.4 Conclusion and Take-Home Message

Feeding represents a complex regulation system. It is one of the most important interactions between a caregiver and a child, which can be affected by many variables. Clinicians should never underestimate feeding difficulties in childhood. They should always carefully consider the medical, dietary and psychosocial history of their young patients to determine any underlying causes for feeding disorders and should utilize anthropometric measurements. Early diagnosis is crucial because FD in infancy may lead up to ED in adolescence and in adulthood and may represent a warning early sign suggesting ASD. Management of a child with FD requires collaborative care of a multi-professional team. Early referral for diagnosis and treatment is mandatory. At present, behavioural therapy is the main supported treatment for FD in childhood. Although recent studies have investigated the efficacy of some drugs, additional studies are needed to provide further evidence for existing treatments.

References

1. Parmeggiani A. Gastrointestinal disorders and autism. In: Patel VB, Preedy VR, Martin CR, editors. Comprehensive guide to autism. Diet and nutrition in autism spectrum disorders. London: Springer; 2014. p. 2035–46.
2. Martini MG, Barona-Martinez M, Micali N. Eating disorders mothers and their children: a systematic review of the literature. Arch Womens Ment Health. 2020 Aug;23(4):449–67.
3. Kabasakal E, Özcebe H, Arslan UE. Eating disorders and needs of disabled children at primary school. Child Care Health Dev. 2020;46(5):637–43.
4. Kerzner B, Milano K, MacLean W, Berall G, Stuart S, Chatoor I. A practical approach to classifying and managing feeding difficulties. Pediatrics. 2015;135(2):344–53.
5. Organic RA. Nonorganic feeding disorders. Ann Nutr Metab. 2015;66(5):16–22.
6. Academy Quality Management Committee and Scope of Practice Subcommittee of Quality Management Committee. Revised 2012 standards of practice in nutrition care and standards of professional performance for registered dietitians. J Acad Nutr Diet. 2013;113(6):S29–45.
7. Goh L, How C, Ng K. Failure to thrive in babies and toddlers. Singapore Med J. 2015;57(06):287–91.
8. Rommel N, van Wijk M, Boets B, Hebbard G, Haslam R, Davidson G, Omari T. Development of pharyngo-esophageal physiology during swallowing in the preterm infant. Neurogastroenterol Motil. 2011;23(10):e401–8.
9. Schieve LA, Tian LH, Rankin K, Kogan MD, Yeargin-Allsopp M, Visser S, Rosenberg D. Population impact of preterm birth and low birth weight on developmental disabilities in US children. Ann Epidemiol. 2016;26(4):267–74.
10. Oskoui M, Coutinho F, Dykeman J, Jetté N, Pringsheim T. An update on the prevalence of cerebral palsy: a systematic review and meta-analysis. Dev Med Child Neurol. 2013;55(6):509–19. Erratum in: Dev Med Child Neurol. 2016;58(3):316.
11. American Psychiatric Association. Diagnostic and statistical manual of mental disorders: diagnostic and statistical manual of mental disorders. 5th ed. Arlington, VA: American Psychiatric Association; 2013.
12. Wittenberg J. Feeding disorders in infancy: classification and treatment considerations. Can J Psychiatry. 1990;35(6):529–33.
13. Reilly S, Skuse D, Wolke D, Stevenson J. Oral-motor dysfunction in children who fail to thrive: organic or non-organic? Dev Med Child Neurol. 2007;41(2):115–22.
14. Manikam R, Perman J. Pediatric feeding disorders. J Clin Gastroenterol. 2000;30(1):34–46.
15. American Psychiatric Association, & American Psychiatric Association. Diagnostic and statistical manual of mental disorders: DSM-IV-TR. Washington, DC: American Psychiatric Association; 2000.
16. American Psychiatric Association. Diagnostic and statistical manual of mental disorders. 4th ed. Washington, DC: American Psychiatric Association; 1994.
17. Chatoor I. Feeding disorders in infants and toddlers: diagnosis and treatment. Child Adolesc Psychiatr Clin N Am. 2002;11(2):163–83.
18. Chatoor I. Diagnosis and treatment of feeding disorders in infants, toddlers, and young children. Washington, DC: Zero to Three; 2009.
19. DC: 0-5 Zero to Three (2016). DC:0-5. Diagnostic classification of mental health and developmental disorders of infancy and early childhood. Washington, DC, Zero to Three (tr. it.: Zero to Three (2018). DC:0-5. Classificazione diagnostica della salute mentale e dei disturbi di sviluppo nell'infanzia Roma, Giovanni Fioriti).
20. Zeanah CH, Carter AS, Cohen J, Egger H, Gleason MM, Keren M, Lieberman A, Mulrooney K, Oser C. Diagnostic classification of mental health and developmental disorders of infancy and early childhood DC:0-5: selective reviews from a new nosology for early childhood psychopathology. Infant Ment Health J. 2016;37(5):471–5.
21. Bryant-Waugh R. Feeding and eating disorders in children. Psychiatr Clin North Am. 2019;42(1):157–67.

22. Claudino A, Pike K, Hay P, Keeley J, Evans S, Rebello T, et al. The classification of feeding and eating disorders in the ICD-11: results of a field study comparing proposed ICD-11 guidelines with existing ICD-10 guidelines. BMC Med. 2019;17(1)
23. Hudson LD, Chapman S. Paediatric medical care for children and young people with eating disorders: achievements and where to next. Clin Child Psychol Psychiatry. 2020;25(3):716–20.
24. Zimmerman J, Fisher M. Avoidant/restrictive food intake disorder (ARFID). Curr Probl Pediatr Adolesc Health Care. 2017;47(4):95–103.
25. Eddy K, Thomas J, Hastings E, Edkins K, Lamont E, Nevins C, et al. Prevalence of DSM-5 avoidant/restrictive food intake disorder in a pediatric gastroenterology healthcare network. Int J Eat Disord. 2014;48(5):464–70.
26. Kurz S, van Dyck Z, Dremmel D, Munsch S, Hilbert A. Early-onset restrictive eating disturbances in primary school boys and girls. Eur Child Adolesc Psychiatry. 2014;24(7):779–85.
27. Zanna V, Criscuolo M, Mereu A, Cinelli G, Marchetto C, Pasqualetti P, Tozzi AE, Castiglioni MC, Chianello I, Vicari S. Restrictive eating disorders in children and adolescents: a comparison between clinical and psychopathological profiles. Eat Weight Disord. 2020;
28. Nicely T, Lane-Loney S, Masciulli E, Hollenbeak C, Ornstein R. Prevalence and characteristics of avoidant/restrictive food intake disorder in a cohort of young patients in day treatment for eating disorders. J Eat Disord. 2014;2(1):21.
29. Norris M, Robinson A, Obeid N, Harrison M, Spettigue W, Henderson K. Exploring avoidant/restrictive food intake disorder in eating disordered patients: a descriptive study. Int J Eat Disord. 2013;47(5):495–9.
30. Fisher M, Rosen D, Ornstein R, Mammel K, Katzman D, Rome E, et al. Characteristics of avoidant/restrictive food intake disorder in children and adolescents: a "new disorder" in DSM-5. J Adolesc Health. 2014;55(1):49–52.
31. Hartdorff C, Kneepkens C, Stok-Akerboom A, van Dijk-Lokkart E, Engels M, Kindermann A. Clinical tube weaning supported by hunger provocation in fully-tube-fed children. J Pediatr Gastroenterol Nutr. 2015;60(4):538–43.
32. Otasowie J, Paraiso A, Bates G. Pervasive refusal syndrome: systematic review of case reports. Eur Child Adolesc Psychiatry. 2020;27:1–13.
33. Ledford J, Gast D. Feeding problems in children with autism spectrum disorders. Focus Autism Other Dev Disabil. 2006;21(3):153–66.
34. Sharp W, Berry R, McCracken C, Nuhu N, Marvel E, Saulnier C, et al. Feeding problems and nutrient intake in children with autism spectrum disorders: a meta-analysis and comprehensive review of the literature. J Autism Dev Disord. 2013;43(9):2159–73.
35. Jacopo Pruccoli, Altea Solari, Letizia Terenzi, Elisabetta Malaspina, Marida Angotti, Veronica Pignataro, Paola Gualandi, Leonardo Sacrato, Duccio Maria Cordelli, Emilio Franzoni, Antonia Parmeggiani. PREPRINT (Version 1) available at Research Square. https://doi.org/10.21203/rs.3.rs-122221/v1.
36. Marí-Bauset S, Zazpe I, Marí-Sanchis A, Llopis-González A, Suárez-Varela M. Anthropometric measurements and nutritional assessment in autism spectrum disorders: a systematic review. Res Autism Spectr Disord. 2015;9:130–43.
37. Parmeggiani A, Corinaldesi A, Posar A. Early features of autism spectrum disorder: a cross-sectional study. Ital J Pediatr. 2019;45(1):144–51.
38. Emond A, Emmett P, Steer C, Golding J. Feeding symptoms, dietary patterns, and growth in young children with autism spectrum disorders. Pediatrics. 2010;126(2):e337–42.
39. Schmitt L, Heiss C, Campbell EA. Comparison of nutrient intake and eating behaviors of boys with and without autism. Top Clini Nutr. 2008;23(1):23–31.
40. Schreck K, Williams K. Food preferences and factors influencing food selectivity for children with autism spectrum disorders. Res Dev Disabil. 2006;27(4):353–63.
41. Allen S, Smith I, Duku E, Vaillancourt T, Szatmari P, Bryson S, et al. Behavioral pediatrics feeding assessment scale in young children with autism spectrum disorder: psychometrics and associations with child and parent variables. J Pediatr Psychol. 2015;40(6):581–90.
42. Cannell J. Autism and vitamin D. Med Hypotheses. 2008;70(4):750–9.

43. Dovey T, Kumari V, Blissett J. Eating behaviour, behavioural problems and sensory profiles of children with avoidant/restrictive food intake disorder (ARFID), autistic spectrum disorders or picky eating: Same or different? Eur Psychiatry. 2019;61:56–62.
44. Benoit S, Davis J, Davidson T. Learned and cognitive controls of food intake. Brain Res. 2010;1350:71–6.
45. Addison L, Piazza C, Patel M, Bachmeyer M, Rivas K, Milnes S, et al. A comparison of sensory integrative and behavioral therapies as treatment for pediatric feeding disorders. J Appl Behav Anal. 2012;45(3):455–71.
46. Peterson C, Becker C, Treasure J, Shafran R, Bryant-Waugh R. The three-legged stool of evidence-based practice in eating disorder treatment: research, clinical, and patient perspectives. BMC Med. 2016;14(1)
47. Arvedson J, Clark H, Lazarus C, Schooling T, Frymark T. The effects of oral-motor exercises on swallowing in children: an evidence-based systematic review. Dev Med Child Neurol. 2010;52(11):1000–13.
48. Edwards C, Walk A, Thompson S, Mullen S, Holscher H, Khan N. Disordered eating attitudes and behavioral and neuroelectric indices of cognitive flexibility in individuals with overweight and obesity. Nutrients. 2018;10(12):1902.
49. Morris N, Knight R, Bruni T, Sayers L, Drayton A. Feeding disorders. Child Adolesc Psychiatr Clin N Am. 2017;26(3):571–86.
50. Brewerton T, D'Agostino M. Adjunctive use of olanzapine in the treatment of avoidant restrictive food intake disorder in children and adolescents in an eating disorders program. J Child Adolesc Psychopharmacol. 2017;27(10):920–2.
51. Sant'Anna A, Hammes P, Porporino M, Martel C, Zygmuntowicz C, Ramsay M. Use of cyproheptadine in young children with feeding difficulties and poor growth in a pediatric feeding program. J Pediatr Gastroenterol Nutr. 2014;59(5):674–8.
52. Sharp W, Volkert V, Scahill L, McCracken C, McElhanon B. A systematic review and meta-analysis of intensive multidisciplinary intervention for pediatric feeding disorders: how standard is the standard of care? J Pediatr. 2017;181:116–124.e4.
53. Couturier J, Isserlin L, Norris M, et al. Canadian practice guidelines for the treatment of children and adolescents with eating disorders. J Eat Disord. 2020;8:4. Published 2020 Feb 1. https://doi.org/10.1186/s40337-020-0277-8.
54. Perrone A, Aruta SF, Crucitti G, et al. Pervasive refusal syndrome or anorexia nervosa: a case report with a successful behavioural treatment. Eat Weight Disord. 2020; https://doi.org/10.1007/s40519-020-00991-8.

Eating Disorders in Males

Giovanni Gravina, Malvina Gualandi, and Emilia Manzato

Eating disorders (EDs) are considered female gender-bound disorders since males appear to be affected by the disease to a lesser extent than females.

Specifically, anorexia nervosa (AN) has been long estimated to be an exclusively female condition, and the diagnostic criteria were tailored on female clinical pictures, considering male AN as a "niche phenomenon."

DSM-5 in 2013 [1] introduced more inclusive and gender-neutral diagnostic criteria especially for AN. In fact, the criterion of amenorrhea (absence of at least three consecutive menstrual cycles) was removed.

Even the evaluation of body mass index was more elastic and evaluated in the context of the nutritional history; therefore, many ED male patients previously included in eating disorders not otherwise specified have been correctly diagnosed and inserted into AN.

Some authors report that 15% AN, 10% bulimia nervosa (BN), and 40% binge-eating disorder (BED) cases involved males. The lifetime prevalence in men is estimated 0.3% for AN, 0.5% for BN, and 2% for BED [2, 3].

G. Gravina (✉)
Eating Disorder Center-Casa di Cura San Rossore Pisa, Pisa, Italy
e-mail: giovagravina@alice.it

M. Gualandi
Day Hospital of Internal Medicine and Eating Disorders, University Hospital S. Anna, Ferrara, Italy
e-mail: malvinagualandi@virgilio.it

E. Manzato
University of Ferrara, Eating and Weight Disorders Center "L'Albero",
Private Hospital "Salus", Ferrara, Italy
e-mail: emilia.manzato@gmail.com

© Springer Nature Switzerland AG 2022
E. Manzato et al. (eds.), *Hidden and Lesser-known Disordered Eating Behaviors in Medical and Psychiatric Conditions*,
https://doi.org/10.1007/978-3-030-81174-7_3

In recent research studies, men represent approximately 10% of the individuals treated for EDs [4], but the percentage of men with EDs may be much higher and underdiagnosed although in recent decades the attention toward EDs in males has grown considerably [5, 6].

Detection of EDs in men is hampered by many factors: the lack of awareness in the family, the scarce training of general practitioners, and the lack of neutrality of diagnostic tools, calibrated on the females.

Furthermore, men may be less likely to seek treatment due to the stereotype that the EDs only affect women [7, 8].

The risk factors, the pathogenesis, and the core symptoms of EDs are quite similar between men and women, even if some significant gender-related differences can be highlighted [9]. These differences mainly concern body image and media pressures, weight history, trauma and sexual abuse, psychiatric comorbidities, and sexual orientation.

In the last decades, the masculine body ideal has changed, due to media exposure to unattainable body images [10] with particular attention to muscle and sculpted body [11, 12] away from the real body, favoring a growing dissatisfaction of the body in males, especially in adolescents. Body dissatisfaction is a relevant risk factor for the ED development in males as well [13, 14].

Furthermore, some research studies suggest that male adolescents can have higher levels of body dissatisfaction than girls [15]. Male ED patients frequently reported overweight or obesity in childhood or in adolescence [16–18]. Compensatory compulsory exercise is used more by men than women, to obtain a muscular body—with a focus particularly on the trunk and shoulders—instead of losing weight as happens in females.

Dieting and compensatory behaviors are the typical symptoms of AN and BN in men, as in females, but physical hyperactivity is more present in males, while laxative and diuretic use as well as self-induced vomiting may be lower than in females [19].

It is important to note that male adolescents have a slower and later pubertal development than females; therefore, occurrence of AN-related malnutrition in adolescence may cause in male gender irreversible complications such as short stature or inadequate peak bone mass.

Psychiatric comorbidity for AN and BN in males has the same high rates of anxiety, depression, and personality disorders than in females, except for more elevated rates of substance abuse in males with BN and BED [20].

Finally, with regard to the sexual orientation, some studies highlighted a much higher prevalence for EDs among gay and bisexual men than in heterosexual men [21], but other studies suggest that being a gay is not, in itself, predictive of ED development in males [22].

"Minority stress theory" posits that stigmatization and social exclusion of sexual and gender minority are ongoing chronic stressors contributing to dysregulation of multiple organ systems in the body and ultimately causing the higher rates of chronic diseases as eating disorders [23].

3.1 Genetic and Epigenetic Factors in Male Anorexia Nervosa

AN is a psychiatric disease prevalently diagnosed in females [24], and the female sex remains the most important risk factor for the development of the disease.

Etiopathogenesis of AN is still unclear, and the reasons for female gender preference are not fully clarified. Nevertheless, in the pathogenetic process of AN, genetic and epigenetic factors play an important role in both genders.

3.2 What Do Genetics and Epigenetics Mean?

Genetics studies genes, their heritance, and their variability in normal and pathological phenotypes.

Epigenetics studies how environmental influences—prenatal or during a person's life—can modify the phenotype, without altering the genotype. Epigenetic action (for instance, through methylation of DNA) modifies the expression of the genes turning it "on or off," i.e., allowing or deleting its activity.

The combined action of genetics and epigenetics—the interaction of genes and the environment ("nature and nurture")—results in the unique individual phenotype.

The history of modern psychiatric genetics is relatively recent, beginning in the 1980s [25].

Studies on genetics aspects of AN begin later than other psychiatric diseases and are difficult due to the low prevalence of AN, specifically in males, a limiting factor for data reliability.

Genetic liability to AN does not follow a Mendelian scheme so that inheritance patterns are much more complex.

An exhaustive review of studies concerning heritability of EDs reports a lifetime prevalence of 3%–12% of AN or subthreshold EDs in first-degree relatives of probands that is much higher than relatives of controls (0%–4%). In detail, relatives of probands with AN were 11.3 times more likely to have AN than relatives of controls [26].

Once familial aggregation was well established, a body of research was directed to distinguish the true genetic influence from environmental familiar factors through twin studies. The heritability estimate for AN, obtained from twin studies, ranged from 0.48 to 0.74, meaning that up to 74% of phenotypic variation could be explained by additive genetic factors [27]. Genetic factors were confirmed as more relevant in "strictly defined anorexia" in comparison with "AN defined through broader criteria" in a research by Dellava [28].

Male patients were too few to give valid information on heritability in a study by Bulik [29].

On the contrary, Strober reported that first-degree female relatives of males with AN full syndrome had an extremely high relative risk, up to 20, to have the disease, demonstrating that the influence of familial-genetic factors on AN is sex-independent [30].

In addition, Raevuori et al. found a strong familial clustering of AN, affective and anxiety disorders, and symptoms of muscle dysmorphia among men in Finnish twin cohorts from the general population [31].

Baker et al. reported that genetic factors showed a stronger contribution in males, whereas shared environment factors contributed more in females than in males to the liability to EDs.

Unique environmental factors appeared to equally contribute in both sexes [32].

Klump adoption study was the first adoption study aiming to differentiate the role of genetics from shared environmental factors in the occurrence of AN in siblings.

Female pairs of biological and adopted siblings were studied through a total score investigating eating behaviors symptoms and not categorical diagnosis. Levels of disordered eating were similar in biological and adoptive siblings (8–29%). The correlation of symptoms between the pairs of biological siblings was present and significant, while no correlation was observed between pairs of adopted sibling. These results indicate the main role of genetic influence, responsible of 59–82% of the variance, while the influence of a shared environment appeared negligible. Even if the study is carried on female sample, Klump affirms that genetic and environmental architecture appears to be similar across the sex and the spectrum of the disease [33].

The preliminary research of genetic factors of AN initially addressed family members, co-twins, and siblings of probands developing an indirect study on inheritance. Subsequently, many studies were oriented to find a direct relation between inheritance of AN and gene variations.

A review on this argument by Manzato et al. reported that the research was initially directed—according to an "a priori hypothesis"—to find variations in candidate genes[1] or to find polymorphic variants of many genes controlling energy homeostasis and eating behaviors such as neurotransmitter systems (reward system) [34].

Identification of a particular candidate gene association or polymorphic variants did not result in a conclusive response. In fact, most results have not been subsequently confirmed by larger samples nor by subsequent genome-wide association studies [35].

In recent decades, modern technology applied to genetic studies allowed to investigate the entire genome by performing genome-wide association studies (GWASs), and this technology was used in many psychiatric diseases, including also AN [36].

Boraska et al. in 2014 reported the global meta-analysis results of single nucleotide polymorphisms (SNPs) in case-control analysis in AN. Although SNPs were involved in AN in multiple chromosomes and positions, the authors concluded that, even though GWASs appear to be the right way versus a better comprehension of

---

[1] Candidate gene is a predefined gene of interest that may be associated with a phenotype or disease of specific most often selected on the basis of a biological hypothesis.

the biological basis of AN, it is mandatory to study larger samples to get reliable and repeatable results [37].

Duncan et al. in 2017 identified a genome-wide significant locus on chromosome 12, in a region associated with type I diabetes and autoimmune disorders as well as insulin metabolism. Positive genetic correlations were found also between AN, neuroticism, and schizophrenia, while significant negative genetic correlations were observed between AN and body mass index, insulin, glucose, and lipid phenotype [38].

Watson et al. recently reported the genome-wide association study of a large sample (16,992 cases) of AN and controls (55,525), combining data from the "AN Genetics Initiative" (ANGI) and the "Eating Disorders Working Group of the Psychiatric Genomics Consortium" (PGC-ED).

In his study, a promising significant genetic correlation was found not only with psychiatric disorders but also with physical activity and metabolic (including glycemic), lipid, and anthropometric traits. In light of these findings, the authors suggest a "rethinking" of AN as a "metabo-psychiatric" disorder [39]. The "genome-wide association studies" appear—different from the previous studies—to give more reliable responses about the associations of genetic variants with AN.

It is important, however, to point out that AN, as well as many other psychiatric diseases, cannot be considered a strictly genetic condition since the expression of genes possibly involved in its etiopathogenesis may or may not be activated. The phenotype of the disease probably represents the result of a dynamic interaction between genotype and multiple environmental factors possibly linked through an epigenetic mechanism according to a recurrent model of many psychiatric diseases [40].

Different from genome sequence, epigenetic mechanisms are dynamic and can vary depending on tissue types, age, and stage of development. Epigenetic mechanisms are also subject to a wide range of confounders by multiple environmental stimuli including medication, stress, and tobacco use.

Hubel in his recent review concludes that "The field of epigenetics in EDs remains 'in its infancy'" and strongly recommends to take into account all environmental variables [41].

Two main environmental factors could act through an epigenetic mechanism: prenatal exposure to androgens and pubertal dysmorphic hormonal cascade.

Going back to the reasons of the sexually dysmorphic prevalence of AN, we have seen that genetics in men has the same or even higher relevance as in women. What is responsible for a sexual dichotomy?

Among environmental factors, the exposure to maternal and fetal testosterone appears to have a critical role by determining a permanent and irreversible morpho-functional organization of the brain and fatty tissue sex oriented.

This complex morpho-functional organization—activation of reward circuits and attitude toward food and regulating energy metabolism and body weight—results in a habitus oriented to anorexia and metabolic anabolism, so that high prenatal exposure to androgens is associated with a reduced incidence of EDs [42, 43].

A research by Culbert on same sex twin males and females and opposite sex twins highlighted how the effects of prenatal testosterone on eating attitudes become evident during puberty and may play a role in sex-differentiated risk for EDs after mid-puberty. Androgens are protective in a female twin of an opposite sex pair, instead males with a female twin are at a higher risk AN than females. This suggests a possible link between intrauterine female hormone exposure and increased ED risk in men. Twin model represents a proxy for differential exposure to androgens since direct measures of overall prenatal testosterone exposure in humans do not currently exist [44]. The only indirect measure of prenatal androgen effects—since the 13th week of pregnancy—is a lower ratio of index finger/ring finger/length. 2D:4D lower ratios are associated with lower levels of body dissatisfaction, drive for thinness, dietary restraint, and binge eating in young adult males [45].

Klump speculates that, in females, the relatively low testosterone level before birth allows their brains to respond to estrogen during puberty, when hormones activate the gene contributors to the greater predisposition to EDs.

Furthermore, Klump observes that a combination of psychosocial risk and hormonal activation could account for puberty's effect in females differently for males where puberty does not activate the genetic risk and psychosocial pressure is generally less strong. Heritability of EDs was 50% in males and constant through the different stages of development (pre-puberty, puberty, and adulthood), while, in females, genetics was activated only at puberty [46]. It is also possible that an environment promoting thinness contributes to the overexpression of genes related to weight and appetite in vulnerable subjects [27]. Many other sex-neutral environmental confounders—such as stress, diet, microbiota, drugs, disease, etc.—complicate epigenetic research, and sample sizes should be as large as those required for GWAS (if not larger) for discovering meaningful and replicable epigenetic risk factors in "epigenome-wide association studies" (EGWASs). Future research should also explore epigenetic mechanisms other than DNA methylation, including—but not limited to—histone modification, chromatin remodeling, and microRNA studies.

Genetics and epigenetics will represent a major field of research on EDs, specifically on AN since GWASs and EGWASs are nowadays recognized as the better tools for understanding the whole etiopathogenetic process of AN.

In conclusion, we quote the sentence of Zerwas and Bulik, who affirm that "Almost all risk and protective factors, both genetic and environmental, are probabilistic, rather than deterministic" [47].

References

1. American Psychiatric Association. Diagnostic and statistical manual of mental disorders. 5th ed. Arlington: American Psychiatric Association; 2013.
2. Hudson J, Hiripi E, Pope H, Kessler R. The prevalence and correlates of eating disorders in the national comorbidity survey replication. Biol Psychiatry. 2007;61:348–58.
3. Raevuori A, Keski-Rahkonen A, Hoek HW. A review of eating disorders in males. Curr Opin Psychiatry. 2014;27(6):426–30.

4. Weltzin T. Eating disorders in men: Update. J Men's Health Gender. 2005;2:186–93.
5. Manzato E, Zanetti T, Gualandi M, Strumia R. Eating disorders in males. New York: Nova Science Publishers Inc; 2011.
6. Jaworski M, et al. Eating disorders in males: a 8-year population-based observational study. Am J Mens Health. 2019;13(4). https://doi.org/10.1177/1557988319860970.
7. Murray SB, et al. The enigma of male eating disorders: a critical review and synthesis. Clin Psychol Rev. 2017;57:1–11.
8. Kostecka B, Kordyńska KK, Murawiec S, Kucharska K. Distorted body image in women and men suffering from Anorexia Nervosa—a literature review. Arch Psychiatry Psychother. 2019;1:13–21.
9. Strother E, Lemberg R, Stanford SC, Turberville D. Eating disorders in men: underdiagnosed, undertreated, and Misunderstood. Eat Disord. 2012;20(5):346–55.
10. Pope H, Phillips K, Olivardia R. The Adonis complex: how to identify, treat, and prevent body obsession in men and boys. New York, NY: Touchstone; 2002.
11. Halliwell E, Dittmar H, Orsborn A. The effects of exposure to muscular male models among men: exploring the moderating role of gym use and exercise motivation. Body Image. 2007;4(3):278–87.
12. Fredericka DA, et al. The happy American body: predictors of affective body satisfaction in two U.S. national internet panel surveys. Body Image. 2020;32:70–84.
13. Manzato E, Gravina G. Body image in males with eating and weight disorders. In: Cuzzolaro M, Fassino S, editors. Body image, eating, and weight. Cham, Switzerland: Springer International Publishing; 2018.
14. Cohane GH, Pope HG Jr. Body image in boys: a review of the literature. Int J Eat Disord. 2001;29:373–9.
15. McCabe MP, Ricciardelli LA. Sociocultural influences on body image and body changes among adolescent boys and girls. J Soc Psychol. 2003;143:5–26.
16. Andersen A. Eating disorders in males: critical questions. In: Lemberg R, Cohn L, editors. Eating disorders: a reference sourcebook. Phoenix, AZ: Oryx Press; 1999. p. 73–9.
17. Gueguen J, Godart N, Chambry J, et al. Severe anorexia nervosa in men: comparison with severe AN in women and analysis of mortality. Int J Eat Disord. 2012;45:537–45.
18. Rastogi R, Rome ES. Restrictive eating disorders in previously overweight adolescents and young adults. Cleve Clin J Med. 2020;88(3):165–71.
19. Shu CY, et al. Clinical presentation of eating disorders in young males at a tertiary setting. J Eat Disord. 2015;3:39–45.
20. Striegel-Moore RH, Garvin V, Dohm FA, Rosenheck RA. Psychiatric comorbidity of eating disorders in men: a national study of hospitalized veterans. Int J Eat Disord. 1999;25:399–404.
21. Strong SM, Williamson DA, Netemeyer RG, Geer JH. Eating disorder symptoms and concerns about body differ as a function of gender and sexual orientation. J Soc Clin Psychol. 2000;19:240–55.
22. Jones WR, Morgan JF. Eating disorders in men: a review of the literature. J Public Ment Health. 2010;9:23–31.
23. Mensinger JL, et al. Sexual and gender minority individuals report higher rates of abuse and more severe eating disorder symptoms than cisgender heterosexual individuals at admission to eating disorder treatment. Int J Eat Disord. 2020;53:541–54.
24. Steinhausen H-C, Jensen CM. Time trends in lifetime incidence rates of first-time diagnosed anorexia nervosa and bulimia nervosa across 16 years in a Danish nationwide psychiatric registry study. Int J Eat Disord. 2015;48:845–50.
25. Gurling H. Candidate genes and favoured loci: strategies for molecular genetic research into schizophrenia, maniac depression, autism, alcoholism and Alzheimer's disease. Psychiatr Dev. 1986;4:289–3091.
26. Thornton LM, et al. The heritability of eating disorders: methods and current findings. Curr Top Behav Neurosci. 2011;(6):141–56. https://doi.org/10.1007/7854_2010_91.
27. Yilmaz Z, et al. Genetics and epigenetics of eating disorders. Adv Genomics Genet. 2015;5:131–50. https://doi.org/10.2147/AGG.S55776.

28. Dellava JE, et al. Impact of broadening definitions of anorexia nervosa on sample characteristics. J Psychiatr Res. 2011;45(5):691–8.
29. Bulik CM, et al. Prevalence, heritability, and prospective risk factors for anorexia nervosa. Arch Gen Psychiatry. 2006;63:305–31.
30. Strober M, et al. Males with anorexia nervosa: a controlled study of eating disorders in first-degree relatives. Int J Eat Disord. 2001;29:263–9.
31. Raevuori A, et al. Lifetime anorexia nervosa in young men in the community: five cases and their co-twins. Int J Eat Disord. 2008;41(5):458–63.
32. Baker JH, et al. Genetic risk factors for disordered eating in adolescent males and females. J Abnorm Psychol. 2009;118(3):576–86. https://doi.org/10.1037/a0016314.
33. Klump KL, et al. Genetic and environmental influences on disordered eating: an adoption study. Abnorm Psychol. 2009;118(4):797–805. https://doi.org/10.1037/a0017204.
34. Manzato E, et al. Anorexia nervosa: an update on genetic, biological and clinical aspects in males. Ital J Gender-Specific Med. 2017;3(2):59–70.
35. Himmerich H, et al. Genetic risk factors for eating disorders: an update and insights into pathophysiology. Ther Adv Psychopharmacol. 2019;9:1–20. https://doi.org/10.1177/2045125318814734.
36. Wang K, et al. A genome-wide association study on common SNPs and rare CNVs in anorexia nervosa. Mol Psychiatry. 2011;16:949–59.
37. Boraska V, et al. A genome-wide association study of anorexia nervosa. Mol Psychiatry. 2014;19:1085–94.
38. Duncan L, et al. Significant locus and metabolic genetic correlations revealed in genome-wide association study of anorexia nervosa. Am J Psychiatry. 2017;174:850–8.
39. Watson H, et al. Genome-wide association study identifies eight risk loci and implicates metabo-psychiatric origins for anorexia nervosa. Nat Genet. 2019;51(8):1207–14. https://doi.org/10.1038/s41588-019-0439-2.
40. Sullivan PF, et al. Genetic architectures of psychiatric disorders: the emerging picture and its implications. Nat Rev Genet. 2012;13:537–51.
41. Hübel C, Marzi SJ, Breen G, Bulik CM. Epigenetics in eating disorders: a systematic review. Mol Psychiatry. 2019;24(6):901–15.
42. Lombardo MV, et al. Fetal programming effects of testosterone on the reward system and behavioral approach tendencies in humans. Biol Psychiatry. 2012a;72:839–47.
43. Procopio M, Marriott P. Intrauterine hormonal environment and risk of developing anorexia Nervosa. Arch Gen Psychiatry. 2007;64(12):1402–7.
44. Culbert KM, et al. The emergence of sex differences in risk for disordered eating attitudes during puberty: a role for prenatal testosterone exposure. J Abnorm Psychol. 2013;122:420–32.
45. Smith AR, et al. The measure of a man: associations between digit ratio and disordered eating in males. Int J Eat Disord. 2010;43:543–8. https://doi.org/10.1002/eat.20736.
46. Klump KL, et al. The effects of puberty on genetic risk for disordered eating: evidence for a sex difference. Psychol Med. 2012;42(3):627–37. https://doi.org/10.1017/S0033291711001541.
47. Zerwas S, Bulik CM. Genetics and epigenetics of eating disorders. Psychiatr Ann. 2011;41(11):532–8.

Eating Disorders in Midlife and in the Elderly

Emilia Manzato and Eleonora Roncarati

EDs often onset in adolescence or in early adulthood, but can persist or arise across lifespan and be present in midlife and in the elderly [1].

"Midlife", the central period of a person's life, is defined as the age between 45 and 60, while "elderly" is defined as the age above 65 [2].

Most research studies have focused on the periods at higher risk for ED onset, and only recently they have paid some interest to EDs in adulthood.

The lack of attention regarding EDs in adults and in the elderly may be due to their reduced presence in both age groups and age-correlated prejudice.

"Ageism" is "the stereotyping of and discrimination against individuals or groups based on their age. Ageism can take many forms, including prejudicial attitudes, discriminatory practices, or institutional policies and practices that perpetuate stereotypical beliefs" [3].

As the elderly population tends to increase (the Census estimates that by 2030, one in five persons in the United States will be over the age of 65 [4]) and as the ideal body image of women proposed by media becomes increasingly thinner, it is therefore natural to expect an increase in the prevalence of EDs both in adulthood and in the elderly population [5].

EDs in adults can be divided into two main groups: early onset (eating disorder (ED) episodes in adolescence which persist or relapse in old age) and late onset (ED episode which appears for the first time later in life). Although there is no complete agreement, ED onset after the age of 40 is generally considered as late onset [6].

Initially, the first descriptions of EDs in adulthood in scientific literature were viewed with much scepticism, and the first data were collected on case reports or on very restricted samples, mostly female.

E. Manzato (✉) · E. Roncarati
University of Ferrara, Eating and Weight Disorders Center "L'Albero", Private Hospital "Salus", Ferrara, Italy
e-mail: emilia.manzato@gmail.com; eleonora.roncarati@unife.it

In 1976, Kellett et al. published the first case of anorexia nervosa (AN) with onset after menopause: a widow of 54 years of age with severe weight loss over a period of 3 years. She reported altered body image; she refused "phobic foods" and used purgative practices such as laxatives, diuretics and self-induced vomiting [7].

In 1979, Carrier in his article used for the first time the term "tardive anorexia" to describe a case of AN with first onset after adolescence [8].

In 1988, Hsu and Zimmer described five cases of EDs in adulthood with phobia of fattening and depressive comorbidity [9].

In 1993, Hall and Driscoll described two ED cases, a 64-year-old man and a 61-year-old woman, with a long persistence of disease—9 and 12 years, respectively—and a long follow-up. The patients showed scarce awareness of their ED, and despite treatment, they died 2 and 5 years later, respectively [10].

In 1996, Beck et al. presented a review of 11 clinical cases of EDs in old age underlining the need "to alert clinicians to the category of late onset eating disorders, especially to clinical features and treatment response" [11].

Scholtz et al. in 2010, in their interesting review on EDs in older women, reported that from 1976 to 2010, only 17 articles had been published on EDs in adults and older women for a total of 37 patients over the age of 50 [12].

Only in 19 patients the onset was really considered late onset occurring after 50 years and not as a continuation of previous episodes.

However, they also emphasized that in most scientific articles, there were not enough anamnestic data to establish with absolute certainty whether the ED was a real late onset or a relapse of a previous episode in adolescence.

Since then, research studies have spread, and the number of samples increased, due to higher presence of EDs in adulthood and in the elderly and to the improved ability to intercept EDs in old people as well.

4.1 What Is the Real Prevalence of EDs or Altered Food Behaviours in Adulthood and in the Elderly?

It is difficult to collect reliable data of the real ED prevalence in these age groups. This is for several reasons, including the higher presence in adulthood and in the elderly of sub-threshold ED symptoms rather than full syndromes.

Data show a prevalence of 11% ED symptoms in females 45–55 years old and a prevalence of 4% of eating disturbed behaviours in females aged between 60 and 70. The most frequent symptom is binge eating [13].

The use of compensatory practices seems to be less frequent than in young people. Vomiting is a rare occurrence (1%); misuse of laxatives/diuretics is self-reported by 2.2% and 2.1%, respectively.

Full ED syndromes that have onset over 40 years have a prevalence of 1.8–3.8% [14].

Mangweth-Matzek et al. assessed the presence of EDs in a large female community sample (475 women) in Austria and estimated that 3.8% of Austrian women

(60–70 years old) presented an ED. "Eating disorders not otherwise specified" were the most frequently reported disorders [15].

A recent study carried out on a large female sample reported the prevalence of 3.25% of EDs (diagnosed according to the DSM-5 criteria).

In this study, binge eating disorder was the most prevalent ED (1.68%), followed by other specified feeding and eating disorders (1.48%) and bulimia nervosa (0.30%) [16].

It is even more difficult to study the ED prevalence on males, because even in old people EDs are more common in women. Furthermore, data are generally derived from studies on mixed samples.

Night eating syndrome (NES) has been included in "other specified feeding and eating disorder" in the fifth edition of the DSM in 2013, and its prevalence in the general population is estimated 1.5% [17].

Andersen et al. found that 9.1% of women aged 55 years and older reported getting up during the night to eat [18].

NES in elderly population seems to link with several normal sleep changes that occur with ageing such as an increase of sleep latency (the time needed to fall asleep), light sleep and a decrease of slow-wave sleep and REM phase. Sleep becomes more fragmented with age, and the number of awakenings intensifies so that the time spent awake during the night increases as well.

Furthermore, older people may also be more prone to suffer from sleep disorders such as insomnia, sleep apnoea and sleep-related movement disorders than younger people.

A growing body of literature has suggested a link between sleep duration and obesity, but the results are mixed, and the nature of this relationship is still unclear. Among the various causes of this link, it has been suggested that sleep disorders in old people could increase hedonic eating, change eating habits and therefore become a risk factor for the onset of NES and obesity [19].

Other disturbed eating behaviours are present in the elderly.

Picking/nibbling is the most prevalent disturbed eating behaviour in adulthood and in the elderly: 36% of women aged 65 years and older reported eating between meals. The prevalence of picking/nibbling increases with age, and it is correlated with obesity [16].

The difficulty in diagnosing an ED in old people is also linked to a presence of many weight variations due to different physical factors. For instance, in menopause, there could be an increase in weight with a redistribution of body fat. Furthermore, in the elderly, there could be a decrease in weight due to muscle mass loss and/or difficulty eating. Finally, there may be many weight fluctuations, related to the onset of physical illnesses that can obscure the presence of an ED.

Up to now, it is not completely clear how specific symptoms or the relationship between symptoms could change across lifespan to maintain an ED. Network analysis—a statistical approach that tends to identify central symptoms such as fear of weight gain, over-evaluation of shape and weight, dietary restrain, etc.—found that some central symptoms remain in ED patients regardless of the developmental stage [20].

Overeating, binge eating, over-evaluation of shape and food avoidance can remain central symptoms across age, but the relationship between these symptoms can present many changes across age [21].

These symptoms could represent important target in the treatment of EDs in midlife and beyond, and the changes in the illness pathway could suggest a tailored treatment to address these changes.

EDs in old people have unique clinical characteristics [22].

In adulthood and the elderly, who suffer from AN achieve weight control mainly with food restriction and physical hyperactivity. The use of evacuative practices is less frequent in the elderly than in younger patients, and, in any case, there is a higher misuse of laxatives rather than self-induced vomiting.

Even in bulimia nervosa (BN), the binge eating episodes are usually accompanied by non-evacuative compensatory behaviours with a lesser use of self-induced vomiting compared to young patients. In addition, in BN, there is a reduced presence of self-injury behaviours, compared to young people.

The most frequent psychiatric comorbidity of EDs in elderly is depression [23, 24].

Other differences between EDs occurring in adulthood and EDs in young people are triggering factors that belong—for the most part—to loss events such as family member's death or onset of physical diseases.

Despite the lower severity of ED symptoms in old people, there are more medical complications than EDs in young patients. There is also a higher mortality risk due to cardiovascular, metabolic and bone complications. Furthermore, dietary restrictions correlate with a higher decrease in cognitive performance that generally accompanies the process of brain ageing [25].

Changes in physical form and consequent body dissatisfaction (BD) are important risk factors for EDs in young people. Many research studies have highlighted the presence of BD as a risk factor for EDs among older women as well [26]. In fact, recent studies on body image showed that BD remains stable across the lifespan and does not decrease with age in both sexes [27]. Higher BD correlates with disturbed eating behaviour (such as increase in binge eating, emotional eating and unhealthy weight control behaviours) and with distress, low self-esteem and depression.

Menopause can be a serious risk factor both for the hormonal oscillation that can cause an alteration of mood and hunger and for the changes in physical form that can push woman to use weight control practices [28].

In menopausal women, BD and depressive experiences could be related to the appearance of signs of ageing and to the redistribution of body fat in specific points (such as the abdomen) considered "focus of concern".

Normal ageing typically moves women body weight/shape further away from the thin-ideal standard of female beauty proposed in Western culture by the media. This change might be promoted by pregnancy, decreased time for exercise, menopause and use of drugs that may increase weight.

BD seems to correlate positively with the fear of ageing and with the intolerance to signs of body ageing [29].

Moreover, in recent decades, pressure by media on midlife women to conform to thinner-ideal body has increased along with focus on an "ideal young body" and devaluation of older women's body.

Thus, midlife and older women might be prone to increased ageing anxiety and both BD and EDs.

Some studies reported that women aged 60 years and older, who show less concerns about weight and shape, have also a more relaxed attitude towards ageing [30].

Within this scope, we cite two old studies carried on midlife and elderly people, which focused on different aspects: one focused on body weight and the other one on dietary restriction. The different results of the two studies highlighted how the attitude and concerns about body shape changed at the end of the last century especially in the elderly population.

The first study, carried out in 1986 on a sample of 207 elderly people, investigated their attitudes towards body image and showed that old people were more tolerant towards overweight and obesity than young people [31]. Elderly people paid less attention to the body shape and showed a lower interest in weight control and physical fitness.

The other study carried out some years later, in 1994, investigated eating behaviours and BD in a sample of 50 normal-weight women aged 60–70 years old. The study showed that about 50% of the sample followed dietary restriction to lose weight. None had started diets in their youth because at the time when they were teenagers, Europe was at war and food was scarce [32].

Part of the sample also reported having started following the first diets around the 1960s, when the media began to propose a leaner ideal body image.

In old people, the protection factors against the ED onset are mainly related to relational aspects that might reduce the sense of fragility often present in the elderly, e.g. having a stable relationship, having children and having financial security. These factors help elderly people to have less concerns about body weight and shape. A study on sample of ED patients aged between 50 and 68 years, focused on relational aspects, highlighted that about half of the sample had no stable relationship and those married reported serious relationship difficulties with the partner. All patients also had a very narrow or no social life [12].

Elderly patients complain of a lack of interest for EDs in old age and an attitude of prejudice (ageism) of therapists towards old people suffering from EDs. The majority of patients considers "group treatment" as the most useful treatment. Social support also plays an important role in ED recovery [33].

Research data on EDs in adulthood and the elderly suggest that, although EDs are not generally the first diagnosis option for patients with altered eating behaviour, these disorders should not be excluded from diagnostic possibility.

Furthermore, it seems essential to make an earlier diagnosis also in elderly people to avoid serious internal complications—favoured by age—and to avoid worse prognosis linked to long duration of illness.

Since the presence of EDs in adulthood and in the elderly is not so sporadic and EDs tend to endure over time or relapse, it is mandatory to maintain contacts with young patients with EDs for a long time, even after their recovery.

In conclusion, we must be aware that every change in weight and in eating behaviour at any age in both sexes could be due to an eating disorder.

4.2 Nutritional Requirements and Eating Disorders in the Elderly

EDs in adulthood and in the elderly are part of a complex organic framework and can lead to more serious complications than in young people [34].

Scientific evidence on nutritional requirements in the elderly are scarce, and there are few guidelines for nutrients according to different ages [35, 36]. Furthermore, it is not correct to compare people aged between 60 and 70 with people aged 80 years and older [37, 38].

The variations in body composition, characterized by loss of active muscle mass and increase of fat mass (FM) in older individuals, lead to a reduction in BMR (basal metabolic rate) [39, 40].

In addition, there is a gradual decrease of physical activity, which could influence the assessment of caloric needs. Therefore, estimating energy requirement in the elderly is complex and depends on the age, on the presence of chronic illnesses and on the level of physical activity as well [41, 42].

An adequate protein intake in the elderly takes on special importance due to the highest prevalence of protein-energy malnutrition, often present in this age, especially in individuals aged 75 years and older. Even in the elderly, there are growth and tissue turnover and metabolic needs.

Protein deficiency can induce tissue wear, delay the healing process of bedsores, increase the risk of anaemia, decrease plasma proteins and immune system reactions and cause oedema [43].

In the elderly, altered eating habits associated with altered processes of digestion and absorption may easily lead to a condition of hypovitaminosis [44, 45].

EDs cause altered food behaviours, such as food restriction or binge eating episodes, and can lead to malnutrition and severe medical complications [46, 47].

Specifically, dietary restrictions to control weight often link to protein-energy malnutrition (PEM) that might impair muscle tissue and essential body fat. PEM is defined as a "Deficiency syndrome caused by insufficient intake or malabsorption of macronutrients that supply energy and proteins to the body" [48, 49]. PEM is a frequent and serious problem in the elderly, and it might influence the underlying pathology and worsen the prognosis as well.

In AN, excessive intake of high-fibre foods along with food restriction might be less tolerated by older individuals. It could lead to gastrointestinal disorders and worsen malabsorption, particularly for some essential nutrients.

The presence of binge eating or picking/nibbling could be associated with overweight and obesity [50, 51]. The correlation between obesity and chronic diseases is heightened in the elderly [52].

The decrease of physical activity, due to "retirement" and physical disabilities, could also play an essential role in obesity development [53]. In the elderly, obesity is also linked to a higher risk of cardiovascular diseases, reduced respiratory efficiency and sleep apnoea syndrome, osteoarthritis, etc.

Furthermore, in the elderly, there is a correlation between obesity and cognitive impairment due to brain damage caused by substances such as adipocytokines, secreted by the adipose tissue and insulin resistance linked to increase of fat mass [54].

References

1. Walsh BT. The enigmatic persistence of anorexia nervosa. Am J Psychiatry. 2013;170(5):477–84.
2. World Health Organisation (WHO). Definition of an older or elderly person; 2010. http://www.who.int/healthinfo/survey/ageingdefnolder/en/index.html.
3. WHO; 2016. http://www.who.int/healthinfo/survey/ageingdefnolder/en/.
4. Census Bureau US. The older population in the United States: 2010 to 2050 population estimates and projections. https://www.census.gov/prod/2010pubs/p25-1138. Accessed 27 Sep 2017.
5. Gadalla TM. Eating disorders and associated psychiatric comorbidity in elderly Canadian women. Arch Womens Ment Health. 2008;11:357–62.
6. Currin L, Schmidt U, Treasure J, Jick H. Time trends in eating disorder incidence. Br J Psychiatry. 2005;86:132–5.
7. Kellett J, Trimble M, Thorley A. Anorexia after the menopause. Br J Psychiatry. 1976;128:555–8.
8. Carrier J. L'anorexia mentale. Paris: Libraire E. Le Francois; 1979.
9. Hsu LKG, Zimmer B. Eating disorders in old age. Int J Eat Disord. 1998;7(1):133–8.
10. Hall P, Driskoll R. Anorexia in the elderly. Int J Eat Disord. 1993;4(4):497–9.
11. Beck D, Casper R, Andersen A. Truly late onset of eating disorders: a study of 11 cases averaging 60 years of age at presentation. Int J Eat Disord. 1996;20(4):389–95.
12. Scholz S, Hill LS, Lacey H. Eating disorders in older women: does late onset anorexia nervosa exist? Int J Eat Disord. 2010;43:393–7.
13. Jenkins PE, Price T. Eating pathology in midlife women: similar or different to younger counterparts? Int J Eat Disord. 2018;51:3–9.
14. Luca A, et al. Eating disorders in late-life. Aging Dis. 2015;6(1):48–55.
15. Mangweth-Matzek, et al. Prevalence of eating disorders in middle-aged women. Int J Eat Disord. 2014;47:320–4.
16. Conceição EM, et al. Prevalence of eating disorders and picking/nibbling in elderly women. Int J Eat Disord. 2017;50:793–800.
17. American Psychiatric Association. Diagnostic and statistical manual of mental disorders. 5th ed. Arlington: American Psychiatric Association; 2013.
18. Andersen GS, Stunkard J, Sørensen TI, Petersen L, Heitmann BL. Night eating and weight change in middle-aged men and women. Int J Obes Relat Metab Disord. 2004;28(10):1338–43.
19. Norton MC. Is poor sleep associated with obesity in older adults? A narrative review of the literature. Eat Weight Disord. 2018;23:23–38.
20. Christian C, et al. Eating disorder core symptoms and symptom pathways across developmental stages: a network analysis. J Abnorm Psychol. 2019; https://doi.org/10.1037/abn0000477.
21. Brown TA, et al. A 30-year longitudinal study of body weight, dieting, and eating pathology across women and men from late adolescence to later midlife. J Abnorm Psychol. 2020;129(4):376–86. https://doi.org/10.1037/abn0000519.
22. Jenkins PE, Price T. Eating pathology in midlife women: similar or different to younger counterpart? Int J Eat Disord. 2018;51:3–9.
23. Midlarsky E, Marotta AK, Pirutinsky S, Morin RT, McGowan JC. Psychological predictors of eating pathology in older adult women. J Women Aging. 2018;30(2):145–57.

24. Henriksen CA, et al. Does age impact the clinical presentation of adult women seeking specialty eating disorder treatment? J Nerv Ment Dis. 2020;208(9):742–5. https://doi.org/10.1097/NMD.0000000000001160.
25. Pérez-Sánchez MC, Torres ND, Morante HJJ. Altered eating attitudes in nursing home residents and its relationship with their cognitive and nutritional status. J Nutr Health Aging. 2018;22(7):869–75.
26. Carrard I, Rothen S. Factors associated with disordered eating behaviors and attitudes in older women. Eat Weight Disord. 2019; https://doi.org/10.1007/s40519-019-00645-4.
27. Matsumoto A, Rodgers RF. A review and integrated theoretical model of the development of body image and eating disorders among midlife and aging men. Clin Psychol Rev. 2020;81:101,903. https://doi.org/10.1016/j.cpr.2020.101903.
28. Thompson KA, Bardone Cone AM. Menopausal status and disordered eating and body image concerns among middle-aged women. Int J Eat Disord. 2019;52(3):314–8.
29. Thompson KA, Bardone Cone AM. Evaluating attitudes about aging and body comparison as moderators of the relationship between menopausal status and disordered eating and body image concerns among middle-aged women. Maturitas. 2019;124:25–31.
30. Black Becker CI. m not just fat, I'm old: has the study of body image overlooked "old talk"? J Eat Disord. 2013;1:6. http://www.jeatdisord.com/content/1/1/6.
31. Harris MB, Furukawa C. Attitudes towards obesity in an elderly sample. J Obes Weight Reg. 1986;5:5–16.
32. Marion M, Hetherington MM, Burnett L. Ageing and the pursuit of slimness: dietary restraint and weight satisfaction in elderly. Women. Br J Clin Psychol. 1994;33:391–400.
33. Mangweth-Matzek B, et al. Never too old for eating disorders or body dissatisfaction: a community study of elderly women. Int J Eat Disord. 2006;39:583–6.
34. Mangweth-Matzek B, et al. Epidemiology and treatment of eating disorders in men and women of middle and older age. Curr Opin Psychiatry. 2017;30(6):446–51.
35. Vandewoude M, Volkert D. ESPEN guidelines on parenteral nutrition. Geriatrics Clin Nutr. 2009;28:461–6.
36. ISSN. Regional guidelines for catering for the elderly in a residential structure. Emilia-Romagna: Emilia-Romagna Regional Health Service; 2017.
37. Streicher M, Themessl-Huber M, et al., editors. Growing older with health and vitality: a nexus of physical activity, exercise and nutrition. Biogerontology. 2016;17(3):529–46.
38. SINU. Nutrient reference intake levels and energy for the Italian population LARN; 2014; IV Ed.
39. Deutz NE, Bauer JM, Barazzoni R, Biolo G, et al. Protein intake and exercise for optimal muscle function with aging: recommendations from the ESPEN Expert Group. Clin Nutr. 2014;33(6):929–36.
40. Fornelli G, Isaia GC, D'Amelio P. Ageing, muscle and bone. JGG. 2016;64:75–80.
41. Baum J, Kim IIY, Wolfe R. Protein consumption and the elderly: what is the optimal level of intake? Nutrients. 2016;8(6):359. https://doi.org/10.3390/nu8060359.
42. Bauer J, et al. Evidence-based recommendations for optimal dietary protein intake in older people: a position paper from the PROT-AGE Study Group. J Am Med Dir Assoc. 2013;14(8):542–59.
43. Donini LM. Control of food intake in the aging. In: Raats MM, De Grrot LCPGM, Van Asselt D, editors. Food for the aging population. Amsterdam: Elsevier Woodhead Publishing; 2017. p. 25–47.
44. Leblanc V, et al. Associations between eating patterns, dietary intakes and eating behaviors in premenopausal overweight women. Eat Behav. 2012;13(2):162–5.
45. Mazzali G, et al. Interrelations between fat distributions, muscle lipid content, adipocytokines, and insulin resistance: effect of moderate weight loss in older women. Am J Clin Nutr. 2006;84:1193–9.
46. European Nutrition for Health Alliance. Malnutrition within an ageing population: a call to action. London: European Nutrition for Health Alliance; 2005.
47. Constans T. Malnutrition in the elderly. Rev Prat. 2003;53:275–9.

48. Agarwala E, Millerb M, Yaxleyb A, Isenringc E. Malnutrition in the elderly: a narrative review. Maturitas. 2013;76(4):296–302.
49. Drobnjak S, Atsiz S, Ditzen B, Tuschen-Caffier B, Ehlert U. Restrained eating and self-esteem in premenopausal and postmenopausal women. J Eat Disord. 2014;2:1–10.
50. Hassing LB, Dahl AK, Thorvaldsson V, Berg S, Gatz M, Pedersen NL, Johansson B. Overweight in midlife and risk of dementia: a 40-year follow-up study. Int J Obes (Lond). 2009;33(8):893–8.
51. Zamboni M, Mazzali G, Fantin F, et al. Sarcopenic obesity: a new category of obesity in the elderly. Nutr Metab Cardiovasc Dis. 2008;18:388–95.
52. Vincent HK, Vincent KR, Lamb KM. Obesity and mobility disability in the older adult. Obes Rev. 2010;11:568–79.
53. Han TS, Tajar A, Lean ME. Obesity and weight management in the elderly. Br Med Bull. 2011;97:169–96.
54. Villareal DT, et al. Weight loss, exercise, or both and physical function in obese older adults. N Engl J Med. 2011;364(13):1218–29.

Eating and Weight Disorders in Sexual and Gender Minorities

Massimo Cuzzolaro

5.1 Introduction

Abnormal eating behaviors and unhealthy weight control practices are more common among girls and women than boys and men [1]. A recent systematic review [2] found that, in 94 studies, based on accurate diagnoses of eating disorders (ED), weighted average lifetime prevalences were:

- 8.4% (range 3.3–18.6%) for women
- 2.2% (range 0.8–6.5%) for men.

As a result, disordered eating behaviors (DEB), starting with anorexia nervosa (AN), have often been considered a woman's illness, which still contributes to delaying the demand for help from male cases, which are increasingly frequent [3]. It should also be remembered that men with ED may present different characteristics compared to female patients, such as muscularity-oriented concerns [4].

As for sexual and gender minorities, the study of ED is in its infancy but overgrowing.

In the United States, in 2018, a national survey found that more than half (about 54%) of lesbian, gay, bisexual, transgender, and genderqueer (LGBTQ) youth surveyed (1034, 13–24-year-olds) had been diagnosed with a full ED syndrome during their lifetime [5].

Many case-control studies have reported higher rates of ED and DEB in LGBTQ individuals compared to their heterosexual and cisgender peers [6, 7].

M. Cuzzolaro (✉)
University of Roma Sapienza, Roma, Italy
e-mail: massimo.cuzzolaro@gmail.com

Several case reports have also been published on the association between eating pathology, gender incongruence, and sexual orientation.

In recent decades, there has been a growing tendency to overcome binary, mutually exclusive classifications: man/woman, homosexuality/heterosexuality, and cisgender/transgender [8].

Even for the biological sex, the idea of distinct categories appears simplistic in light of a broad spectrum of variants [9].

As to the psychosocial concept of gender, empirical data show that there are more than two categories, and the term should instead indicate a dimensional psychological variable that lies on a continuum [10].

The concept of gender identity appears today as a shifting landscape that spans nations and cultures [11].

The January 2017 issue of *National Geographic* magazine was dedicated to the theme "Gender revolution" [12]. Many Millennials—the generation that became adults around the third-millennium turn—reject male/female and heterosexual/homosexual labels and challenge traditional gender stereotypes. They argue that sexual orientation and gender identity are much more fluid than previously thought and include various options [13].

However, social stigma, discrimination, bullying, homophobia, transphobia, and violence still affect gender and sexual minorities, with greater vulnerability in childhood and adolescence and persistent healthcare use difficulties.

Health services and healthcare professionals must acknowledge changes in both social customs and theoretical models. Recognition of the complexity of phenomena related to sex, gender, and sexuality is essential to provide respectful and appropriate care for all, particularly in adolescence and young adulthood [14, 15].

5.2 Definitions and Acronyms

Sex at birth: anatomical-biological categorical variable. The legal sex is attributed at birth primarily based on the morphology of the external genitals and, if necessary, the karyotype, gonads, and hormones. An individual is classified as male, female, or intersex if it presents a mixture of biological characteristics (genitals, gonads, chromosomes) male and female. The concept of *sex spectrum* has been remembered in the previous lines.

Gender role: set of social and cultural norms that indicate how men and women, respectively, should feel, think, behave, dress, talk, and interact. An individual may correspond more or less to the gender role that the society to which he or she belongs considers appropriate for his or her gender.

Gender non-conformity: to express gender, consistently and persistently, in ways that differ from the cultural norms associated with natal sex. For example, cross-dressing or transvestitism indicates the habit of dressing in clothes that one's culture associates with the opposite sex.

Gender: the term is sometimes used categorically, as a synonym for sex. But, strictly speaking, it refers to social and cultural characteristics rather than biological ones. Therefore, it includes beliefs, values, feelings, attitudes, and behaviors learned from the paradigms of masculinity/femininity (gender role) of one's own culture. For these norms, every human being builds, in the course of life, a particular way of being a man or a woman and testifies it every day through physical appearance, hairstyling, clothing, behavior, voice, and language (*gender expression*).

Gender identity: the consistent and persistent feeling and awareness that an individual has of being male or female. The term *trans-identity* appeared in the early twentieth century to indicate a legal and social problem more than a medical one. The following terms are in use:

- *Cisgender*: individuals whose subjective gender identity coincides with the gender assigned at birth
- *Transgender*: individuals whose subjective gender identity does not coincide with the sex assigned at birth: FtM (female-to-male) or MtF (male-to-female) transgender depending on whether the sex assigned at birth is female or male, respectively
- *Agender*: people who do not identify with any gender and feel genderless or gender-neutral
- *Genderqueer*: individuals who feel their gender unstable (from time to time, bigender, genderfluid, agender)
- *Pangender/omnigender*: people who identify with all genders.

Gender incongruence: the transgender condition.

Gender dysphoria: living the transgender condition in a conflicting way and with a deep malaise.

Gender transition: the process (clothing, hairstyle, medical/surgical interventions) through which transgender individuals try to make the appearance and functions of their body similar to the gender they feel they belong to.

Gender confirmation medical and surgical treatments: interventions aimed at realizing the physical characteristics of the gender that a transgender person feels is appropriate. The Danish painter Einar Magnus Andreas Wegener (better known as Lili Elbe) was among the first cases of sex reassignment surgery (male-to-female) [16]. At the age of 48, between 1930 and 1931, Lili Elbe underwent four experimental surgeries in Germany, under the supervision of Magnus Hirschfeld, a sexologist who was a defender of sexual minorities. Lili Elbe died after the last surgery (construction of a vaginal canal and uterus transplantation). Only later, in the second half of the twentieth century, did developments in endocrinology and surgery make gender transition pathways possible and more and more frequent.

Gender confirmation surgery: surgery performed by a multi-specialist team to give transgender people the physical appearance and functions of the gender they feel they belong to.

Sexual orientation: an individual may feel sexually attracted to people of the opposite sex (*heterosexual*), of the same sex (*homosexual*), or of both sexes (*bisexual*) or feel no sexual attraction (*asexual*). Homosexuality and bisexuality can be associated with both cisgender and transgender conditions.

LGBT: acronym for lesbian, gay, bisexual, and transgender.
LGBTI: acronym for lesbian, gay, bisexual, transgender, and intersexual.
LGBTQ: acronym for lesbian, gay, bisexual, transgender, and genderqueer.
LGBTQ+: abbreviated acronym for LGBTQIP2SAA (lesbian, gay, bisexual, transgender, genderqueer, questioning, intersex, pansexual, two-spirit, asexual, ally). *Two-spirit* refers to Native Americans who feel inhabited by two spirits, one male and the other female. *Ally* refers to those who support the community while not being part of it.
TGNC: acronym for transgender and gender non-conforming.

5.3 Gender Identity and Sexual Orientation in DSM and ICD

Medical and psychiatric taxonomies are deeply affected by the evolution of scientific knowledge and treatment techniques and the customs and normative values of each society and historical era. This case is especially evident for sexuality, gender identity, and gender expression.

Current classifications oscillate between *nosologomania* [17]—with a continuous proliferation of diagnostic categories—and *depathologization* in the name of human rights and the defense of minorities from discrimination and social stigma [8].

Some historical references to the two globally used classification systems—ICD (all diseases) and DSM (mental disorders)—may help understand the changes over time.

The search for a universal catalog of diseases for statistical purposes dates back to the mid-nineteenth century. Medical statisticians such as Jacob Marc d'Espine, William Farr, and Jacques Bertillon laid the foundations [18].

In the beginning, it was a matter of nomenclature of the only causes of death.

In 1900, to build a globally used diagnostic tool, the French government organized in Paris the first International Conference for the revision of the *Bertillon or International Classification of Causes of Death*. The first *International List of Causes of Death* (sometimes referred to as ILCD-1) was produced. Four other revisions followed, respectively, in 1909, 1920, 1929, and 1938.

In 1948, the French government and the newly formed World Health Organization (WHO) set up in Paris the International Conference for the Sixth Decennial Revision of the International Lists of Diseases and Causes of Death. This sixth revision—*International Statistical Classification of Diseases, Injuries, and Causes of Death*, later named *ICD-6*—extended the catalog to all diseases, injuries, and causes of death, including non-fatal diseases and mental illnesses [19].

Homosexuality was among the latter as "a sexual deviation" within the diagnostic cluster "Disorders of character, behavior, and intelligence" (Fig. 5.1).

From that time, WHO was responsible for periodic revisions of the official and internationally shared medical nomenclature. The three subsequent reviews—1955 (ICD-7), 1965 (ICD-8), and 1975 (ICD-9)—continued to classify sexual deviance as psychiatric disorders.

```
BULLETIN OF THE WORLD HEALTH ORGANIZATION
            SUPPLEMENT 1

              MANUAL
               OF THE
           INTERNATIONAL
       STATISTICAL CLASSIFICATION
         OF DISEASES, INJURIES,
          AND CAUSES OF DEATH

    Sixth Revision of the International Lists
      of Diseases and Causes of Death
             Adopted 1948
                                      (320–326) Disorders of character, behaviour, and intelligence
              Volume 2                  320      Pathological personality
         ALPHABETICAL INDEX              320.0        Schizoid personality
                                         320.1        Paranoid personality
                                         320.2        Cyclothymic personality
                                         320.3        Inadequate personality
        WORLD HEALTH ORGANIZATION        320.4        Antisocial personality
             Geneva, Switzerland         320.5        Asocial personality
                  1949                   320.6        Sexual deviation
                                         320.7        Other and unspecified
```

Fig. 5.1 Sixth revision of the international lists of diseases and causes of death (WHO 1948)

In 1992, the tenth edition (ICD-10) replaced homosexuality with the "ego-dystonic sexual orientation" category, explicitly stating that sexual orientation by itself is not to be considered a disorder [20].

In 2019, the eleventh revision (ICD-11) was presented. It is expected to be implemented on January 1, 2022 [21]. In the ICD-11, the term homosexuality has disappeared.

As for the *Diagnostic and Statistical Manual of Mental Disorders* (DSM), published by the American Psychiatric Association (APA), homosexuality was classified among the mental disorders both in the first edition of 1952 [22] and in the second edition of 1968 [23].

The year 1973 was the turning point, mainly due to gay and lesbian activism and the anti-psychiatry movement. The APA Board of Trustees decided to remove homosexuality from the DSM. A 58% majority of APA members voted in support of this decision, and the DSM-II replaced the word homosexuality with the ambiguous expression "sexual orientation disturbance" to be applied when a person is in painful conflict with the direction of his/her sexual urges. As a result, the DSM no longer considered homosexuality disease per se but continued to consider sexual conversion therapies legitimate (in theory from homosexuality to heterosexuality and vice versa).

Seven years later, in an attempt to make the nomenclature less vague, the DSM-III [24] replaced "sexual orientation disturbance" with "ego-dystonic homosexuality," a psychiatric diagnostic category to be applied to people in conflict with their homosexuality.

Finally, in the subsequent revision (DSM-III-R) [25], homosexuality fell out of the DSM [8].

For the variants of gender identity—an emerging twenty-first-century problem—the taxonomy has followed a similar path [26].

In DSM-III (1980), DSM-III-R (1987), and DSM-IV (1994), the transgender condition was considered a psychiatric disease with a specific diagnosis, "gender identity disorder."

In 2013, DSM-5 abolished that diagnosis and introduced the diagnostic category "gender dysphoria" [27]. The phenomenon considered pathological is not the transgender condition itself, but the possible clinically significant distress.

The ICD-11 made a different choice and eliminated the diagnostic categories "gender identity disorder of children" and "transsexualism" that were in Chap. 5 ("Mental and Behavioral Disorders") of ICD-10 [20]. Instead, two new diagnostic categories were introduced: "gender incongruence of childhood" and "gender incongruence of adolescence and adulthood." Furthermore, they were not included in Chap. 6 ("Mental and Behavioral Disorders") but placed in a new chapter, "Conditions Related to Sexual Health" [21].

The ICD-11, therefore, *depsychiatrized* trans-identities but maintained a medical diagnosis, independent of dysphoria, to allow transgender people adequate health insurance coverage for gender-affirming treatments (psychological, social, medical, and surgical).

Table 5.1 shows the changes from DSM-I to DSM-5 and in ICD-11.

The *depathologization/depsychiatrization* of variants of sexual orientation and gender identity is an achievement in terms of human rights, considering the weakness of psychiatric diagnoses based essentially on syndromic descriptive criteria.

However, one must not believe that this passage is sufficient to simplify the complexity of sexual and gender issues and to solve the deep psychological conflicts, conscious and unconscious, which often accompany them and which are not only the effect of social discrimination and internalized stigma.

Table 5.1 Gender identity and sexual orientation in DSM (from DSM-I to DSM-5) and ICD-11

DSM-I	DSM-II	DSM-III	DSM-III-R	DSM-IV	DSM-5	ICD-11
1952 [22]	1968 [23]	1980 [24]	1987 [25]	1994 [28]	2013 [27]	2018 [21]
Homosexuality	Homosexuality (sexual orientation disturbance)[a]	Ego-dystonic homosexuality	–	–	–	–
–	–	Gender identity disorders	Gender identity disorders	Gender identity disorders	Gender dysphoria	Gender incongruence[b]

[a]The American Psychiatric Association (APA) removed the diagnostic category *Homosexuality* from DSM-II in 1973 but retained the category "sexual orientation disturbance" (ego-dystonic sexual orientation)

[b]The ICD-11 diagnostic categories *Gender incongruence of childhood* and *Gender incongruence of adolescence and adulthood* are not included in the chapter on *Mental and Behavioral Disorders*, but they appear in a new section, *Conditions Related to Sexual Health*

5.4 Eating-Related Pathology in Sexual Minorities

Studies on ED in gay and lesbian adults are the oldest and most numerous. Those on adolescents and bisexuals are more recent and still limited.

According to a thorough review of the literature, data on prevalence rates of DEB and ED among lesbian adolescents and adults are more heterogeneous and uncertain than other LGBT subgroups [7].

In the past, some research has led to the hypothesis that female homosexuality was even a protective factor for eating psychopathology, as opposed to the male one, recognized as a risk factor [29]. Feldman and Meyer, using the WHO Composite International Diagnostic Interview, found that there were no differences in eating disorder prevalence between lesbian, bisexual, and heterosexual women [30]. Other studies supported the idea that lesbians and heterosexual women showed more similarities than differences in eating attitudes and behaviors.

However, in the Pittsburgh Girls Study, sexual minority women reported higher BMI values and higher eating psychopathology levels than heterosexual peers. Body dissatisfaction mediated the relationship between BMI and eating pathology, and sexual minority status did not mitigate association levels [31].

According to other recent studies, eating pathology rates are higher in both gay and lesbian adolescents and adults than their heterosexual peers [32, 33].

In the Healthy Minds Study (36,691 cisgender men and 81,730 cisgender women), 15.7% of participants self-identified as sexual minorities. The self-reported lifetime ED diagnosis rates were higher in gay and bisexual men and lesbian, bisexual, and questioning women than heterosexual men and women, respectively [34].

In a sample of public high school adolescents, gay men performed intense physical activity, ate little, vomited to lose weight, and took diet pills more often than heterosexual peers [35].

An online survey examined 2733 sexual minority males in Australia and New Zealand. Almost all (98.2%) used pornography (median use 5.33 h per month). The intensity of the use of pornography was correlated with body dissatisfaction (particularly with height, fat, muscularity), eating disorder symptoms, drive for muscularity, and thoughts around the use of anabolic-androgenic steroids [36].

Homosexuality seems to be a risk factor for ED in males, also in non-Western countries [37].

In recent years, some research has also evaluated food addiction symptoms (irresistible craving for highly rewarding foods): Rainey et al. found a double prevalence in sexual minorities compared to heterosexual counterparts [38].

5.5 Eating-Related Pathology in Gender Minorities

The scientific literature on eating pathology in transgender and gender nonconforming individuals is more recent, and studies with adequate samples and robust methodology are still few.

Several studies report, in general, a higher prevalence of mental disorders among transgender people than among cisgender ones.

Data from the 2015 to 2017 Healthy Minds Study (65,213 students, including 1237 gender minority persons) report a higher prevalence of psychopathological symptoms in transgender and gender non-conforming students than in others (78% versus 45%). The symptoms were depression, anxiety, DEB, self-injurious behaviors, and suicidality [39].

As regards, in particular, the psychopathology of nutrition—full-syndrome ED, subclinical ED, and DEB—transgender adolescents and adults usually report eating pathology rates higher than their cisgender peers [5–7, 40, 41, 33].

Only a few articles presented contradictory results, e.g., lower levels of binge eating and excessive exercise in transgender individuals than in cisgender peers [42].

The case reports on MtF transgender people typically indicate a powerful drive for thinness aimed to make the body thinner and more feminine [43].

Hepp et al. described the case of male twins at birth, monozygotic, who during childhood both showed gender incongruent behaviors [44]. Later, one called himself MtF transgender and asked for gender confirmation treatment. The other maintained a male identity but with a non-conforming gender expression (effeminate appearance and clothing). The orientation of both twins was homosexual. In adolescence, both had developed AN. The article raised questions about the interweaving of hereditary and environmental factors.

The case reports on ED in FtM transgender people are less numerous.

A 13-year-old FtM transgender person with AN said she wanted to increase muscle and block breast growth [43].

Strandjord and Rome discussed the case of a 16-year-old girl with AN (BMI 14.9 kg/m^2) who had started outpatient family-based therapy without any doubt about her gender identity [45].

Only after a few months, when she had recovered a healthy weight, she revealed that she felt like a boy in a girl's body (FtM transgender) and asked for additional counseling regarding gender.

An intense drive for thinness is typical of MtF transgender people. In this case, according to the patient, the restrictive behaviors aimed to make the forms of a female body disappear.

The patient undertook individual psychotherapy and hormone therapy (testosterone) and underwent a bilateral mastectomy at age 19. This transgender man reported an improvement in anxiety and discomfort for the body, openly assumed the male identity, and began a romantic relationship with a woman. However, 10 months after surgery, he resumed restrictive eating and excessive exercise (BMI 17.9 kg/m^2).

This case report was the first to describe the effects of gender confirmation treatment on eating behaviors, albeit with a brief follow-up.

5.6 Health Problems in Sexual and Gender Minorities

The prevalence of physical and mental health problems—including ED—is higher in gender and sexual minorities than in the general population [39, 46, 47].

In China, a recent no-school-based study involved over 12,108 adolescents and found that transgender and gender non-conforming (TGNC) individuals, compared with their cisgender counterparts, reported lower overall health and poorer mental health with a higher rate of self-harm and suicidal ideation [47]. The Chinese research has the merit of examining the differences in mental health risk among the different subgroups of young transgender individuals and found that the risk for ideas and suicide attempts was uniformly high.

5.7 What Factors Contribute to the Increased Vulnerability of These Populations?

First of all, it is useful to recall the minority stress model (MSM), which was initially applied to lesbian, gay, and bisexual populations [48] and then extended to transgender and gender non-conforming persons [49].

This conceptual framework gives an essential role to the effects of prejudice, social stigma, discrimination, parental rejection, and peer victimization (defined *distal stressors*). Such distal stressors interact with internal factors (*proximal stressors*): hiding/concealing sexual orientation and gender identity issues, expectations of rejection, internalized stigma, internalized homophobia, and internalized transphobia. Of course, in the MSM application, it is necessary to consider each culture's specific characteristics [50].

Secondly, in sexual and gender minorities, body image dissatisfaction (BID) is a core stressor and represents, as is known, a significant risk factor for the development of eating pathology [51].

A multicenter European study confirmed that discomfort and shame are mainly focused on parts and characteristics of the body more related to the natal sex in male-to-female (MtF) and female-to-male (FtM) young gender dysphoric adults [52].

In a matched control study, transgender participants (MtF and FtM) reported greater body dissatisfaction not only for sex-identifying body parts but also for body shape and weight. MtF transgender individuals appeared to be at particular risk for eating pathology [53].

Appearance ideals are inspired by family, social media, LGBT-specific media, LGBT communities, and dating apps. Stereotypes correspond to one's gender and sexual subjective identity but do not differ substantially from heterosexual and cisgender peers. Many MtF transgender individuals have a thin ideal. Instead, a muscle ideal is more common among FtM transgender persons. Many gay men aspire to a muscular and lean body [54, 7].

An updated systematic review with meta-analysis concluded that gay men report, on average, more BID than heterosexual men, while lesbian women have less body image dissatisfaction (BID) than heterosexual women but more compared to gay men [55].

There are few studies on body image and bisexual orientation. An Italian online survey on the role of sexual orientation in cisgender people found that gay men and bisexual women reported higher body weight dissatisfaction and distorted body shape perception than other groups [56].

Thirdly, childhood traumatic experiences have a potential impact on mental health. An online cross-sectional survey of 3508 LGBTQ+ youth (age 14–18) found significantly higher rates of adverse childhood experiences than the general population [57].

An American study examined 2818 patients treated for ED. 471 (17%) belonged to sexual and gender minorities. At the beginning of treatment, LGBT patients reported experiences of sexual abuse and other trauma (bullying, verbal/physical/emotional abuse) with a significantly higher frequency than others [58].

Parker and Harriger tried to extract from the empirical literature the risk factors for ED and DEB distinguishing them for each of the different subgroups (lesbians, gay males, female bisexuals, male bisexuals, MtF and FtM transgender and gender non-conforming people) and, in each subgroup, for two age groups (adolescents and adults) [7].

However, it seems difficult to derive sufficiently specific indications, useful to differentiate treatment and prevention programs. Several factors are shared with many or all subgroups, and most of them are recognized as risk factors for the development of eating pathology in cisgender and heterosexual individuals as well. A list of the main risk factors includes, in alphabetical order [41, 7]:

- Anxiety
- Body image dissatisfaction
- Body shame
- Bullying
- Childhood traumatic experiences
- Depression
- Higher BMI
- History of childhood sexual abuse
- Low self-esteem
- Low support from family and friends
- Pornography use
- Reaching sexual minority developmental milestones at a younger age (in particular, first identifying as a sexual minority in early adolescence is associated with worse mental health [59])
- Sexual objectification experiences
- Shame
- Weight-based victimization.

Many factors appear to be mutually intertwined.

For example, bullying and sexual abuse are shared risk factors for obesity and ED.

This event also happens in heterosexual and cisgender people. A large Australian study recently confirmed that lifetime histories of bullying and/or sexual abuse were associated with an increased risk of obesity and ED symptoms [60].

Weight-based victimization (WBV, a form of bullying) and, in particular, weight teasing from different sources (family, friends, peers, teachers) affect many young people with overweight/obesity and promote the development of internalized weight bias, negative emotions, and avoidance behaviors [61].

According to the interpersonal model of eating disorders [62], negative social interactions (in particular, feeling devalued) lead to self-disorders (low self-esteem and negative affect) which, in turn, initiate and maintain disturbed eating behaviors (e.g., dieting to improve self-esteem and binge eating to soothe unpleasant emotions).

In the case of sexual and gender minorities, overweight/obesity can produce a double stigma.

Himmelstein et al. recently investigated WBV in a large national sample of LGBTQ adolescents (LGBTQ Teen Study, 9679 participants, mean age 15.6 years, 37.2% overweight/obesity). More than half of the participants reported WBV experiences from peers and family. WBV was associated with more unhealthy eating and weight control behaviors and less physical activity [63].

The literature on protective factors for eating psychopathology is limited both in general and for sexual and gender minorities. A protective role is recognized for factors such as [7, 41, 64, 65]:

- Being in a stable relationship
- Masculinity (gender role), regardless of natal sex
- Self-compassion
- Family support
- Social support.

As for attending LGBT-specific community spaces, for some individuals, it has protective effects on their acceptance of themselves and their physical appearance, but in others it increases the sense of inadequacy compared to ideal stereotypes [54].

5.8 Concluding Remarks and Clinical Suggestions

Gender identity and sexual orientation issues are often associated with unhealthy eating and weight control behaviors.

Beyond the distal and proximal stressors identified by the minority stress model, other individual risk factors are at stake. They are related to life history, family dysfunction, traumatic experiences, body image, intrapsychic functioning, socioeconomic status, ethnicity, and culture.

Usually, DEB arise during or after assuming a transgender identity. Sometimes, however, gender incongruity comes to light only after the diagnosis of an eating disorder [45].

The symptoms do not differ significantly from cisgender and heterosexual patients [7, 38]: fasting, binge eating, self-induced vomiting, craving for addictive foods, body weight and shape overconcern, excessive exercise, and misuse of diet pills, laxatives, and steroids.

In clinical practice, recent guidelines [66, 67] recommend considering gender and sexual orientation issues in the evaluation and treatment of patients with ED.

It should be noted that gender and sexual minority individuals with ED start, on average, later an appropriate treatment and have more severe initial symptoms [58].

The effectiveness of therapies available for eating and weight disorders should be evaluated including individuals who are gender variant or gender nonconforming. For example, the Canadian 2020 guidelines suggest studying the effects of family-based treatments for children and adolescents across the gender spectrum [66].

Suicidal ideation and self-injurious behavior are particularly frequent [47]. In the American study mentioned above, 58% of LGBTQ youth with a lifetime diagnosis of ED reported suicidal ideation [5].

Regarding gender-confirming treatments in adolescents with gender incongruence, in November 2017, the Endocrine Society published a guideline suggesting that most individuals have the mental capacity to give informed consent to these irreversible interventions by age 16 years old. However, hormone treatment is not recommended before puberty, and special attention is required during adolescence [68].

Nonetheless, in the case report of Ristori et al., two adolescents with gender dysphoria and AN symptoms were treated with gonadotropin-releasing analogs (GnRHa). The therapy resulted in pubertal suppression with an improvement in psychological functioning and DEB. In these cases, the authors suggest that the fear of weight gain and disturbed eating behaviors should be considered symptoms of gender incongruence and not AN symptoms and treated accordingly [69].

However, the improvement of gender dysphoria after gender-confirming treatment does not always lead to an improvement in associated psychopathological disorders. The body image issues do not always improve [70]. As for DEB some patients continue to need the help of an ED team [45].

Reliable studies with adequate samples on the long-term evolution of eating-related pathology after gender confirmation therapy in adolescents and adults are still lacking. Accurate, multidimensional research with long follow-ups before, during, and after gender-confirming treatments is needed.

Furthermore, the analysis of separate data by subgroups—lesbian women, gay men, bisexual women and men, MtF and FtM transgender people, and genderqueer persons—is still insufficient and is recommended in future studies on gender and sexual minorities [7, 71].

References

1. Hoek HW. Review of the worldwide epidemiology of eating disorders. Curr Opin Psychiatry. 2016;29(6):336–9. https://doi.org/10.1097/YCO.0000000000000282.
2. Galmiche M, Dechelotte P, Lambert G, Tavolacci MP. Prevalence of eating disorders over the 2000-2018 period: a systematic literature review. Am J Clin Nutr. 2019;109(5):1402–13. https://doi.org/10.1093/ajcn/nqy342.
3. Raisanen U, Hunt K. The role of gendered constructions of eating disorders in delayed help-seeking in men: a qualitative interview study. BMJ Open. 2014;4(4):e004342. https://doi.org/10.1136/bmjopen-2013-004342.
4. Nagata JM, Ganson KT, Murray SB. Eating disorders in adolescent boys and young men: an update. Curr Opin Pediatr. 2020;32(4):476–81. https://doi.org/10.1097/MOP.0000000000000911.

5. The Trevor Project, National Eating Disorders Association, Reasons Eating Disorder Center. Eating disorders among LGBTQ youth: a 2018 national assessment; 2018. https://www.nationaleatingdisorders.org/sites/default/files/nedaw18/NEDA%20Trevor%20Project%202018%20Survey%20-%20Full%20Results.pdf. Accessed 30 Oct 2020.
6. Nagata JM, Ganson KT, Austin SB. Emerging trends in eating disorders among sexual and gender minorities. Curr Opin Psychiatry. 2020;33(6):562–7. https://doi.org/10.1097/YCO.0000000000000645.
7. Parker LL, Harriger JA. Eating disorders and disordered eating behaviors in the LGBT population: a review of the literature. J Eat Disord. 2020;8:51. https://doi.org/10.1186/s40337-020-00327-y.
8. Drescher J. Out of DSM: depathologizing homosexuality. Behav Sci (Basel). 2015;5(4):565–75. https://doi.org/10.3390/bs5040565.
9. Ainsworth C. Sex redefined. The idea of two sexes is simplistic: biologists now think there is a wider spectrum than this. Nature. 2015;518(7539):288–91. https://doi.org/10.1038/518288a.
10. Castleberry J. Addressing the gender continuum: a concept analysis. J Transcult Nurs. 2019;30(4):403–9. https://doi.org/10.1177/1043659618818722.
11. Malalagama A. The shifting landscape of gender identity and the situation in Sri Lanka. Sri Lanka J Sex Health HIV Med. 2017;3:45–50. https://doi.org/10.4038/joshhm.v3i0.63.
12. Goldberg S. We are in the midst of a gender revolution. National Geographic; January 2017, pp. 3–4. https://www.nationalgeographic.com/pdf/gender-revolution-guide.pdf. Accessed 19 Oct 2020.
13. Marsh S. The gender-fluid generation: young people on being male, female or non-binary. The Guardian; 23 Mar 2016. https://www.theguardian.com/commentisfree/2016/mar/23/gender-fluid-generation-young-people-male-female-trans. Accessed 19 Oct 2020
14. Kidd KM, Thornburgh C, Casey CF, Murray PJ. Providing care for transgender and gender diverse youth. Prim Care. 2020;47(2):273–90. https://doi.org/10.1016/j.pop.2020.02.006.
15. Goldenberg T, Kahle EM, Stephenson R. Stigma, resilience, and health care use among transgender and other gender diverse youth in the United States. Transgend Health. 2020;5(3):173–81. https://doi.org/10.1089/trgh.2019.0074.
16. Hérault L. La chirurgie de transsexuation: une médecine entre réparation et amélioration (halshs-01242019). In: Bujon T, Dourlens C, Le Naour G, editors. Aux frontières de la médecine. Paris: Editions des archives contemporaines; 2014. p. 209–20.
17. van Praag HM. Nosologomania: a disorder of psychiatry. World J Biol Psychiatry. 2000;1(3):151–8. https://doi.org/10.3109/15622970009150584.
18. Lewes FM. Dr Marc d'Espine's statistical nosology. Med Hist. 1988;32(3):301–13. https://doi.org/10.1017/s0025727300048250.
19. World Health Organization. Manual of the international statistical classification of diseases, injuries, and causes of death. Sixth revision of the International Lists of Diseases and Causes of Death. Adopted 1948 (ICD-6). Geneva: World Health Organization; 1949.
20. World Health Organization. The ICD-10 classification of mental and behavioural disorders. Clinical descriptions and diagnostic guidelines. Geneva: World Health Organization; 1992.
21. World Health Organization. ICD-11, International Classification of Diseases for mortality and morbidity statistics. Geneva: World Health Organization; 2019. https://icd.who.int/browse11/l-m/en. Accessed 9 Aug 2020.
22. American Psychiatric Association. Diagnostic and statistical manual of mental disorders (DSM-I). Washington, DC: American Psychiatric Association Mental Hospital Service; 1952.
23. American Psychiatric Association. DSM-II. Diagnostic and statistical manual of mental disorders. 2nd ed. Washington, DC: American Psychiatric Association; 1968.
24. American Psychiatric Association. Diagnostic and statistical manual of mental disorders, DSM-III. 3rd ed. Washington, DC: American Psychiatric Association; 1980.
25. American Psychiatric Association. Diagnostic and statistical manual of mental disorders. DSM-III-R (3rd edition revised). Washington, DC: American Psychiatric Association; 1987.
26. Davies RD, Davies ME. The (slow) depathologizing of gender incongruence. J Nerv Ment Dis. 2020;208(2):152–4. https://doi.org/10.1097/NMD.0000000000001119.

27. American Psychiatric Association DSM-5 Task Force. Diagnostic and statistical manual of mental disorders, DSM-5™. 5th ed. Arlington, VA: American Psychiatric Publishing, Inc.; 2013.
28. American Psychiatric Association, editor. Diagnostic and statistical manual of mental disorders, DSM-IV. 4th ed. Washington, DC: American Psychiatric Association; 1994.
29. Siever MD. Sexual orientation and gender as factors in socioculturally acquired vulnerability to body dissatisfaction and eating disorders. J Consult Clin Psychol. 1994;62(2):252–60. https://doi.org/10.1037//0022-006x.62.2.252.
30. Feldman MB, Meyer IH. Eating disorders in diverse lesbian, gay, and bisexual populations. Int J Eat Disord. 2007;40(3):218–26.
31. Jones CL, Fowle JL, Ilyumzhinova R, Berona J, Mbayiwa K, Goldschmidt AB, Bodell LP, Stepp SD, Hipwell AE, Keenan KE. The relationship between body mass index, body dissatisfaction, and eating pathology in sexual minority women. Int J Eat Disord. 2019;52(6):730–4. https://doi.org/10.1002/eat.23072.
32. Matthews-Ewald MR, Zullig KJ, Ward RM. Sexual orientation and disordered eating behaviors among self-identified male and female college students. Eat Behav. 2014;15(3):441–4. https://doi.org/10.1016/j.eatbeh.2014.05.002.
33. Simone M, Askew A, Lust K, Eisenberg ME, Pisetsky EM. Disparities in self-reported eating disorders and academic impairment in sexual and gender minority college students relative to their heterosexual and cisgender peers. Int J Eat Disord. 2020;53(4):513–24. https://doi.org/10.1002/eat.23226.
34. Hazzard VM, Simone M, Borg SL, Borton KA, Sonneville KR, Calzo JP, Lipson SK. Disparities in eating disorder risk and diagnosis among sexual minority college students: findings from the national healthy minds study. Int J Eat Disord. 2020;53(9):1563–8. https://doi.org/10.1002/eat.23304.
35. Zullig KJ, Matthews-Ewald MR, Valois RF. Relationship between disordered eating and self-identified sexual minority youth in a sample of public high school adolescents. Eat Weight Disord. 2019;24(3):565–73. https://doi.org/10.1007/s40519-017-0389-6.
36. Griffiths S, Mitchison D, Murray SB, Mond JM. Pornography use in sexual minority males: associations with body dissatisfaction, eating disorder symptoms, thoughts about using anabolic steroids and quality of life. Aust N Z J Psychiatry. 2018;52(4):339–48. https://doi.org/10.1177/0004867417728807.
37. Boon E, Zainal KA, Touyz SW. Perceptions of eating disorder diagnoses and body image issues in four male cases in Singapore. J Eat Disord. 2017;5(33) https://doi.org/10.1186/s40337-017-0159-x.
38. Rainey JC, Furman CR, Gearhardt AN. Food addiction among sexual minorities. Appetite. 2018;120:16–22. https://doi.org/10.1016/j.appet.2017.08.019.
39. Lipson SK, Raifman J, Abelson S, Reisner SL. Gender minority mental health in the U.S.: results of a national survey on college campuses. Am J Prev Med. 2019;57(3):293–301. https://doi.org/10.1016/j.amepre.2019.04.025.
40. Diemer EW, Grant JD, Munn-Chernoff MA, Patterson DA, Duncan AE. Gender identity, sexual orientation, and eating-related pathology in a national sample of college students. J Adolesc Health. 2015;57(2):144–9. https://doi.org/10.1016/j.jadohealth.2015.03.003.
41. Bell K, Rieger E, Hirsch JK. Eating disorder symptoms and proneness in gay men, lesbian women, and transgender and non-conforming adults: comparative levels and a proposed mediational model. Front Psychol. 2019;9:2692. https://doi.org/10.3389/fpsyg.2018.02692.
42. Nagata JM, Murray SB, Compte EJ, Pak EH, Schauer R, Flentje A, Capriotti MR, Lubensky ME, Lunn MR, Obedin-Maliver J. Community norms for the eating disorder examination questionnaire (EDE-Q) among transgender men and women. Eat Behav. 2020;37:101381. https://doi.org/10.1016/j.eatbeh.2020.101381.
43. Couturier J, Pindiprolu B, Findlay S, Johnson N. Anorexia nervosa and gender dysphoria in two adolescents. Int J Eat Disord. 2015;48(1):151–5. https://doi.org/10.1002/eat.22368.
44. Hepp U, Milos G, Braun-Scharm H. Gender identity disorder and anorexia nervosa in male monozygotic twins. Int J Eat Disord. 2004;35(2):239–43. https://doi.org/10.1002/eat.10247.

45. Strandjord SE, Ng H, Rome ES. Effects of treating gender dysphoria and anorexia nervosa in a transgender adolescent: lessons learned. Int J Eat Disord. 2015;48(7):942–5. https://doi.org/10.1002/eat.22438.
46. Flentje A, Heck NC, Brennan JM, Meyer IH. The relationship between minority stress and biological outcomes: a systematic review. J Behav Med. 2020;43(5):673–94. https://doi.org/10.1007/s10865-019-00120-6.
47. Wang Y, Yu H, Yang Y, Drescher J, Li R, Yin W, Yu R, Wang S, Deng W, Jia Q, Zucker KJ, Chen R. Mental health status of cisgender and gender-diverse secondary school students in China. JAMA Netw Open. 2020;3(10):e2022796. https://doi.org/10.1001/jamanetworkopen.2020.22796.
48. Meyer IH. Prejudice, social stress, and mental health in lesbian, gay, and bisexual populations: conceptual issues and research evidence. Psychol Bull. 2003;129(5):674–97. https://doi.org/10.1037/0033-2909.129.5.674.
49. Hendricks ML, Testa RJ. A conceptual framework for clinical work with transgender and gender nonconforming clients: an adaptation of the minority stress model. Prof Psychol Res Pract. 2012;43(5):460–7. https://doi.org/10.1037/a0029597.
50. Sun S, Hoyt WT, Tarantino N, Pachankis JE, Whiteley L, Operario D, Brown LK. Cultural context matters: testing the minority stress model among Chinese sexual minority men. J Couns Psychol. 2020. https://doi.org/10.1037/cou0000535.
51. Cuzzolaro M, Milano W. Gender identity, sexual orientation, body image, eating, and weight. In: Cuzzolaro M, Fassino S, editors. Body image, eating, and weight. Cham: Springer; 2018. p. 261–72.
52. Becker I, Nieder TO, Cerwenka S, Briken P, Kreukels BP, Cohen-Kettenis PT, Cuypere G, Haraldsen IR, Richter-Appelt H. Body image in young gender dysphoric adults: a European multi-center study. Arch Sex Behav. 2016;45(3):559–74. https://doi.org/10.1007/s10508-015-0527-z.
53. Witcomb GL, Bouman WP, Brewin N, Richards C, Fernandez-Aranda F, Arcelus J. Body image dissatisfaction and eating-related psychopathology in trans individuals: a matched control study. Eur Eat Disord Rev. 2015;23(4):287–93. https://doi.org/10.1002/erv.2362.
54. Gordon A, Austin S, Pantalone D, Baker A, Eiduson R, Rodgers R. Appearance ideals and eating disorders risk among LGBTQ college students: the being ourselves living in diverse bodies (BOLD) study. (Poster Symposia Vi: gender/sexual minority youth health). J Adolesc Health. 2019;64(2 Suppl):S43–4. https://doi.org/10.1016/j.jadohealth.2018.10.096.
55. Dahlenburg SC, Gleaves DH, Hutchinson AD, Coro DG. Body image disturbance and sexual orientation: an updated systematic review and meta-analysis. Body Image. 2020;35:126–41. https://doi.org/10.1016/j.bodyim.2020.08.009.
56. Meneguzzo P, Collantoni E, Bonello E, Vergine M, Behrens SC, Tenconi E, Favaro A. The role of sexual orientation in the relationships between body perception, body weight dissatisfaction, physical comparison, and eating psychopathology in the cisgender population. Eat Weight Disord. 2021;26(6):1985–2000. https://doi.org/10.1007/s40519-020-01047-7.
57. Craig SL, Austin A, Levenson J, Leung VWY, Eaton AD, D'Souza SA. Frequencies and patterns of adverse childhood events in LGBTQ+ youth. Child Abuse Negl. 2020;107:104,623. https://doi.org/10.1016/j.chiabu.2020.104623.
58. Mensinger JL, Granche JL, Cox SA, Henretty JR. Sexual and gender minority individuals report higher rates of abuse and more severe eating disorder symptoms than cisgender heterosexual individuals at admission to eating disorder treatment. Int J Eat Disord. 2020;53(4):541–54. https://doi.org/10.1002/eat.23257.
59. Katz-Wise SL, Rosario M, Calzo JP, Scherer EA, Sarda V, Austin SB. Associations of timing of sexual orientation developmental milestones and other sexual minority stressors with internalizing mental health symptoms among sexual minority young adults. Arch Sex Behav. 2017;46(5):1441–52. https://doi.org/10.1007/s10508-017-0964-y.
60. Mitchison D, Bussey K, Touyz S, Gonzalez-Chica D, Musker M, Stocks N, Licinio J, Hay P. Shared associations between histories of victimisation among people with eating disor-

der symptoms and higher weight. Aust N Z J Psychiatry. 2019;53(6):540–9. https://doi.org/10.1177/0004867418814961.
61. Himmelstein MS, Puhl RM. Weight-based victimization from friends and family: implications for how adolescents cope with weight stigma. Pediatr Obes. 2019;14(1). https://doi.org/10.1111/ijpo.12453.
62. Rieger E, Van Buren DJ, Bishop M, Tanofsky-Kraff M, Welch R, Wilfley DE. An eating disorder-specific model of interpersonal psychotherapy (IPT-ED): causal pathways and treatment implications. Clin Psychol Rev. 2010;30(4):400–10. https://doi.org/10.1016/j.cpr.2010.02.001.
63. Himmelstein MS, Puhl RM, Watson RJ. Weight-based victimization, eating behaviors, and weight-related health in sexual and gender minority adolescents. Appetite. 2019;141:104321. https://doi.org/10.1016/j.appet.2019.104321.
64. Cella S, Iannaccone M, Cotrufo P. Influence of gender role orientation (masculinity versus femininity) on body satisfaction and eating attitudes in homosexuals, heterosexuals and transsexuals. Eat Weight Disord. 2013;18(2):115–24. https://doi.org/10.1007/s40519-013-0017-z.
65. Meyer C, Blissett J, Oldfield C. Sexual orientation and eating psychopathology: the role of masculinity and femininity. Int J Eat Disord. 2001;29(3):314–8. https://doi.org/10.1002/eat.1024.
66. Couturier J, Isserlin L, Norris M, Spettigue W, Brouwers M, Kimber M, McVey G, Webb C, Findlay S, Bhatnagar N, Snelgrove N, Ritsma A, Preskow W, Miller C, Coelho J, Boachie A, Steinegger C, Loewen R, Loewen T, Waite E, Ford C, Bourret K, Gusella J, Geller J, LaFrance A, LeClerc A, Scarborough J, Grewal S, Jericho M, Dimitropoulos G, Pilon D. Canadian practice guidelines for the treatment of children and adolescents with eating disorders. J Eat Disord. 2020;8:4. https://doi.org/10.1186/s40337-020-0277-8.
67. National Institute for Health and Care Excellence (NICE). Eating disorders: recognition and treatment. NICE guideline [NG69]; Published date: 23 May 2017. https://www.nice.org.uk/guidance/ng69.
68. Hembree WC, Cohen-Kettenis PT, Gooren L, Hannema SE, Meyer WJ, Murad MH, Rosenthal SM, Safer JD, Tangpricha V, T'Sjoen GG. Endocrine treatment of gender-dysphoric/gender-incongruent persons: an endocrine society* clinical practice guideline. J Clin Endocrinol Metabol. 2017;102(11):3869–903. https://doi.org/10.1210/jc.2017-01658.
69. Ristori J, Fisher AD, Castellini G, Sensi C, Cipriani A, Ricca V, Maggi M. Gender dysphoria and anorexia nervosa symptoms in two adolescents. Arch Sex Behav. 2019;48(5):1625–31. https://doi.org/10.1007/s10508-019-1396-7.
70. Becker I, Auer M, Barkmann C, Fuss J, Moller B, Nieder TO, Fahrenkrug S, Hildebrandt T, Richter-Appelt H. A cross-sectional multicenter study of multidimensional body image in adolescents and adults with gender dysphoria before and after transition-related medical interventions. Arch Sex Behav. 2018;47(8):2335–47. https://doi.org/10.1007/s10508-018-1278-4.
71. Thoma BC, Choukas-Bradley S. Mental health of transgender adolescents around the globe—a call for comprehensive assessment of gender identity. JAMA Netw Open. 2020;3(10):e2023412. https://doi.org/10.1001/jamanetworkopen.2020.23412.

Food and Addictions

Umberto Nizzoli

6.1 Human Development

Everything that is loved grows, Father Vincenzo Sorce used to repeat [1], which is equivalent to observing that those who are not loved, that is the unwelcome child, suffer damage to the development of the brain architectures that expose them to developmental disorders, like ADHD, during childhood and can further develop into behaviour disorders and drug use disorders during adolescence as evidenced by research conducted at Harvard Child Development Institute [2].

Our biological structures are predisposed to welcome. When we are born, we are in a state of absolute dependence, and we are biologically built to live the condition of dependence, which in the initial stages of life is the most total. The quality of the mother–child interaction is the tool that lays the foundation for later emotional regulation and cognition [3], the qualities that are most involved in the formation of addiction.

Human history starts from a condition of radical dependence and develops a trajectory aimed at a progressive, even if never completely realized, autonomy.

This is the direction of the human development process.

The paths from dependence to autonomy is far from linear.

A text by Ogden [4] talks about unlived lives; the hypothetical lives that the individual could have developed and followed if in certain circumstances, such as suffering an accident or met someone other, he would have had other occurrences. Inside the individual there remains a memory of unlived lives, memories of sketched hypotheses and for some reason that did not happen. Those memories give rise to an emotional background of melancholy for the renunciations that are inherent in them.

U. Nizzoli (✉)
Azienda Sanitaria Reggio Emilia, SISDCA, Reggio Emilia, Italy
e-mail: nizzoliumberto@gmail.com

© Springer Nature Switzerland AG 2022
E. Manzato et al. (eds.), *Hidden and Lesser-known Disordered Eating Behaviors in Medical and Psychiatric Conditions*,
https://doi.org/10.1007/978-3-030-81174-7_6

Growth is the mixture between opportunities, accidents and choices. Therefore between decisions, openings, conquests and renunciations, where from a numerical point of view the latter far outweigh the former, there are always many more hypotheses that could have been explored than realities.

The process of building the human person that passes from the most absolute dependence to an autonomy, never completed, is the meaning of growing up and becoming a person. The arrow of growth is sustained with a series of renunciations.

Learning to bear frustration is one of the major skills that is required for the human being. The strength of resilience to frustration is a buildable quality, which helps to face the defeats and losses in life by keeping hope high and knowing how to resist frustrations. [5]

As human beings we have to face an existential enigma: even if you are well trained to consider one's limitations due to the continuous renunciation of impossible evolutionary hypotheses, it can happen that the individual becomes so continuously fixated on his need to own a certain object or to assume a behaviour so that that evolutionary trajectory, made up of achievements flanked by multiple frustrations, seems to be interrupted. He fixes his attention on an object or behaviour and starts wanting that object in every way.

It seems that the development process no longer receives the signal to stop. The individual can continue to carry out a series of human tasks but an object or behaviour appears in his existential trajectory and becomes, for him, the source of all desire for a paralysing fixation. He wants that object, he desires that object, he has become addicted to that object.

We enter into that phenomenology that became so widespread over the last few decades: addiction, or rather addictions, due to the many expressive declinations that it can assume [6].

On the perspective of the WHO (1948) health is a positive condition not limited to the absence of disease that measures the level of psychic, physical, relational and, according to some authors, spiritual well-being, addiction is what is on the opposite end.

In fact, while health is the level of equilibrium that the individual has in terms of calm and inner safety, of experience, immersed in the historical-social and relational contexts of his vital expression, addiction is the escape from oneself from the control point of the inner balance/imbalance. Human vitality is the continuous transfer of energies through neural pathways. The impetus for those innumerable processes comes from the stimuli. The basins of the stimuli are the external world, made up of nature and people, the body with its signals and the memories stored in us; in a word, reality. It continually launches its stimuli to human beings. In people with addiction, the addictive substance or behaviour is the underlying trigger for the behaviour.

6.2 Addiction

When the International Society of Addiction Journals Editors was founded in 2001, part of the discussion led by Edward Griffith centred on the choice of the term that defined the field of scientific interest and which ended up in the society's acronym, ISAJE. https://www.isaje.net/

For the Italian, the reflection could seem distant, given that in any case in my language I would have used "pathological addictions", but Addiction was chosen instead of Dependence to underline the neurobiological and psychic internal aspect that pushes the subject to addictive behaviours towards the object/behaviour without which existence seems meaningless. The fundamental vector would therefore be the pathology in the subject rather than the force of the external object.

The construct of Addiction, despite an overwhelming literature, is still controversial. Its implications are pervasive. For this reason, various descriptions and theories have followed on the subject of pathological dependence, addiction.

Although it is not accepted within the DSM-5 [7] because it is considered not sufficiently supported by research evidence, it is too polluted by its media use, the practical use of the term Addiction is found more and more frequently in thesis, publications, titles and reports, including this article.

The term Addiction is therefore used both from the point of view of the phenomenological description of behaviours that go under the banner of compulsiveness and impulsivity both for neurobiological configuration and even more openly for its clinical value.

The fate of this name is really strange also because the journal that has the highest Impact Factor in the field of addiction is exactly called Addiction (https://www.addictionjournal.org)

The first edition of Addiction dates back to 1884 as a scientific journal of the Society for the Study on Addiction: the start of publication however occurs before the release of the first DSM. Addiction is therefore the most historic, the most titled and the most authoritative journal in the sector. Its policy recognizes all behaviours marked by impulsiveness and loss of control, from legal drugs to illegal ones to additive drug-free behaviours of which, however, the DSM-5 recognizes only pathological gambling for now.

The gap that exists between seeing it always everywhere and stabilizing its data is even more open, if it is possible, in relation to alcohol of which our civilization has millennia of experience with [8], and the food that is an important part of everyone's daily life.

For a long time the term drug dependence has been used and subsequently often replaced by pathological dependence; Drug Abuse or Substance Abuse or Dependence, again in DSM IV to switch to Drug Related Disorders and Addictive Disorders in DSM-5

Addiction makes some experiences easier and more rewarding and, conversely, other different experiences increasingly difficult and less rewarding. Either due to initial difficulties or thanks to gratifications, the person ends up favouring certain habits (of drug use or behaviour) at the expense of others. Addiction is a disease of the brain that structures itself following its experiences.

The National Institute of Drug Abuse (NIDA) [9] uses the term Addiction to describe compulsive drug seeking despite the negative behaviours and negative consequences of which the subject is aware. Addiction is a chronic disorder with relapses characterized by compulsive and continuous research, despite the negative consequences and with effects of modification of the brain architectures; therefore it is considered both as a complex brain disorder and as a mental illness at the same time.

Although controversial, addiction theories recognize the etiological importance of environmental and cognitive factors in addition to neuro-biological predispositions. There is a great power of the environment (family, friends, education, media, language, market, culture) to facilitate or compromise the delicate balance between pleasure and addiction [10].

The aforementioned definition appears inadequate when referring to the evolution of the "market for substances and lifestyles". Both the consumption of legal or illegal or prescription drugs and the impulsive-compulsive behaviours are so prevalent that they can be considered common.

It would therefore not be possible to argue that addictive behaviours are widespread if we include only those that are continuously activated by craving.

We therefore fell into the dilemma: is addiction just the severe degree of impulsive-compulsive disorders sedated/modulated by drugs or behaviours or does it embrace all consumption and impulsive-compulsive behaviours?

I believe we have to accept that the term Addiction ends up defining both the most severe degree of disorder from the use of legal or illegal substances and the plethora of all forms in which human conduct is declined in terms of dependence on an object (drugs, food, money, objects) or behaviour (gambling, video-chat Internet, shopping, sex). Addictions that can coexist, can follow each other according to an unpredictable pathway, order, forcing the clinician to follow even sudden diagnostic migrations.

In fact, individual stories do not require any predefined path within the spectrum, leaving all evolutionary possibilities open to the person.

Goodman [11] proposed criteria for defining addictive behaviours (with or without substances):
1. The inability to resist the urge to adopt that behaviour
2. The growing internal tension before starting the behaviour
3. Pleasure or relief at the moment of action
4. The loss of control from the very beginning of the behaviour
5. At least five of the following eight criteria:
   – Frequent preoccupation with behaviour
   – The commitment due to that more intense or longer than expected behaviour
   – Repeated efforts to reduce or quit
   – The considerable time spent realizing the behaviour or recovering from its effects
   – The reduction of social, professional, family activities determined by behaviour
   – Engagement in behaviour prevents the fulfilment of social, family or professional obligations
   – Perseverance in behaviour despite physical, social or financial problems
   – A state of agitation and irritability if it is possible to implement the behaviour

Inside these criteria there are an enormous quantity of human behaviours that can be considered as addictive.

The complication of the Addiction construct increases because, alongside the disorders related to substance use, a new category is introduced that already absorbs previous frameworks and criteria disseminated above the chapter of loss of control and forms a new dimension: Addictive Behaviours. There are addictive behaviours without the use of substances. The DSM-5 declares them to be equivalent in terms of the neuronal process. Curiously, he recognizes only one form of Addiction, pathological gambling: the implicit is that, once some epidemiological steps have been overcome, other forms of addiction will come.

Addiction is a disease of the brain that structures itself following its experiences. According to this model, the concept of addiction as a disease has emerged [12] for the maintenance of which craving is fundamental [13], that is the basic syndromic condition of all addictions, characterized by appetitive urge to seek pleasure and an irrepressible implementation, even to the disadvantage of the very will of the subject. A visceral and overwhelming "hunger" that underestimates the damage [14].

Because it focuses on biologic factors rather than moral arguments, it has helped reduce stigma faced by those with addictions and their families, at least in some aspects. It is very important to reduce internal or external harms induced by stigma. Addiction as a brain disease is not accepted by all authors.

Addiction is the result of the intersection of at least three determining matrices. They are pathogenetic: all three are needed, albeit in varying proportions and they are pathoplastic: they are capable of shaping the expressiveness of the addictive phenomenon. Indeed, a phenomenon of addiction occurs because:

– A substance (or a human habit) that carries within it the possibility of addiction
– A person and therefore a personality open to addiction
– A socio-environmental context

All three aspects are necessary, but none alone is sufficient to determine the condition [15].

Addiction is conceived as behaviour learned by a mind that is structured in a continuous dialogue with environmental stimuli. Addiction makes some experiences easier and more rewarding and, conversely, the others increasingly difficult and less rewarding. Either due to initial difficulties or thanks to gratifications, the person ends up favouring certain habits at the expense of others [16].

Hence the need to overcome the Manichean dimension of the inside or the outside. In fact, it is necessary that the "object/behaviour" likely to give addiction meets the "right person": someone with characteristics capable of interacting with it (second matrix factor). These characteristics can be biological, but also personological. Often the two aspects overlap and interconnect [17]. That is, a tropism takes place between "object" and personality. Not less important is the socio-cultural-environmental factor (third matrix factor). The context in which a "substance or a behaviour" and a "personality" meet is not irrelevant. There can be favouring or impeding effects, triggered by a certain socio-economic and cultural environment.

Because the disease model focuses on brain change, it has helped explain why persons with addictions find it difficult to change their thoughts and behaviours quickly or easily. Learning models propose that addiction, though disadvantageous, is a natural, context-sensitive response to challenging environmental contingencies, not a disease [18, 19].

6.3 Craving

The point that we could consider as a conjunction between the definition of the DSM-5 and the definition of the NIDA Guide is craving (since 2013 an unavoidable criterion of the DSM-5 for the diagnosis of substance use related disorder), i.e. the basic syndromic condition of all addictions [14], characterized by the appetitive urge to seek pleasure and an irrepressible implementation, even to the disadvantage of the very will of the subject. A visceral and overwhelming "hunger" that underestimates the damage [20].

According to ASAM [21], the American Society of Addiction Medicine, addiction is a chronic neurobiological disease with genetic, psychosocial and environmental factors that influence its development and its manifestations.

Addiction is characterized by behaviours that include one or more of the following:

- Impaired control over drug use
- Compulsive use
- Continued use despite the damage
- Craving

It would therefore be necessary to detect the frequency of the craving to establish whether the subject is affected by mild, medium or severe degree, so addicted.

According to West and Brown [22], addiction is that condition in which individual needs the immediate and full satisfaction of what a craving.

The construct of craving appears central. The DSM-5 describes craving as "a strong desire or urge".

Craving is a complex phenomenon related to the inability to feel emotions, boredom, dissociative mental states, impulsivity and loss of control. Its measure is subjective.

Even today we do not know whether to consider craving as a completely subjective experience or a physiological need for a substance or a behaviour.

Although the association between overwhelming desire and addiction has been known from antiquity, it is only the study on the effects of drugs that has put craving at the centre of the scientific debate.

When what is missing becomes too disturbing a presence, the individual can lose control. I want it, I want it, I want it now, whatever its cost, can't live without it, I absolutely must have it.

A pressure grows, like a wave, an emotional tsunami, it's craving.

Obviously there are genetic bases of craving. Nothing can be done outside of the genetic basis.

But craving is a powerful, overwhelming experience that shakes the body and stirs the mind and that grows out of all proportion and becomes everything for that individual at that moment.

One can desire a person, a thing; but one can also experience the shock of craving itself as an experience of individual devastation.

Usually individuals overestimate the duration and intensity of the craving. But after the wave it gradually calms down, as explained by the beautiful figure described by Marlatt & Gordon [23].

The visualization of the desired object or another sensory stimulus is the trigger point of the craving. This has been observed for drugs but occurs in a similar way for a wide range of situations or substances, including food.

Craving compromises the processing capacity and in particular the working memory, which is the cognitive process linked to decision-making activities.

Breaking the craving means (almost an impossible task, as breaking it once triggered is very difficult work) trying to turn off the drive capable of generating the continuous search.

The continued search, the "hunger" of the other: craving can be considered the point of passage in which an experience of appetition becomes a disease. To stop it is to stop the hunger of addiction.

6.4   Addiction and Autonomy

Individual life begins with a separation: the original unity is broken forever and the new reality arises: the "object" one [24]. Nourishment is no longer provided for free and relentlessly, but in an exchange between two separate subjects, one in need who asks for it and the other who may or may not be there depending on many factors, not least its availability. From that separation derives the condition of lack and the correlated addiction.

The pain of separation and the inspiration of reunion give life in Aristophanes in the Platonic Symposium to the myth of the halved apple: halved human beings in the never-ending search for the missing half [25].

The word addiction is not synonymous with constitutional weakness or disease. Dependence is a state of mind and originally also of the body, which underlies the movement of our drives towards a goal and which attests our ability to bond with others and objects. When it is not expressed in a pathological way, addiction is the very essence of human relationships and appears, moreover, natural. We know how to depend on children and parents for countless aspects. On our closest friends, on the work we do, on society and even on the routine acts of our life whose interruption is a source of discomfort and disharmony. In evolutionary terms, a relationship of dependence is aimed at acquiring the skills that allow you to become yourself and explore the world with confidence. We depend in order to learn, explore and subsequently become creative, feeling that we can count on a secure basis [26] first external and then introjected.

The mind is relational [27] which is structured starting from a genetic and on neurobiological correlates on the basis of the relationships that the person establishes; therefore it is diffused not only in the whole human body but in the whole context from which the sensory stimulations come and from the whole context from which the relational fields come.

The human mind tends to repeat the circuits and experiences that have gratified it in the absence of some reason that motivates a change. The human mind is doomed to habit and to the progressive limitation of its associative abilities [28].

Desires characterize the life of human beings. At any age, one does not stop desiring and implementing choices that help their realization. This dynamism arises from an experience of incompleteness that asks to be filled for the awareness of the limit, to be historical, embodied, relational. Only if we perceive ourselves in this way, we can desire new horizons. However, not all wishes are possible. Some are impossible claims, impositions that trample the reality of things and relationships. People should be satisfied despite having unfulfilled desires [29].

6.5 Food and Addiction

Drugs have always been used for some precise purposes in the history of humanity:

(a) For religious purposes
(b) For medical purposes
(c) For initiation rites

A passage from Euripides' Bacchae is emblematic: "The son of Semele who taught that juice drawn from grapes, the drink that to the unhappy beings that are men, soothes all pain and gives sleep, and with sleep the oblivion of all evils of the day; there is no medicine other than this for those whith suffering and pain".

The relationship between eating disorders and substance use disorders is one of the many possible comorbidities, and although many times underestimated and insufficiently investigated in clinical practice, the presence of substance use disorders in people with eating disorders and vice versa is significant.

It is common to encounter concomitant addictions with another diagnosis of mental disorder.

It is common to encounter ED concomitant with another diagnosis of mental disorder.

Food and Addiction records the concomitance of the presence of these two diagnostic categories. The "double diagnosis" of both is more frequently combined with personality disorder (mainly borderline personality disorder).

ED and SUD have various similarities: neuro-biological, emotional and behavioural mechanisms seem to bring them together. The disease histories must clarify which of the two disorders arose first or whether the onset is contemporary.

In one clinical area as in the other, disorders are often underestimated, not sought after, they do not emerge in practices centred on the disorder being treated. Given the frequency, they should instead be included in the explorations already along first assessment and after and receive appropriate care.

Psychoactive substances such as alcohol, illicit drugs and prescription drugs can be used for emotional regulation or as a pattern of impious behaviour.

The misuse of substances such as caffeine, tobacco, insulin, thyroid drugs, stimulants or others (laxatives, diuretics) may have the aim of helping weight loss and/or providing energy.

There are high rates of comorbidity between ED and SUD [30].

In individuals with ED, the prevalence of SUD is roughly 50%, against 7–9% in the general population, while in people with SUD about 35% have ED against about 3–7% of the general population. The literature highlights the concomitance of ED subtypes with SUD types [31–35].

6.6 Food Addiction

In DSM-5 alongside the disorders related to the use of substances, a new category is introduced, Addictive behaviours. The DSM-5 declares them to be equivalent in terms of the neuronal process.

The term "food addiction" (FA) was originally coined in 1956 by Randolph [36], who associated it with addictive drinking.

Food addiction, especially activated by refined and manipulated, palatable foods, would override the cortical inhibitory processes that signal satiety to cause the compulsive consumption of food in large quantities. The loss of control and compulsive behavioural patterns of food consumption replicate the patterns of drug use observed in the SUD [37, 38]. The salience of food incentives is a key factor, in particular for the one rich in sugars and fats that triggers the desire and pleasure of its use ("wanting" and "liking") as components of the reward [36] causing a real and own dependence [38–40].

The study of food addiction has been corroborated by research carried out with the use of the Yale Food Addiction Scale—YFAS, validated to identify food patterns with characteristics similar to the typical behaviours of classic addiction [41, 42], the original version of which was recently updated [43].

The concept of food addiction remains subject of discussion. In fact, it has been recalled that the different forms of obesity and eating disorders are too varied and complex in their phenotypic manifestations and their neurobiological characteristics to be traced simply to the addiction model [44]. Some authors have underlined the evident difficulty of comparing food to a substance of abuse [45], recalling the complex nutritional and sensory properties of food, which in addition to taste include other elements (taste, smell, texture), and underlining how nutrition is intrinsically an activity that generates gratification and reinforcement. Any food, regardless of its chemical/nutritional composition, can activate the brain system of the reward, but it does not necessarily follow that the activation of the system takes place in a form of addiction understood as a serious pathology. Each subject derives enjoyment and desire from intrinsic food cues that act as triggers for them. In fact, there are subjects who have binge access to non-hyper-palatable foods. More than the sensory and nutritional properties of foods is the ways in which they are consumed that define addiction [46, 47].

However, if a cut-off is not set that allows those who do not perform it to be excluded from Food addiction, it can be seen that practically every ED framework struggles between impulse and control. The expansion would be such that every picture of ED would belong to food addiction, thus making it, in its ubiquity, a useless diagnosis.

6.7 Addiction Again

Over a short period of time, almost all ways of life can express a pathology: playing, sport, the Internet, chat, TV, sex, shopping, work, stealing, money, power, exercise, … You get to understand the phenomenon of love addiction [48] although for a long time [49] it was the subject of poetry and literature.

As mentioned, the Addiction construct is complicated and controversial. Its success can turn into a further complication. Since addiction has to do with the repetition of acts which are considered pleasant by the subject, it is possible to spread it in its less intense forms in all life activities that the person does not only with pleasure but also with insistence.

It would paradoxically be possible to find addiction in reading the newspaper, leafing through magazines, eating pasta, and strolling around the streets, provided these things were done with insistent desire. All these activities, all those done with passion, stimulate the reward system.

But how many people usually don't eat an extra biscuit after completing dinner, even when they know they shouldn't? Or get lost in thought or immerse themselves in some pleasant reading even though they should be working? Can they be considered suffering from a mild form of Addiction?

If these habits are excessive, they can be classified as addiction; but what is excessive? Is the "negative effect for the subject" that is his experience in establishing whether his conduct has exceeded the limit to deserve the diagnosis? Affected individuals would have difficulty learning from the consequences of their previous behaviours. I know that the slice of cake after I get up from the table makes me sleep worse; but I don't hold back; I reduce it by one part and eat it, and after that I reduce a smaller part again and I eat it.

The era we live in of increasing overstimulation in the name of the speed of exchanges (information) and the processes of outsourcing. Conducted even more accentuated in this period of pandemic where the spread of network connections creates an overcrowding of stimuli in the real and in the virtual world which affect the individual.

The increase in environmental and social pressure requires that the reactions to the stimuli received be made more sudden, aiming at the immediacy of the need. Outsourcing creates a great theatre of appearance, with serious implications for the image and its management.

This global context leads to the slipping of identities and the inability to lead oneself, reflecting before acting; instead it induces impulsiveness, speed with a propensity to rob objects that can satisfy desires and any kind of pleasure. The race for increasing immediacy clears customs inhibitions that could have been deeply rooted in the value system of some time ago.

Any object or any behaviour, regardless of its conformation, can activate the brain system of the reward.

In his latest work on food addiction Melchionda [39] explains one of the essences of life: the struggle between regulation and dysregulation of behaviour, above all food. But the same struggle can be re-proposed on every relationship that the individual establishes. Melchionda argues that food is a more dangerous drug than cocaine because it is ubiquitous and inevitable for anyone.

The struggle between accepting and letting go has at its root the ontological incompleteness of the human person. The lack alludes to the absence of something that was there, that could be there, that should have been there. At the root there was an act of separation and rupture. A large part of religions and theogonies are structured to explain the original absence.

The point is that today the hybris of modernity, with the indefinite expansion of individualism, comes to idolize themselves as "gods on earth".

We are currently in a new phase in the history of addiction: globalization has led, among other things, to mass consumption of drugs for hedonistic and performance-enhancing reasons. There is a widespread demand for pleasure and power: drugs tease on the one hand and respond to this request on the other. Pleasure, if considered the supreme end, reveals itself as a master so tyrannical to lockdown man in selfishness and such a liar as to not keep what he promises to the point of even leading to self-destruction, as happens in addiction behaviours.

The frenzy quivers to leave behind boredom and tiredness that comes from the ordinary life. In the spasmodic search for an elsewhere that never exists, for a future that does not exist. Which is not thought, sought or planned; so there is no sacrifice: it must be here now, immediately, in a present that must give the taste of the future. The clash between control and loss of control is pervasive and ubiquitous. Here then is the craving, structurally related to all those situations in which the absence of the possibility of exercising the behaviour is dependent on dominates. Excess of a kind of mass craving. Craving is a very complex phenomenon that correlates on several fronts with the inability to feel emotions, boredom, dissociative mental states and impulsivity and loss of control.

An environment full of stimuli related to the object of too much desire, which can be drugs, food, sex, play, the Internet, shopping, work, power and, why not, the beloved, stimulates the desire to take drugs, eat, have sex, play and so on until you are always with your loved one. Desire is formed before acting, creating a state of expectation that can become poignant, tearing and craving.

It is in the struggle and integrative abilities between pleasure-enjoyment and control-enjoyment that the game is played that gives life to individual expression (behaviour). Feeling pleasure without losing control, becoming aroused by remaining in control of yourself: this is the fine line that prolongs pleasure into happiness and prevents pleasure from falling into addiction. Good doses of self-awareness and self-control are required; it's not for everyone. Helping people achieve this balance is the real goal of those with clinical duties.

Assaggioli (1888–1974), founder of Psychosynthesis [50], who used to communicate through metaphors, coined a very suitable one to describe the theme covered by this article. He said: the human being is like a dog on a chain. If he's attracted to what he sees and hears out of range of the chain, he ends up choking. But if he is clear about the circle in which he can move and thinks only about that, he feels like a king.

By continuously expanding the addictive behaviours and triggering the overwhelming appetite desire we can find an integrative reading in the writings of Dante Alighieri.

On his 700th death anniversary, it might seem suggestive to connect the subject of this article with the path taken by Dante Alighieri accompanied by Virgil in the Divine Comedy in the descent into hell "I do not say well why I enter there; I was so confused and slept that I lost the right way "(Inferno c I ° 9) and even more when in The Vita Nova Dante debates with his friend Guido Cavalcanti whom he contrasts the way of ascent with that of passions [51].

To be able to use the construct of Addiction appropriately in the clinical setting, there is still a lot of digging to do if we don't want to retrace the essential human dilemma of the struggle between desires and limits, between dreams and reality.

References

1. Stornello S. Oltre le pieghe dell'anima, Ordine Psicologi Sicilia 2020; 2020. https://www.oprs.it/psicologi-e-psicologia-in-sicilia/oltre-le-pieghe-dellanima-la-mia-storia-come-psicologo-di-comunita-al-tempo-del-coronavirus/
2. National Scientific Council on the Developing Child (2012). The science of neglect: the persistent absence of responsive care disrupts the developing brain: working paper no. 12. www.developingchild.harvard.edu.
3. Murray L, de Pascalis L, Bozicevic L, Hawkins L, Sclafani V, Ferrari PF. The functional architecture of mother-infant communication, and the development of infant social expressiveness in the first two months. Sci Rep. 2016;6:39019. https://doi.org/10.1038/srep39019.
4. Ogden TH. Vite non vissute. Esperienze in psicoanalisi (Traduttore: S. Boffito). Cortina Raffaello: Psicologia clinica e psicoterapia; 2016.
5. Cyrulnik B. il dolore meraviglioso, Frassinelli ed.; 2000.
6. Nizzoli U, Il tempo del craving, drugs and addictions, vatican dicastery for promoting integral human development, Libreria editrice Vaticana; 2020, 78-91.
7. APA. DSM-5 Diagnostic and statistical manual of mental disorders. 5th ed. Arlington, VA: APA; 2013.
8. Gregory T. Noè ovvero della sobria ebbrezza. In L'ebbrezza di Noè, il Vicolo Cesena; 2003.
9. NIDA, The science of drug use and addiction, guide; 2018
10. Volkow ND, Koob GF, McLellan AT. Neurobiologic advances from the brain disease model of addiction. N Engl J Med. 2016;374(4):363–71.
11. Goodman A. Addiction: definition and implications. Addiction. 2006;85(11):1403–8.
12. O'Brien CP, McLellan AT. Myths about the treatment of addiction. Lancet. 1996;347:237–40.
13. Isbell H. Craving for alcohol. QJ Stud Alcohol. 1955;16:38–42.

14. Nizzoli U, Margaron H, Caretti V, Croce M, Lorenzi P, Zerbetto R. Craving. Mucchi: Alla base di tutte le dipendenze; 2011.
15. Olievenstein C. La Vie du toxicomane: Séminaire de l'Hôpital Marmottan—Paris. PUF; 1982.
16. Volkow ND, Morales M. The brain on drugs: from reward to addiction. Cell. 2015;162(4):712–25. https://doi.org/10.1016/j.cell.2015.07.046.
17. Dagher A, Robbins TW. Personality, addiction, dopamine: insights from Parkinson disease. Neuron. 2009;61:502–10.
18. Lewis M. Addiction and the brain: development, not disease. Neuroethics. 2017;10:7–18.
19. Heather N, Best D, Kawalek A, et al. Challenging the brain disease model of addiction: European launch of the Addiction Theory Network. Addict Res Theory. 2018;26:249–55.
20. Rosenberg H. Clinical and laboratory assessment of the subjective experience of drug craving. Clin Psychol Rev. 2009;29:519–34.
21. Definition of Addiction, American Society on Addiction Medicine. https://www.asam.org/docs/default-source/quality-science/asam's-2019-definition-of-addiction-(1).pdf?sfvrsn=b8b64fc2_2
22. West R, Brown J. Theory of addiction. Chichester: John Wiley & Sons, Ltd; 2013.
23. Marlatt GA, Gordon JR. Relapse prevention. New York: Guilford; 1985.
24. Malher M, Pine MM, Bergman A. The psychological birth of the human infant. New York: Basic Books; 1973.
25. Plato, Symposium, written 360 B.C.E.
26. Bowlby J. Attachment and loss. New York: Basic Books; 1969.
27. Siegel D. The developing mind, third edition: how relationships and the brain interact to shape who we are. Brilliance corp.; 2012.
28. Edelman GM. Seconda natura. Scienza del cervello e conoscenza umana. Milano: Raffaello Cortina; 2007.
29. Bonhoeffer D. Gli scritti. Brescia: Queriniana; 1979. p. 1928–44.
30. Brownell KD, Gold MS. Food and addiction, a comprehensive handbook. New York: Oxford University Press; 2014.
31. Calero-Elvira A, Krug I, Davis K, López C, Fernández-Aranda F, Treasure J. Meta-analysis on drugs in people with eating disorders. Eur Eat Disord Rev. 2009;17(4):243–59. https://doi.org/10.1002/erv.936.
32. Conason AH, Brunstein-Klomek A, Sher L. Recognizing alcohol and drug abuse in patients with eating disorders. QJM. 2006;99:335–9.
33. Courbasson CM, Smith PD, Cleland PA. Substance use disorders anorexia, bulimia, and cocurrent disorders. Can J Public Health. 2005;96(2):102–6.
34. Fouladi F, Mitchell JE, Crosby RD, Engel SG, Crow S, Hill L, et al. Prevalence of alcohol and other substance use in patients with eating disorders. Eur Eat Disord Rev. 2015;23(6):531–6.
35. Tinghino B, Lugoboni F, Amatulli A, et al. The FODRAT study (FOod addiction, DRugs, Alcohol and Tobacco): first data on food addiction prevalence among patients with addiction to drugs, tobacco and alcohol. Eat Weight Disord. 2021;26:449–55. https://doi.org/10.1007/s40519-020-00865-z.
36. Randolph TG. The descriptive features of food addiction; addictive eating and drinking. Q J Stud Alcohol. 1956;17(2):198–224.
37. Blum K, Oscar-Berman M, Barh D, et al. Dopamine genetic and function in food and substance abuse. J Genet Syndr Gene Ther. 2013;4:100–21.
38. The National Center on Addiction and Substance Abuse at Columbia University. Food for thought: substance abuse and eating disorders. Nancy Reagan Linda Johnson Rice Georg Rupp 2003;12:73.
39. Melchionda N. Food Addiction. Sviluppo dei Disturbi Alimentari e delle Obesità. Modena: Mucchi; 2014.
40. Kenny PJ. Common cellular and molecular mechanisms in obesity and drug addiction. Nat Rev Neurosci. 2011;12(11):638–51.
41. Pelchat ML. Food addiction in humans. J Nutr. 2009;139:620–2.

42. Schulte EM, Avena NM, Gearhardt AN. Which foods may be addictive? The roles of processing, fat content, and glycemic load. PLoS One. 2015;10:e0117959.
43. Gearhardt AN, Corbin WR, Brownell KD. Preliminary validation of the Yale food addiction scale. Appetite. 2009;52(2):430–6.
44. Manzoni GM, Rossi A, Pietrabissa G, et al. Validation of the Italian Yale Food Addiction Scale in postgraduate university students. Eat Weight Disord. 2018;23(2):167–76.
45. Gearhardt AN, Corbin WR, Brownell KD. Development of the Yale Food Addiction Scale Version 2.0. Psychol Addict Behav. 2016;30(1):113–21.
46. Hebebrand J, Albayrak O, Adan R, et al. "Eating addiction", rather than "food addiction", better captures addictive-like eating behavior. Neurosci Biobehav Rev. 2014;47:295–306.
47. Ziauddeen H, Fletcher PC. Is food addiction a valid and useful concept? Obes Rev. 2013;14:19–28.
48. Alavi SS, Ferdosi M, Jannatifard F, et al. Behavioral addiction versus substance addiction: Correspondence of psychiatric and psychological views. Int J Prev Med. 2012;3:290–4.
49. Burrows T, Skinner J, McKenna R, et al. Food addiction, binge eating disorder, and obesity: is there a relationship? Behav Sci. 2017;7:pii: E54. https://doi.org/10.3390/bs7030054.
50. Assaggioli R. L'atto di Volontà. Roma: Astrolabio; 1978.
51. Malato E. Dante e Guido Cavalcanti: il dissidio per la «Vita nuova» e il «Disdegno» di Guido. Salerno editore; 2004.

Post-Traumatic Eating Disorder

Romana Schumann, Valentina Fasoli, and Chiara Mazzoni

7.1 Background

The association between feeding and eating disorders (FED) [1] and trauma represents a central object of study for clinical practice [2, 3]. A distinction between different types of trauma constitutes the starting point. The traumatic event can be described as simple or complex [4], and the psychopathological outcomes of such events can produce many disorders due to their disruptive characteristics (post-traumatic stress disorder, PTSD; complex post-traumatic stress disorder, C-PTSD; dissociative disorders). It is equally important to circumscribe the relationship between trauma and FED development.

The term "post-traumatic eating disorder" [5–7] was introduced to describe the clinical conditions (similar to post-traumatic stress disorder) in which the refusal to eat in childhood is structured following one or more traumatic episodes involving the oropharynx or oesophagus. In Chatoor's article [5, 6], traumatic episodes related to the risk of suffocation increased the child fear (already present) of dying and separating from parents and produced refusal to eat. It might be interesting to propose an adaptation and addition to the term "post-traumatic eating disorder" and describe the circular relationship between trauma and FED using this term.

It is essential to illustrate the existing functional relationships between trauma and eating disorders (EDs). There are two main hypotheses emerging from literature. The first is that the function of ED as a self-healing factor of PTSD symptoms (with a function of emotional regulation and management of post-traumatic flashbacks). In this perspective, the way in which trauma precedes and activates

R. Schumann (✉) · V. Fasoli · C. Mazzoni
Psychotherapeutic Unit of Centro Gruber, Outpatient Treatment Center for Eating and Weight Disorders, Anxiety and Psychosomatic Disorders, Bologna, Italy
e-mail: romana.schumann@centrogruber.org; valentina.fasoli@centrogruber.org; chiara.mazzoni@centrogruber.org

post-traumatic symptoms and the way in which the eating disorder itself can represent a traumatic and maintenance factor are both central. Secondly, the relationship between trauma and dissociation will be discussed, in particular how ED symptomatology connects to the field of studies on trauma and dissociation.

Because of this specific clinical complexity, "hidden" interactions need to be explored in order to improve clinical practice. First of all, as Stolorow states [8], pain is not a pathology itself [9]. Addressing the theme of trauma implies the need to define it and the effort to identify the paths in which pain acquires psychopathological forms.

7.2 The Definition of Trauma and Its Relational Implications

The *Substance Abuse and Mental Health Services Administration* [10] proposes a definition of trauma based on the interaction of the concepts of "Event, Experience, Effect": "Individual trauma results from an event, series of events, or set of circumstances that is experienced by an individual as physically or emotionally harmful or threatening and that has lasting adverse effects on the individual's functioning and physical, social, emotional, or spiritual well-being. Events and circumstances may include the actual or extreme threat of physical or psychological harm or the withholding of material or relational resources essential to healthy development. These events and circumstances may occur as a single occurrence or repeatedly over time. The individual's experience of these events or circumstances helps to determine whether it is a traumatic event. A particular event may be experienced as traumatic for one individual and not for another" (SAMHSA, cited in [11]). The subjective meaning of trauma (*experience*) and the associated emotions shaping the experience itself are central, as well as socio-cultural beliefs, the presence of social support and age. Another fundamental element concerns the consequences of trauma (*effect*) in terms of personal suffering or psychopathological outcomes [11]. As already mentioned, post-traumatic stress disorder is one of the main consequences of traumatic events and traumatic experience. The DSM-5 [1] reserves a chapter to disorders related to traumatic and stressful events (Trauma- and Stressor-Related Disorders) as a consequence of exposure to one or more traumatic or stressful events. Specifically, this category—which was absent in the previous version and which included PTSD in the section dedicated to anxiety disorders—includes the following disorders: reactive attachment disorder, disinhibited social engagement disorder, post-traumatic stress disorder (PTSD), acute stress disorder, adjustment disorders and other specified and unspecified trauma- and stressor-related disorder. More extensively, it is possible to describe traumatic events according to two types: single and complex traumatic events.

Single traumatic events appear as specific and highly intense experiences such as road accidents, isolated incidents of violence, earthquakes and other natural disasters. Differently, complex trauma refers to cumulative traumatic events that occur repeatedly, characterized by the interpersonal nature, such as abuse or mistreatment.

They tend to occur during early caregiver-child relationships from which the victim cannot escape [4, 12]. This condition seems to have an impact on neurobiological development and the ability to integrate sensory, emotional and cognitive information. Regarding this, the disorder called complex PTSD has been introduced by clinicians in the literature [13].

The impact of interpersonal traumatic experiences (abuse, neglect, violence) has been highlighted in the literature, especially concerning the victim's ability to develop and maintain future relationships [14]. This is particularly relevant when traumatic experiences develop in childhood and when they are provoked by significant figures who should ensure safety and protection. The attachment theory introduced by John Bowlby [15, 16] explores the importance of early infant-caregiver relational attachment. Attachment is an innate system that motivates specific behaviours in children, such as seeking proximity to the attachment figure when upset or threatened. In this theory, the caregiver role includes responding sensitively and appropriately to the child's needs, ensuring safety, responsiveness and protection. It is within these relationships that internal working models (IWM) are encoded in the implicit memory system. IWM consist in stable representations of oneself and others, which act at an implicit level of awareness and serve as a framework for future relationships—the way people live in their own world, regulate their emotions and face danger. Attachment based on these assumptions can take the following forms:

1. Secure attachment
2. Insecure-ambivalent attachment
3. Insecure-avoidant attachment
4. Insecure-disorganized attachment

The impact of such attachment patterns has been investigated [17]. Concerning disorganized attachment pattern in the context of trauma, the behavioural characteristics of children with this pattern seem to show similarities with dissociative responses in adults. This clinical pattern occurs especially in the case of patients with complex traumatic personal pathways where the caregiver is both the source of the threat and the source of care [18–21]. Therefore, trauma cannot be conceived outside a situated relational context. The entwined bond of pain produced by events, combined with the emotional pain produced by neglect or emotional reactions (i.e. anger, shame, denial) expressed by caregivers, results in the traumatic condition. It is the absence or scarcity of adequate parental sensitivity that transforms the child's emotional reactions and configures them as unmanageable and thus becomes the source of the psychopathological form of trauma. In a relational context in which pain cannot be integrated, the victims dissociate the emotions that can manifest in psychosomatic and physical states. The child structures his or her own implicit, non-reflective knowledge on the basis of the exclusion of disruptive emotions mainly in order to preserve the bond with the caregiver and to avoid re-traumatization [8].

7.3 ED and Trauma: The Dimensions of the Phenomenon

Several randomized controlled trials indicate that about half of patients receiving standard treatment for eating disorders (EDs) do not achieve full remission. Indeed, specific and registered treatments for EDs cannot act on all the psychopathological factors contributing to maintain the disorder. The literature [3] shows that among these factors the comorbidity with post-traumatic stress disorder (PTSD) deserves special attention as a potential maintenance factor. In fact, FEDs seem associated with a wide presence of PTSD, ranging from 4 to 52%. Table 7.1 illustrates the literature data concerning these associations. Furthermore, the literature shows a more severe ED symptomatology in patients with comorbid PTSD [22]. When discussing about PTSD, it is fundamental to distinguish the specific type of trauma. Although childhood sexual abuse is a risk factor for the development of psychopathology, it does not seem to be a specific risk factor for the development of an ED. Other more common forms of trauma are physical and emotional abuse, teasing and bullying, parental separation and loss of a family member [2]. However, despite these premises, several studies highlight that trauma is more present in patients affected by bulimia nervosa [23].

In a recent meta-analysis conducted by Caslini [24], the relationship between child abuse and FED and the impact of different forms of sexual and non-sexual abuse on the development of anorexia nervosa (AN), bulimia nervosa (BN) and binge eating disorder (BED) were evaluated [2]. In this publication, the literature has been evaluated by coding the different types of trauma into distinct categories of abuse in childhood: sexual abuse[1], physical abuse[2] and emotional abuse[3]. The results show a positive association between childhood sexual abuse, BN and BED, while it does not appear significant for AN. The same relationship is found for emotional abuse with BN and BED. Physical abuse is linked to all EDs [2].

Together with these findings, it was also investigated whether there was any form of association between the number, different types of compensatory behaviour, different traumatic history, PTSD and other comorbidities [25]. It resulted that 60% of women who used all the compensatory behaviours (self-induced vomiting, laxatives and diuretics) also met the criteria for three or more psychiatric disorders.

Overall, a greater presence of interpersonal trauma has been observed in patients with BN and BED. Moreover, depending on the subject's protective or harmful nature of the interpersonal matrix, PTSD seems to impact negatively on the sense of coherence—intended as the subject's ability to cope with traumatic events—and PTSD is more likely to develop in the absence of social support. Precisely because

---

[1] Under the age of 18: (1) physical sexual relationship with a family member; (2) unwanted or forced physical sexual relations with an adult non-family member; and (3) sexual relations with a person at least 5 years older [21].

[2] Continuous physical attack by a person over the age of 18 leading to identifiable pain in a person under the age of 18 [22].

[3] An act of omission and commission perpetrated by significant adults or parents that makes the child vulnerable [23].

Table 7.1: Different types of trauma associated with eating disorder

References	Single trauma	Complex trauma
Faravelli, C. et al. (2004) [27] Tagay, S. et al. (2010) [28]	Sexual assault (35%)	
Mahon, J. et al. (2001) [29]	Parental break-up and loss of a family member (6%)	
Carmassi, C. et al. (2015) [30] Reyes-Rodrigurez, M.L. et al. (2011) [31] Masedu, F. et al. (2016) [32]	Massive earthquake and natural disaster (4%)	
Aoun, A. et al. (2019) [33]		Refugee's conditions (5.79%)
White, A.A., Pratt, K.J., Cottrill, C. (2018) [34]		Bullying (9.9%)
Caslini, M. et al. (2016) [24] Carratero-Garcia, A. et al. (2012) [35] Rorty, M. et al. (1994) [36] Kent, A. et al. (1999) [37]		Physical abuse (6.2%)
Carratero-Garcia, A. et al. (2012) [35] Caslini, M. et al. (2016) [24]		Sexual abuse by family members (6.8%)
De Groot, G & Rodin, G.M. (1999) [38] Wonderlich, S.A. et al. (2001) [39] Carratero-Garcia, A. et al. (2012) [35]		Other sexual abuse (13.7%)
Carratero-Garcia, A. et al. (2012) [35] Caslini, M. et al. (2016) [24] Rorty, M. et al. (1994) [36] Kent, A. et al. (1999) [37] Doyle, C. (1997) [40]		Emotional abuse (30.1%)
Carratero-Garcia, A. et al. (2012) [35] Wonderlich, S.A. et al. (1997) [41]		Childhood sexual abuse (40.8%)
White, A.A., Pratt, K.J., Cottrill, C. (2018) [34] Treuer, T. et al. (2005) [42]	Sexual abuse (8.3%)	

of this relational value of trauma, it is not surprising that patients with EDs with traumatic history are more at risk of drop-out and show lower therapeutic results and higher relapse rates [23]. In addition to the perpetrators of traumatic events, the way people react to trauma revelation also seems to be crucial. A Waller and Ruddock study [26] shows that family members' reactions perceived as negative or hostile seem to have an impact on the severity of ED and are associated with increased frequency of vomiting and intensified symptoms of borderline personality disorder.

7.4 ED as a "Pseudo-management Strategy" for Handling PTSD Symptoms

The relationship between trauma and eating disorder relates to the presence of traumatic events in patients with FED, to the functional relationship between PTSD symptoms and ED as well as to the high presence of comorbid disorders.

As previously mentioned, it seems that ED symptoms (intense self-induced binge eating and vomiting, severe restriction) can play a "pseudo-management strategy" role in the handling of PTSD symptoms, thus structuring themselves as a type of maintenance mechanism. Literature shows that although exposure to traumatic events is a predisposing factor for psychopathology in general, there is no direct correlation with the traumatic history; it does, however, seem to be linked with PTSD symptoms [43].

A recent qualitative study [44] highlights a "pseudo-management strategy" value of the disordered eating behaviours. The research consists in the thematic analysis of focus groups/interviews of 20 veteran women. First, it emerges that disordered eating, triggered by negative emotions and maladaptive thoughts, can represent a "method" used to manage both negative emotions (such as anger for having suffered from a trauma) and post-traumatic flashbacks. However, disordered eating seems to provide relief from negative emotions only in the short term. Subsequently, it seems to generate in the patient the feeling of having increased one's discomfort and perpetrating a vicious circle. Finally, a disordered diet can "offer" a mechanism to circumvent unwanted attention from potential and past trauma sufferers. The latter highlights a further defensive value against traumas perpetuated by others. Some women reported that the transformation of their bodies as a result of overfeeding could make them less attractive and less visible to the eyes of possible assailants. One in particular said that the weight gain might discourage perpetrators. In fact, the literature seems to reveal the existence of a relationship between child abuse, symptoms of PTSD and BMI. From the results of Roenholt and colleagues' research of 2012 [45], it emerges that the presence of traumatic events in childhood correlates to BMI imbalances both in defect and in excess. In fact, it emerges that participants in normal-weight condition show a lower presence of symptoms related to PTSD, unlike underweight or overweight participants. These authors also suggest a similar interpretation of this data, particularly for obesity, a condition that could represent a type of defence mechanism to minimize the risks of future abuse by members of the opposite sex.

So, in people with past traumas, the impulsive eating and vomiting behaviours characteristic of BN could play the role of a powerful regulator of negative emotions. A recent study by Karr [46] investigated this relationship with interesting results. Confronting two groups of patients, it emerged that the group diagnosed with bulimia nervosa and PTSD showed a higher frequency and emotional intensity of binge eating and self-induced vomiting behaviours. Also, in the group of patients with BN without PTSD, it seemed that binge eating and self-induced vomiting have a regulatory function, but in this group negative emotions seemed to increase and decrease before and after binge eating and vomiting episodes less rapidly than in the group of people with BN and PTSD. Difficulties in emotional regulation may also be related to the characteristics of the attachment style that characterizes the original dyadic relationship with the attachment figure [47]. Insecure attachment seems to contribute to the development of dysfunctional strategies for the affection regulation which can lead to the development of the eating disorder symptomatology. Literature suggests that patients with an eating disorder and anxious-resistant attachment live their emotions with an unmanageable form of activation, such as binges or compensatory behaviours, as a way to cope with emotional states dysregulation. On the contrary, ED patients with avoidant attachment style interrupt their emotional experience due to the extreme dietary restriction [48]. The post-traumatic conditions following environmental disasters, such as earthquakes, seem to share the hypothesis of eating as an emotional regulator [49]. Women already sensitive to emotional eating reported an increase in excess food consumption after the earthquake related to the post-event stress level.

7.5 Trauma, Dissociation and ED

Another important factor that seems to emerge from the literature is the mediating role of the dissociation between traumatic history and eating disorders. As mentioned by Liotti and Farina [4], the term "dissociation" in psychopathology refers to different contents. Primarily, it refers to a specific diagnostic category, dissociative disorders, as described in the *Diagnostic and Statistical Manual of Mental Disorders* [1]. In addition to the diagnostic value, both dissociative symptoms and psychopathogenic processes that interfere with integrated psychic functioning refer to the term dissociation. The American Psychiatric Association in DSM-5 [1] defines dissociative disorders as a discontinuity in the normal integration of consciousness, memory, identity, perception, body representation and behaviour. The relationship between dissociative symptoms and FED has been examined in some studies such as the recent study by Belli et al. in 2019 [50] which investigated, in a sample of 241 women with obesity, the presence of BED and the relationship between traumatic history and dissociative symptoms. A percentage of 31.1% of the sample fulfilled the diagnosis of BED. In addition, it was found that patients with BED showed higher dissociative symptoms than those without BED. The results also showed that the most represented traumas were physical abuse and emotional abuse, more present in patients with BED. It must be highlighted that many ED patients often experience dissociative states while binge drinking or vomiting. Dissociation is also a symptom of PTSD that predominantly characterizes the experience of those with ED and a traumatic history. Psychopathological overlaps seem to correlate with the likelihood that eating disorder symptomatology arises as an attempt to manage the consequences of the traumatic experience. ED could represent an extreme way to handle the psychological, or even physical, damage of the trauma [51, 52].

The relationship between the established coexistence of traumatic and dissociative experiences is still objet of research. Vanderlinden and Palmisano [53] highlight that two different theories try to define it: the "escape from self-awareness" theory

[54] and the "blocking model" theory [55]. The first theory suggests that people with BN could use binge eating as a mechanism to avoid negative emotions related to expectations about themselves. In particular, it seems to be the negativity of the self-image perceived by others, anxiety and negative emotions (abstract functioning) to produce a lowering of the state of awareness (uncontrolled feeding) to the point of producing a more basic functioning, similar to a dissociative experience. This mechanism could cause a loosening of inhibitions and therefore represents a dissociative form that precedes the binge. According to the "blocking model" theory, instead, binge eating could have an anaesthetic effect on the pain and guilt felt as a result of childhood trauma; in this condition, it seems that dissociation occurs during binge [53].

Vanderlinden and Vandereycken in their famous text *Trauma, Dissociation and Impulse Dyscontrol in Eating Disorders* [56] suggest that in order to understand the relationship between childhood violence and psychological problems, it is important to refer to a multifactorial model. The model results are characterized by specific mediation factors such as the developmental phase in which the trauma occurs, the nature of the trauma, the response that the person received when he or she first revealed the trauma, characteristics of the family (i.e. high conflict or disorganization), life events with risk of re-victimization and characteristics of the self-image. The integration of traumatic experiences is protective for the mental health of the patient in relation to the associated dissociative risk. In the continuum between integration and dissociation, the eating disorder can be evaluated in different ways, but always as a defence mechanism against feelings, memories and feelings associated with trauma. FED can also be conceptualized as a way to manage a negative physical experience related to abuse.

7.6 Discussion

The existing relationship between trauma and eating disorders seems to be characterized by a difficulty in identifying the interactions between the complex factors that play a role in the symptomatologic structuring of patients with these sufferings.

Starting from the previous elements, what is "hidden" in the existing relationship between trauma and ED?

1. The symptomatologic presentation of the ED can hide the complex interaction between PTSD and ED and the traumatic impact of the ED itself.

    Any research reflection in the literature must start from a reflection on the characteristics of the difficult experiences of people who, coming from life paths studded with traumatic experiences, develop an eating disorder. On the one hand, ED can represent a way to manage flashbacks and traumatic symptomatology by configuring itself as a self-care factor in the functional direction that develops from PTSD to ED. But it is also possible to identify a different direction between ED and PTSD and configure a type of traumatic eating disorder. Especially in the bulimic phase, the failure of rigid control system can lead to feelings of helpless-

ness and feelings of danger of death, linked to extreme intensity experiences of binge eating and vomiting. Literature advises that this phase can be related to suicide attempts [57]. Also treatment may constitute a source of re-traumatization. Tube feeding, which in some cases is necessary, could produce a traumatic experience. In fact, being forced to be fed can represent a terrifying experience for ED patients. Other traumatic aspects could be related to inpatient treatment: sudden separation from family and friends (especially for children and young patients) can present a traumatic risk. Medical examinations, because of their physical contact characteristics, may also reactivate traumatic experiences: specific training and a high level of competence are important to the medical management of these patients. Finally, patients requiring intensive care may need a long time to build a trusting therapeutic relationship and then experience the reactivation of past traumas of being abandoned during the discharge [58].
2. ED as "pseudo-management strategy" and maintenance of PTSD symptoms.

ED development as an attempt to self-care for PTSD symptoms represents a critical issue. First of all, this pattern risks becoming a maintaining factor for PTSD symptoms. The symptomatologic "camouflage" produces both subjective and physical fatigue for the patient. It is well known that in AN the amygdala activation—whose activity is also connected to the PTSD symptomatology—is amplified by the starvation condition [59], thus configuring a vicious circle difficult to interrupt during the treatment. The association between PTSD and a higher frequency of "poorly defined" medical symptoms, more than other psychiatric disorders, seems to contribute to maintain the vicious circle [60]. The most frequent medical conditions associated with PTSD in both adults [61, 62] and children [63] are cardiovascular disorders, respiratory disorders, musculoskeletal disorders, neurological disorders, gastrointestinal disorders, diabetes, chronic pain, sleep disorders and other immune-mediated disorders. The risk of underestimating this complex pattern is therefore high. This condition, hidden under the complex symptomatology of PTSD, requires specific attention and medical management in order to achieve an integrated care of the patient.

Conditions of overweight or obesity in childhood and adolescence represent the first "cause" of teasing by the peer group that could cause, in some cases, traumatic experiences. Research found that at least 84% of students observed episodes in which overweight peers were mocked and teased [64]. Unfortunately, weight stigma is socially widespread and tolerated because of misconceptions, such as the fact that stigma and shame will motivate people to lose weight. However, rather than motivating positive change, stigma contributes to behaviours such as binge eating, social isolation, lack of medical care and health services, decreased physical activity and weight gain, which worsen obesity and create additional barriers to change [65]. There is evidence that stigmatization regarding weight and body shape can lead to the development of important patterns of psychological, physical and social malaise and traumatic reactivations with psychophysical activations that drastically compromise the quality of life, especially for young people [65, 66], generating the food consuming as a sedative [67].

3. The type of trauma: "hidden" trauma.

   The classic DSM trauma definition of involvement or witnessing an event involving death, serious injury and sexual assault associated with feelings of helplessness does not account for the complexity of traumatic developmental pathways characterized by insecure or disorganized attachment, mistreatment, emotional abuse and lack of protection or neglect. The consequences of these complex traumas, which can occur in a non-explicit way in patients' reports, can be multiple if present in childhood and adolescence and can produce symptoms of post-traumatic stress disorder, deficits in the regulation of emotions, impulsiveness, serious relational problems, somatization or dissociation [4].

4. ED and dissociation as "lack of integration".

   Dissociation, as already mentioned, can refer to different contents. The singular aspect is represented by the fact that, although the category of dissociative disorders is present in the DSM-5, dissociation is defined both on the basis of the discontinuities of consciousness [68] and on the basis of the lack of integration of those functions which, if present in a harmonic form, constitute a good personal functioning and represent in themselves a possibility to cope with critical life experiences.

5. Theory of attachment, internal working model and therapeutic relationships.

   We have tried to explain how the attachment theory, in particular the effects on the construction of the internal working models, represents an explanatory framework of the effects of a specific development path. However, IWMs, as stable representations of themselves and others, act at an implicit level of awareness in relationships even in adulthood. This configuration does not manifest itself in an explicit way but is acted out in the therapeutic relationship. Starting from these aspects, in fact, one cannot but underline the fact that the therapeutic relationship is also a relationship in which it is probable that the same cognitive and experiential modalities are put into action, in which patient and therapist interact with their personal characteristics. The therapist has the task of involving the patient in the construction of a context of security and trust. What declines the complexity of clinical work in the experience of therapy is the need to maintain an empathic attitude [69]. The difficulty in maintaining such a radical inner attitude is influenced by the reactions that the therapist himself might feel when confronted with the traumatic experiences of the people in therapy. The therapist's experiences could oscillate between opposite poles: on the one hand an over-identification that could configure a loss of boundary and hyper-involvement and provoke a condition of mutual dependence and a feeling of vulnerability and on the other hand an attitude of avoidance as a distancing from the experience of others, denial and withdrawal [70]. It is evident how the therapist's awareness and ability to tune in play a far from marginal role in understanding and handling the traumatic experience of the other with respect, in a significant relational context. Sometimes a conscious attitude of one's own limits in grasping what for the other has meant living the experiences that emerge in therapy.

7.7 Conclusions and Implications for Treatment

In conclusion, we would like to suggest some reflections for clinical practice. It is essential that the acute symptoms of post-traumatic anxiety in patients with FED are recognized not only by psychotherapists and psychiatrists but also by the medical and nutritional professionals, who are involved in the multidisciplinary and integrated treatment of patients with ED [71]. In many cases, the severe psychic symptomatology leads to treatments that exclude or marginalize the medical-nutritional aspect which plays an important role in these conditions. The consequences may be an increased risk of acute complications for the patient, maintenance of the effects of dietary restriction, persistence of debilitating effects of elimination behaviours, compensatory behaviours and physical and psychic prostration related to binge eating. As already highlighted, patients with PTSD in comorbidity show lower therapeutic results and higher drop-out rates. Researchers' and clinicians' efforts to understand how, when and which evidence-based focused trauma therapy can be integrated in the ED treatment are shown in literature [48]. International guidelines for the treatment of EDs [72–74] and PTSD [75] do not describe how to integrate the specific treatment of these comorbidities. Appropriate treatment in these cases should also address the aspects of comorbid PTSD in order to ensure the best outcome and needs to consider the centrality of the therapeutic relationship as a restorative experience for the patient.

Suffering from the effects of complex and interpersonal traumatic experiences implies the structuring of a perception of the world and the other characterized by distrust, fear of being betrayed or not being believed. Beyond the specific implications related to the symptomatology of the disorder, it is important to point out the centrality of the therapeutic relationship as a reparative experience. The therapeutic attitude should be based on the awareness of how these patients present difficulties to stay in a honest, and not threatening, relationship.

References

1. American Psychiatric Association. Diagnostic and statistical manual of mental disorders (DSM-5®). Am Psychiatric Pub. 2013;
2. Grogan K, et al. Family-related non-abuse adverse life experiences occurring for adults diagnosed with eating disorders: a systematic review. J Eat Disord. 2020;8:36. https://doi.org/10.1186/s40337-020-00311-6.
3. Rabito-Alcon MF, et al. Mediating factors between childhood traumatic experiences and eating disorders development: a systematic review. Children (Basel). 2021;8(2). https://doi.org/10.3390/children8020114.
4. Liotti G, Farina B. Sviluppi traumatici. Eziopatogenesi, clinica e terapia della dimensione dissociativa; 2011.
5. Chatoor I, Conley C, Dickson L. Food refusal after an incident of choking: a posttraumatic eating disorder. J Am Acad Child Adolesc Psychiatry. 1988;27(1):105–10.
6. Chatoor I. Eating disorders in infancy and early childhood. In: The Oxford handbook of child and adolescent eating disorders: developmental perspectives; 2012.

7. Celik G, Diler RS, Tahiroglu AY, and Avci A. Fluoxetine in posttraumatic eating disorder in 2-year-old twins. J Child Adolesc Psychopharmacol. 2007;17(2):233–6.
8. Stolorow RD. Trauma and human existence: Autobiographical, psychoanalytic, and philosophical reflections. New York: Routledge; 2011.
9. Stolorow RD, Atwood GE, Ross JM. The representational world in psychoanalytic therapy. Int Rev Psycho-Analysis. 1978;5:247–56.
10. Substance Abuse and Mental Health Services Administration (SAMHSA). SAMHSA's working definition of trauma and principles and guidance for a trauma-informed approach; 2012
11. Brewerton TD, Brady K. The role of stress, trauma, and PTSD in the etiology and treatment of eating disorders, addictions, and substance use disorders. In: Brewerton TD, Dennis AB, editors. Eating disorders, addictions and substance use disorders. Berlin, Heidelberg: Springer; 2014. p. 379–404.
12. Van der Kolk BA. Assessment and Treatment. Treating trauma survivors with PTSD. Amer Psychiatric Pub Inc; 2008. p. 127–156.
13. Van der Kolk BA. The assessment and treatment of complex PTSD. Treating trauma survivors with PTSD 2002;127:156.
14. Pearlman LA, Courtois CA. Clinical applications of the attachment framework: Relational treatment of complex trauma. J Trauma Stress. 2005;18(5):449–59.
15. Bowlby J. Attachment and loss: attachment. John Bowlby. Basic books; 1969.
16. Bowlby J. Clinical applications of attachment: A secure base, vol. 85. London: Routledge; 1988.
17. S Kuipers G, HJ Bekker M. Attachment, mentalization and eating disorders: a review of studies using the adult attachment interview. Curr Psychiatry Rev. 2012;8(4):326–36.
18. Torem MS, Curdue K. PTSD presenting as an eating disorder. Stress Med. 1988;4(3):139–42.
19. Liotti G. La dimensione interpersonale della coscienza. Roma: Nis; 1994.
20. Tambelli R, Cimino S, Cerniglia L, Ballarotto G. Early maternal relational traumatic experiences and psychopathological symptoms: a longitudinal study on mother-infant and father-infant interactions. Sci Rep. 2015;5(1):1–1.
21. Williamson V, Creswell C, Fearon P, Hiller RM, Walker J, Halligan SL. The role of parenting behaviors in childhood post-traumatic stress disorder: a meta-analytic review. Clin Psychol Rev. 2017;53:1–3.
22. Vierling V, Etori S, Valenti L, Lesage M, Pigeyre M, Dodin V, Cottencin O, Guardia D. Prevalence and impact of post-traumatic stress disorder in a disordered eating population sample. Presse Medicale (Paris, France: 1983). 2015;44(11):e341–52.
23. Tagay S, Schlottbohm E, Reyes-Rodriguez ML, Repic N, Senf W. Eating disorders, trauma, PTSD, and psychosocial resources. Eat Disord. 2014;22(1):33–49.
24. Caslini M, Bartoli F, Crocamo C, Dakanalis A, Clerici M, Carrà G. Disentangling the association between child abuse and eating disorders: a systematic review and meta-analysis. Psychosom Med. 2016;78(1):79–90.
25. Brewerton TD. Stress, trauma, and adversity as risk factors in the development of eating disorders. Wiley handbook of eating disorders. New York: Guilford; 2015. p. 445–60.
26. Waller G, Ruddock A, Pitts C. When is sexual abuse relevant to bulimic disorders? The validity of clinical judgements. Eur Eat Disord Rev. 1993;1(3):143–51.
27. Faravelli C, Giugni A, Salvatori S, Ricca V. Psychopathology after rape. Am J Psychiatry. 2004;161(8):1483–5.
28. Tagay S, Schlegl S, Senf W. Traumatic events, posttraumatic stress symptomatology and somatoform symptoms in eating disorder patients. Eur Eat Disord Rev. 2010;18(2):124–32.
29. Mahon J, Bradley SN, Harvey PK, Winston AP, Palmer RL. Childhood trauma has dose-effect relationship with dropping out from psychotherapeutic treatment for bulimia nervosa: a replication. Int J Eat Disord. 2001;30(2):138–48.
30. Carmassi C, Bertelloni CA, Massimetti G, Miniati M, Stratta P, Rossi A, Dell L. Impact of DSM-5 PTSD and gender on impaired eating behaviors in 512 Italian earthquake survivors. Psychiatry Res. 2015;225(1-2):64–9.
31. Reyes-Rodríguez ML, Ann Von Holle T, Thornton LM, Klump KL, Brandt H, Crawford S, Fichter MM, Halmi KA, Huber T, Johnson C, Jones I. Post traumatic stress disorder in anorexia nervosa. Psychosom Med. 2011;73(6):491.

32. Masedu F, Monti AC, Pietro MD, Gileno L, Valenti M. Eating disorders risk profiles in the adolescents in the Abruzzo's region in Italy: a cross-sectional survey in the aftermath of an earthquake. J Nutr Health Food Sci. 2016;4(4):1–6.
33. Aoun A, Joundi J, El Gerges N. Prevalence and correlates of a positive screen for eating disorders among Syrian refugees. Eur Eat Disord Rev. 2019;27(3):263–73.
34. White AA, Pratt KJ, Cottrill C. The relationship between trauma and weight status among adolescents in eating disorder treatment. Appetite. 2018;129:62–9.
35. Carretero-García A, Planell LS, Doval E, Estragués JR, Escursell RR, Vanderlinden J. Repeated traumatic experiences in eating disorders and their association with eating symptoms. Eat Weight Disord. 2012;17(4):e267–73.
36. Rorty M, Yager J, Rossotto E. Childhood sexual, physical, and psychological abuse. Am J Psychiatry. 1994;151(8):1122–6.
37. Kent A, Waller G, Dagnan D. A greater role of emotional than physical or sexual abuse in predicting disordered eating attitudes: The role of mediating variables. Int J Eat Disord. 1999;25(2):159–67.
38. De Groot J, Rodin GM. The relationship between eating disorders and childhood trauma. Psychiatric Anna. 1999;29(4):225–9.
39. Wonderlich SA, Crosby RD, Mitchell JE, Thompson KM, Redlin J, Demuth G, Smyth J, Haseltine B. Eating disturbance and sexual trauma in childhood and adulthood. Int J Eat Disord. 2001;30(4):401–12.
40. Doyle C. Emotional abuse of children: Issues for intervention. Child Abuse Rev. 1997;6(5):330–42.
41. Wonderlich SA, Brewerton TD, Jocic Z, Dansky BS, Abbott DW. Relationship of childhood sexual abuse and eating disorders. J Am Acad Child Adolesc Psychiatry. 1997;36(8):1107–15.
42. Treuer T, Koperdák M, Rózsa S, Füredi J. The impact of physical and sexual abuse on body image in eating disorders. Eur Eat Disord Rev. 2005;13(2):106–11.
43. Trottier K, MacDonald DE. Update on psychological trauma, other severe adverse experiences and eating disorders: state of the research and future research directions. Curr Psychiatry Rep. 2017;19(8):45.
44. Breland JY, Donalson R, Dinh J, Nevedal A, Maguen S. Women veterans' treatment preferences for disordered eating. Womens Health Issues. 2016;26(4):429–36.
45. Roenholt S, Beck N, Karsberg S, Elklit A. Post-traumatic stress symptoms and childhood abuse categories in a national representative sample for a specific age group: associations to body mass index. Eur J Psychotraumatol. 2012;3(1):17188.
46. Karr TM, Crosby RD, Cao L, Engel SG, Mitchell JE, Simonich H, Wonderlich SA. Posttraumatic stress disorder as a moderator of the association between negative affect and bulimic symptoms: an ecological momentary assessment study. Compr Psychiatry. 2013;54(1):61–9.
47. Tasca GA, Szadkowski L, Illing V, Trinneer A, Grenon R, Demidenko N, Krysanski V, Balfour L, Bissada H. Adult attachment, depression, and eating disorder symptoms: the mediating role of affect regulation strategies. Personal Individ Differ. 2009;47(6):662–7.
48. Tasca GA, Ritchie K, Balfour L. Implications of attachment theory and research for the assessment and treatment of eating disorders. Psychotherapy. 2011;48(3):249.
49. Kuijer RG, Boyce JA. Emotional eating and its effect on eating behaviour after a natural disaster. Appetite. 2012;58(3):936–9.
50. Belli H, Ural C, Akbudak M, Sagaltıcı E. Levels of childhood traumatic experiences and dissociative symptoms in extremely obese patients with and without binge eating disorder. Nord J Psychiatry. 2019;73(8):527–31.
51. Vanderlinden J, Vandereycken W, Van Dyck R, Vertommen H. Dissociative experiences and trauma in eating disorders. Int J Eat Disord. 1993;13(2):187–93.
52. Strickler HL. The interaction between post-traumatic stress disorders and eating disorders: a review of relevant literature. J Trauma Treat. 2013;3(183):1–5.
53. Vanderlinden J, Palmisano GL. Trauma and eating disorders: the state of the art. In: Andrew Seubert NC, Virdi P, editors. Trauma-informed approaches to eating disorders. New York: Springer Publishing Company; 2018. p. 28.

54. Heatherton TF, Baumeister RF. Binge eating as escape from self-awareness. Psychol Bull. 1991;110(1):86.
55. Lacey J, Downey LJ, Malkin JC. Pathogenesis. In: Downey L, Malkin J, editors. Current approaches. Southampton: Duphar; 1986. p. 17–27.
56. Vanderlinden J, Vandereycken W. Trauma, dissociation, and impulse dyscontrol in eating disorders (No. 9). Psychology Press; 1997.
57. Pisetsky EM, Thornton LM, Lichtenstein P, Pedersen NL, Bulik CM. Suicide attempts in women with eating disorders. J Abnorm Psychol. 2013;122(4):1042.
58. Andrew Seubert NC, Virdi P, editors. Trauma-informed approaches to eating disorders. In: Springer Publishing Company. New York; 2018.
59. Joos AA, Saum B, van Elst LT, Perlov E, Glauche V, Hartmann A, Freyer T, Tüscher O, Zeeck A. Amygdala hyperreactivity in restrictive anorexia nervosa. Psychiatry Res. 2011;191(3):189–95.
60. Andreski P, Chilcoat H, Breslau N. Post-traumatic stress disorder and somatization symptoms: a prospective study. Psychiatry Res. 1998;79(2):131–8.
61. Pietrzak RH, Whealin JM, Stotzer RL, Goldstein MB, Southwick SM. An examination of the relation between combat experiences and combat-related posttraumatic stress disorder in a sample of Connecticut OEF–OIF Veterans. J Psychiatr Res. 2011;45(12):1579–84.
62. Stam R. PTSD and stress sensitisation: a tale of brain and body: Part 1: Human studies. Neurosci Biobehav Rev. 2007;31(4):530–57.
63. Seng JS, Graham-Bermann SA, Clark MK, McCarthy AM, Ronis DL. Posttraumatic stress disorder and physical comorbidity among female children and adolescents: results from service-use data. Pediatrics. 2005;116(6):e767–76.
64. Sahoo K, Sahoo B, Choudhury AK, Sofi NY, Kumar R, Bhadoria AS. Childhood obesity: causes and consequences. J Fam Med Primary Care. 2015;4(2):187.
65. Pont SJ, Puhl R, Cook SR, Slusser W. Stigma experienced by children and adolescents with obesity. Pediatrics. 2017;140(6):e20173034.
66. Fox CL, Farrow CV. Global and physical self-esteem and body dissatisfaction as mediators of the relationship between weight status and being a victim of bullying. J Adolesc. 2009;32(5):1287–301.
67. Palmisano GL, Innamorati M, Vanderlinden J. Life adverse experiences in relation with obesity and binge eating disorder: a systematic review. J Behav Addict. 2016;5(1):11–31.
68. Liotti G, editor. La discontinuità della coscienza. Etiologia, diagnosi e psicoterapia dei disturbi dissociativi. FrancoAngeli; 1993.
69. Stein E. On the problem of empathy, tr. it. Il problema dell'empatia; 1917.
70. Wilson JP, Lindy JD. Empathic strain and countertransference. In: Horowitz MJ, editor. Essential papers on post traumatic stress disorder, vol. 14. New York: NYU Press; 1999.
71. Ballardini D, Schumann R. La riabilitazione psiconutrizionale nei disturbi dell'alimentazione. Carocci Faber; 2011.
72. Yager J, Devlin M, Halmi K, Herzog DB, Mitchell JE, Powers P. American Psychiatric Association practice guideline for the treatment of patients with eating disorders. Am J Psychiatry. 2006;163(7 Suppl):4–54.
73. National Institute for Health and Care Excellence. Eating Disorders: recognition and treatment, NICE Guidelines (NG69).
74. Hay P, Chinn D, Forbes D, Madden S, Newton R, Sugenor L, Touyz S, Ward W. Royal Australian and New Zealand College of Psychiatrists clinical practice guidelines for the treatment of eating disorders. Aust N Zeal J Psychiatry. 2014;48(11):977–1008.
75. American Psychological Association. Clinical practice guideline for the treatment of post-traumatic stress disorder (PTSD) in adults. Washington, DC: American Psychological Association; 2017.

Psychotropic Drug-Induced Disordered Eating Behaviors

8

Enrica Marzola, Maria Musso, and Giovanni Abbate-Daga

8.1 Introduction

Anorexia nervosa and bulimia nervosa are usually mainly described when referring to eating disorders (EDs); nevertheless, also other forms of EDs exist, although somehow neglected. For example, binge eating disorder, namely, the most frequent ED [1], was introduced in the DSM only in 2013 [2]. The influence of drugs on body weight and food drive is complex and multi-faceted. Multiple brain areas are involved in the regulation of eating behaviors [3], and in some cases, psychotropic drugs influence the same areas (e.g., midbrain and striatum). The dopaminergic activity of many medications is also connected to the complex mechanisms of reward in the brain. From this perspective, a shared mechanism of reward pathways between EDs and substance abuse disorders has been proposed. Describing all the potential connections between medications and eating behaviors goes beyond the scope of this work, so this chapter will focus on those psychotropic agents that (a) increase appetite and weight and (b) decrease appetite and weight.

8.2 Psychotropic Drug-Induced Increased Appetite and Weight

Several pharmacological classes, entailing different pathways, are known to increase appetite and weight: mainly antipsychotics, mood stabilizers, antidepressants, and cannabinoid agents.

E. Marzola · M. Musso · G. Abbate-Daga (✉)
Eating Disorders Center for Treatment and Research, Department of Neuroscience, University of Turin, Turin, Italy
e-mail: enrica.marzola@unito.it; maria.musso@edu.unito.it; giovanni.abbatedaga@unito.it

8.2.1 Antipsychotics

Antipsychotics (APs) represent the gold standard for the treatment of many psychiatric disorders, including schizophrenia and bipolar disorder. APs are associated with weight gain [4] over the short- and long-term use [5]. Second-generation antipsychotics (SGAs)—especially olanzapine, risperidone, and quetiapine—show major effects on weight gain and exert their action on body weight and food intake in several ways. Firstly, SGAs interact with many different central receptors: antagonism on striatum D2 receptors determines hyperphagia and increased appetite via impairment of the reward circuitry [6], while antagonism on hypothalamus D2 impairs the regulation of hunger/satiety mechanisms. Furthermore, 5HT2c receptors' blockade contributes to hyperphagia: in particular, olanzapine shows the highest ability to induce weight gain, since it is an inverse agonist of 5HT2c [7]. Antagonism on H1 causes increased appetite, while blockade on M3 and alfa2 receptors lead to inhibition of insulin release [8]. Furthermore, SGAs have been shown to have negative effects on metabolic balance, impairing glucose [9] and lipidic [10] homeostasis and causing hyperleptinemia [11] and increased ghrelin levels [12]. Additionally, recent studies have found a negative correlation between SGA treatment and gut microbiota which may lead to weight gain [13].

8.2.2 Mood Stabilizers

Overweight and obesity are common in patients with bipolar disorders (BDs). Since the beginning of their utilization, mood stabilizers can cause weight gain, even in the first 6 months of treatment [14].

The 25% of patients using lithium showed an increase in weight ranging from 4.5 up to 12 kg, potentially leading to low compliance to therapy. This may be due to different mechanisms: firstly, lithium can increase appetite and cause hyperphagia; secondly, kidney damage can cause fluid retention and polydipsia, which may lead to increased consumption of sweet and high caloric drinks; finally, thyroid toxicity, a well-known side effect of lithium, may lead to lower metabolic rate and weight gain.

Valproate acid (VPA), an antiepileptic drug used as a mood stabilizer, has been shown to increase insulin/glucose ratio, which may be the reason for increased appetite [15] and thirst, with higher consumption of caloric drinks. Furthermore, VPA-induced hyperinsulinemia in some cases leads to polycystic ovary syndrome [16], commonly associated with overweight and obesity.

Also, the literature showed that overweight and BDs are intertwined since overeating, reduced physical activity, and impulsivity are part of these mental illnesses independent of medications [17]. From this perspective, patients affected by a BD report greater hunger and more unhealthy eating habits than controls, and BED is common comorbidity [18].

8.2.3 Antidepressants

Antidepressant drugs (ADs) could entail weight gain, loss, or neutrality, depending on the specific spectrum of activity. Broadly speaking, a review on this topic [19] found that 55.2% of patients on ADs gained weight, 48.8% reported increased appetite, and 39.5% reported a craving for carbohydrates. The drug mostly associated with weight gain was mirtazapine (88.2%), followed by paroxetine (73.8%), venlafaxine (64.6%), escitalopram (64.5%), citalopram (52.6%), duloxetine (41.7%), and sertraline (33.8%). Young women with a lower body mass index at the beginning of therapy, a lower degree of education, and a family history of obesity seem to be at higher risk of significant weight gain. Another review [20] concluded that TCAs (amitriptyline, imipramine, and nortriptyline) are mostly associated with weight gain, followed by mirtazapine and paroxetine. However, two elements should be taken into account when evaluating the effects of ADs on body weight: firstly, loss of appetite is a major symptom of depression so the observed weight gain may be a sign of clinical improvement; therefore, former body mass index should be taken into account when measuring weight gain. Secondly, AAPs are frequently co-prescribed for treatment-resistant depression, so they may represent a confounding bias.

8.2.4 Cannabinoids

Studies on the effects of cannabinoids led to the discovery of the endocannabinoid system, represented by autacoid endocannabinoids (eCB) and their receptors CB1 and CB2. CB1 is mainly located in the hypothalamus, limbic forebrain, stomach, and gut, and its activation determines increased food intake, hyperphagia, craving for food (the so-called "munchies", especially for sweet and highly palatable foods), and adipogenesis [21]. Nevertheless, in the long term, chronic use of cannabis has been associated with lower body mass index and lower prevalence of obesity potentially inducing loss of appetite [22]: this is probably due to a downregulation of CB1 [22], resulting in weight loss. Similarly, rimonabant, a CB1 antagonist, decreases appetite. It is noteworthy that rimonabant has been withdrawn from the market for the increased suicide risk. So, CB receptors seem to have biphasic effects, increasing food intake at lower doses of cannabis and reducing it at higher doses [23]. CB1 receptor exerts its effects in many ways: in CNS, it is found in the paraventricular nucleus, where it causes hyperphagia both in hungry and satiated animals via interactions with ghrelin and in both nucleus accumbens and ventral tegmental area, where it modulates dopaminergic signaling, thus influencing salience to general and food stimuli. Peripherally, CB1 activation influences glucose intake, glucose tolerance, and lipogenesis; moreover, it seems to increase the perception of food smell and taste, mostly for sweets and fatty foods [23].

8.3 Psychotropic Drug-Induced Reduced Appetite and Weight

8.3.1 Mood Stabilizers

Topiramate (TPM) is currently an FDA-approved medication for the treatment of epilepsy and the prophylaxis of migraine. As side effects, TPM induces weight loss, loss of appetite, decreased food and macronutrient intake, and increased energy expenditure. In CNS, TPM alters the rewarding properties of food [24], modulates the GABA receptors, and blocks glutamatergic transmission (thus antagonizing the orexigenic effects of glutamate) [25]. Furthermore, clinical research suggests that TPM may exert metabolic effects, including reduced leptin levels; increased adiponectin levels (determining increased lipid oxidation and insulin sensitivity), insulin sensitization, and glucose tolerance (consequently decreasing blood glucose levels); and reduced total cholesterol levels. Furthermore, TPM has been shown to inhibit carbonic anhydrase, an enzyme involved in *de novo* lipogenesis pathways [24]. The use of TPM has been suggested for the treatment of binge eating episodes in both bulimia nervosa and binge eating disorder [25].

8.3.2 Antidepressants

Bupropion and fluoxetine at high doses have been associated with weight loss in short-term treatments, while in long-term use, only bupropion has clearly shown persisting effects on body weight [26], mostly in obese people [20]. Though bupropion effective mechanism of action is still partially unknown, it is supposed to block dopamine and norepinephrine transporters, which results in dopaminergic and noradrenergic potentiation and mild psychostimulant effects. Given this, it is not surprising that bupropion can cause weight loss, probably influencing appetite/satiety and feeding behavior.

Regarding fluoxetine, it is effective in reducing the frequency and severity of binge-purging episodes in bulimia nervosa and approved for such a diagnosis since 1994. Its serotoninergic effects may reduce appetite and affect food choice; besides, 5-HT potentiation may enhance the melanocortin system's effects and block NPY signaling, thus leading to reduced caloric intake [27]. However, a recent Cochrane work [27] concluded that scarce evidence is at present available on the effects of weight loss of fluoxetine in obesity; therefore, fluoxetine should not be considered as a weight loss agent for obese people.

8.3.3 Cannabinoid-1 Receptor Antagonists

Given the aforementioned appetite-stimulating properties of cannabinoids (see earlier section), CB1 antagonism has been studied as a mechanism for suppressing food intake. The first drug to be marketed as rimonabant, a CB1 reverse agonist, was shown to be effective in reducing body weight and waist circumference in obese patients. Nevertheless, it had a short life: after being commercialized in 2006 for obesity treatment, rimonabant soon revealed serious psychiatric side effects, since around 25% of treated individuals developed anxiety and depressive symptoms and suicidal ideation. For this reason, it was withdrawn from the European market in 2009 [28]. Currently, other CB1 antagonist molecules that do not pass the brain-blood barrier, to avoid or minimize the CNS effects, are being studied [29].

8.3.4 Amphetamines

Appetite and weight loss effects of amphetamines, both as drugs and as recreational substances of abuse, have been known since the first decades of the twentieth century. Phentermine was approved in 1959 for obesity treatment and is still used for short-term treatments (up to 3 months) in the USA [30]. More recently, in 2015, lisdexamfetamine, a pro-drug of d-amphetamine, was approved for BED treatment in the USA. Though its mechanism of action remains still unknown, it is supposed to be due to its ability to modulate dopamine and norepinephrine circuits involved in food choice, eating behavior, and reward mechanisms. Different from other amphetamines, it has been shown to have a high profile of safety and low liability of inducing addiction and abuse [31].

8.3.5 Thyroid Hormones

Thyroid hormones (THs) T3 and T4 physiologically induce increased basal metabolism, energy expenditure, and catabolic state, which lead to weight loss; for this reason, exogenous THs have been (mis)used for decades among obese people and patients with eating disorders, often leading to thyrotoxicosis *factitia*.

Besides the abuse of thyroid drugs, often bought illegally by abusers, clinicians should pay attention to the consumption of nutraceutical products, since many cases of adulteration and/or mislabelling of "natural" products and herbs with TH have been reported. In the USA, 20.6% of women and 9.7% of men have been taking some of these supplements to lose weight, and often the consumer is not aware of the exact content of these products.

Moreover, levothyroxine is a second-line treatment for drug-resistant depression, so weight loss should be considered as a side effect [32].

8.3.6 Cocaine

Cocaine, through its inhibition of monoamine reuptake, acts as a powerful psychostimulant, subjectively increasing energies and cognitive performance. Furthermore, its consumption is often related to the intent of controlling weight, especially among women [33], given cocaine appetite suppressant properties due to dopamine stimulation. Cocaine induces CART (cocaine- and amphetamine-regulated transcript) upregulation: this peptide is involved in both feeding behaviors and reward mechanisms induced by psychostimulants, and its levels are proportional to leptin levels, showing anorexigenic effects [34]. Some authors [35] have underlined how eating habits in cocaine abusers consist of higher consumption of fatty foods and carbohydrates despite the lower fat mass/lean mass ratio, suggesting that, while increasing drive for fatty foods, cocaine activation of CART may lead to lipidic mobilization and inhibition of fat deposition [35]. The well-known weight gain associated with cocaine discontinuation could be then due to the loss of CART effects on metabolism [35].

8.3.7 Opiates

Since the 1970s when heroin dependence became a social and medical problem all over the world, it has been noticed that opiate abusers showed lower body weight and poorer dietary habits than non-abusers, consuming fewer vegetables and fruits and more junk food [36]. Heroin abusers' risk of being underweight is 3.4-fold higher than amphetamine abusers [37]. Heroin is an appetite suppressant, delaying gastric emptying and causing hyperkalemia (which can cause nausea, vomiting, and diarrhea); frequent comorbidities in heroin addicts, such as HIV or HCV infections, can worsen nutritional status and feeding behaviors. Ex-heroin abusers report how, during active abuse, they lost interest and pleasure in feeding, found food tasteless, and preferred low-cost snacks, mostly sweet foods; furthermore, choice of drugs over food had a primary role [36]. The preference for sweet foods seems to be mediated by the central actions of opioids on mu-receptors (nucleus accumbens, hypothalamus, and paraventricular nucleus of the hypothalamus) [38]. Moreover, heroin use has been associated with glucose metabolism impairment and insulin resistance, which can predispose to the development of diabetes [39]. Conversely, naltrexone and naloxone reduce caloric intake and search for sweet foods and suppress NPY-induced feeding behaviors [40]. In 2014, the FDA approved the association naltrexone/bupropion extended release for the treatment of obesity in the USA. Methadone treatment is associated with weight gain [41]: this may be directly due to the detoxification and renewed interest in food [36] or to the recovery of a normal body mass index or sweet food craving associated with mu-receptor agonist.

8.3.8 Tobacco

It is commonly known how smoking tobacco correlates with low body weight and that its cessation may lead to weight gain, although the underlying mechanisms are still not well understood. The common risk of incurring weight gain after smoking cessation may represent a maintaining factor for smoking habits, mostly in women. Many hypotheses have been raised about the way nicotine suppresses food intake and increases energy balance. Different nAChR subtypes (namely, α3β4, α7, and α4β2) have been correlated with the role of nicotine in the regulation of body weight, via their interactions with POMC and melanocortin system, pro- and anti-inflammatory cytokines, and mesolimbic pathway of dopamine release. Furthermore, chronic exposure to nicotine upregulates NPY mRNA and peptide but downregulates its hypothalamic receptors, while α3β4 activation on POMC neurons leads to melanocortin system activation and appetite suppression. Concerning peripheral hormones, nicotine modulates ghrelin and leptin, thus influencing appetite, food intake, and fat mass deposition [42].

8.4 Anecdotal Remarks

8.4.1 Pica

Pica is defined as an abnormal craving for non-nutritive substances such as sand, dirt, clay, or hair. Anecdotal cases of psychotropic drug-induced pica have been reported in the literature. Initiation of olanzapine has been related to transient pica in two cases of women with schizophrenia [43], while risperidone only in one case (a 50-year-old psychotic woman [44]). Also, tramadol has been reported inducing pica in a 17-year-old boy who was recovering from heroin abuse [45]. However, the underlying mechanisms are still unknown.

8.4.2 Sleep-Related Eating Disorder (SRED)

SRED is a kind of parasomnia characterized by abnormal eating patterns during the night, usually followed by complete or partial amnesia of the episodes. Many psychotropic drugs have been found to cause SRED. The most commonly associated drug is zolpidem: 37 cases of zolpidem-induced SRED have been reported [46], typically in middle-aged women, and usually, the disorder is quickly remitted after the cessation of the medication. Other case reports of psychotropic drug-induced SRED include olanzapine, quetiapine, risperidone, and aripiprazole.

8.4.3 Conclusions

While prescribing a psychotropic drug, its effects on body weight and appetite should be carefully considered. Weight gain could determine reduced compliance to therapy, especially for those patients who present a comorbid ED or have a history of overweight or obesity. Conversely, drugs that exert a negative effect on appetite could worsen a situation of malnutrition and/or underweight co-occurring or determined by the disease itself. Also, medications that cause weight loss could be used by patients as a pathological way to control their weight. The same attention should be paid to patients recovering from substance abuse, as the majority of illicit substances determine underweight and their discontinuation could cause an undesired weight gain and, consequently, relapse.

> **Box 1 Rainbow Pills**
> Between the 1940s and the 1960s, preparations including thyroid hormone, amphetamines, and other substances like diuretics, laxatives, and benzodiazepines were commercialized for weight loss with the name of "Rainbow Pills," given their variety of colors. These pills became very popular, mostly in the USA. Nonetheless, because of their side effects, which caused more than 60 deaths in the USA, in 1968, they were withdrawn from the market [47].

References

1. Kessler RC, Berglund PA, Chiu WT, et al. The prevalence and correlates of binge eating disorder in the World Health Organization World Mental Health Surveys. Biol Psychiatry. 2013;73(9):904–14.
2. American Psychiatric Association. Diagnostic and statistical manual of mental disorders. 5th ed. 2013. https://doi.org/10.1176/appi.books.9780890425596.744053.
3. Trinko R, Sears RM, Guarnieri DJ, DiLeone RJ. Neural mechanisms underlying obesity and drug addiction. Physiol Behav. 2007;91(5):499–505. Epub 2007 Jan 16.
4. Bak M, Fransen J, Janssen J, van Os J, Drukker M. Almost all antipsychotics result in weight gain: a meta-analysis. PLoS One. 2014;9(4):e94112. https://doi.org/10.1371/journal.pone.0094112.
5. Tarricone I, Ferrari Gozzi B, Serretti A, Grieco D, Berardi D. Weight gain in antipsychotic-naive patients: a review and meta-analysis. Psychol Med. 2010;40:187–200.
6. Nielsen MØ, Rostrup E, Wulff S, Glenthøj B, Ebdrup BH. Striatal reward activity and antipsychotic-associated weight change in patients with schizophrenia undergoing initial treatment. JAMA Psychiat. 2016;73:121–8.
7. Leucht S, Corves C, Arbter D, Engel RR, Li C, Davis JM. Second-generation versus first-generation antipsychotic drugs for schizophrenia: a meta-analysis. Lancet. 2009;373:31–41.
8. Coccurello R, Moles A. Potential mechanisms of atypical antipsychotic-induced metabolic derangement: clues for understanding obesity and novel drug design. Pharmacol Ther. 2010;127:210–51. https://doi.org/10.1016/j.pharmthera.2010.04.008.
9. Albaugh VL, Singareddy R, Mauger D, Lynch CJ. A double blind, placebo-controlled, randomized crossover study of the acute metabolic effects of olanzapine in healthy volunteers. PLoS One. 2011;6:e22662.
10. Takeuchi Y, Kajiyama K, Ishiguro C, Uyama Y. Atypical antipsychotics and the risk of hyperlipidemia: a sequence symmetry analysis. Drug Saf. 2015;38:641–50.
11. Potvin S, Zhornitsky S, Stip E. Antipsychotic-induced changes in blood levels of leptin in schizophrenia: a meta-analysis. Can J Psychiatry. 2015;60:S26.
12. Zhang Q, Deng C, Huang XF. The role of ghrelin signalling in second-generation antipsychotic-induced weight gain. Psychoneuroendocrinology. 2013;38(11):2423–38. https://doi.org/10.1016/j.psyneuen.2013.07.010. Epub 2013 Aug 14. Review.
13. Kanji S, Fonseka TM, Marshe VS, Sriretnakumar V, Hahn MK, Müller DJ. The microbiome-gut-brain axis: implications for schizophrenia and antipsychotic induced weight gain. Eur Arch Psychiatry Clin Neurosci. 2018;268:3–15.

14. Bond DJ, Kauer-Sant'Anna M, Lam RW, Yatham LN. Weight gain, obesity, and metabolic indices following a first manic episode: prospective 12-month data from the Systematic Treatment Optimization Program for Early Mania (STOP-EM). J Affect Disord. 2010;124(1–2):108–17. https://doi.org/10.1016/j.jad.2009.10.023. Epub 2009 Nov 14
15. Kanemura H, Sano F, Maeda Y, Sugita K, Aihara M. Valproate sodium enhances body weight gain in patients with childhood epilepsy: a pathogenic mechanisms and open-label clinical trial of behavior therapy. Seizure. 2012;21(7):496–500. https://doi.org/10.1016/j.seizure.2012.05.001. Epub 2012 Jun 12
16. Torrent C, Amann B, Sanchez-Moreno J, Colom F, Reinares M, Comes M, Rosa AR, Scott J, Vieta E. Weight gain in bipolar disorder: pharmacological treatment as a contributing factor. Acta Psychiatr Scand. 2008;118:4–18.
17. McElroy SL, Keck PE Jr. Obesity in bipolar disorder: an overview. Curr Psychiatry Rep. 2012;14:650–8.
18. McElroy SL, Crow S, Cuellar-Barboza AB, Prieto ML, Veldic M, Winham SJ, Bobo WV, Geske J, Seymour LR, Mori N, Bond DJ, Biernacka JM, Frye MA. Clinical features of bipolar spectrum with binge eating behaviour. J Affect Disord. 2016;201:95–8.
19. Uguz F, Sahingoz M, Gungor B, Aksoy F, Askin R. Weight gain and associated factors in patients using newer antidepressant drugs. Gen Hosp Psychiatry. 2015;37(1):46–8. https://doi.org/10.1016/j.genhosppsych.2014.10.011. Epub 2014 Oct 31
20. McElroy SL, Guerdjikova AI, Mori N, Keck PE. Managing comorbid obesity and depression through clinical pharmacotherapies. Expert Opin Pharmacother. 2016;17(12):1599–610.
21. Kirkham T. Endocannabinoids and the neurochemistry of gluttony. J Neuroendocrinol. 2008;20:1099–100.
22. Hirsch S, Tam J. Cannabis: From a Plant That Modulates Feeding Behaviors toward Developing Selective Inhibitors of the Peripheral Endocannabinoid System for the Treatment of Obesity and Metabolic Syndrome. Toxins. 2019;11:275.
23. Tarragon E, Moreno JJ. Cannabinoids, chemical senses, and regulation of feeding behavior. Chem Senses. 2019;44(2):73–89. https://doi.org/10.1093/chemse/bjy068.
24. Verrotti A, Scaparrotta A, Agostinelli S, Di Pillo S, Chiarelli F, Grosso S. Topiramate-induced weight loss: a review. Epilepsy Res. 2011;95:189–99.
25. Kushner RF. Weight loss strategies for treatment of obesity: lifestyle management and pharmacotherapy. Prog Cardiovasc Dis. 2018;61:246–52.
26. Arterburn D, Sofer T, Boudreau DM, Bogart A, Westbrook EO, Theis MK, Simon G, Haneuse S. Long-term weight change after initiating second-generation antidepressants. J Clin Med. 2016;5(4)
27. Serralde-Zúñiga AE, Gonzalez Garay AG, Rodríguez-Carmona Y, Melendez G. Fluoxetine for adults who are overweight or obese. Cochrane Database Syst Rev. 2019;10:CD011688. https://doi.org/10.1002/14651858.CD011688.pub2. [Epub ahead of print] Review.
28. Krentz AJ, Fujioka K, Hompesch M. Evolution of pharmacological obesity treatments: focus on adverse side-effect profiles. Diabetes Obes Metab. 2016;18(6):558–70. https://doi.org/10.1111/dom.12657. Review.
29. Fulp A, Zhang Y, Bortoff K, Seltzman H, Snyder R, Wiethe R, Amato G, Maitra R. Pyrazole antagonists of the CB1 receptor with reduced brain penetration. Bioorg Med Chem. 2016;24:1063–70.
30. Saunders KH, Umashanker D, Igel LI, Kumar RB, Aronne LJ. Obesity pharmacotherapy. Med Clin North Am. 2018;102(1):135–48.
31. Amodeo G, Cuomo A, Bolognesi S, Goracci A, Trusso MA, Piccinni A, Neal SM, Baldini I, Federico E, Taddeucci C, Fagiolini A. Pharmacotherapeutic strategies for treating binge eating disorder. Evidence from clinical trials and implications for clinical practice. Expert Opin Pharmacother. 2019;20(6):679–90. https://doi.org/10.1080/14656566.2019.1571041. Epub 2019 Jan 29. Review.
32. Bernet VJ. Thyroid hormone misuse and abuse. Endocrine. 2019;66:79–86.
33. Cochrane C, Malcolm R, Brewerton T. The role of weight control as a motivation for cocaine abuse. Addict Behav. 1998;23(2):201–7.

34. Vicentic A, Jones DC. The CART (cocaine- and amphetamine-regulated transcript) system in appetite and drug addiction. J Pharmacol Exp Ther. 2007;320(2):499–506. Epub 2006 Jul 13.
35. Ersche KD, Stochl J, Woodward JM, Fletcher PC. The skinny on cocaine: insights into eating behavior and body weight in cocaine-dependent men. Appetite. 2013;71:75–80. https://doi.org/10.1016/j.appet.2013.07.011. Epub 2013 Aug 3.
36. Neale J, Nettleton S, Pickering L, Fischer J. Eating patterns among heroin users: a qualitative study with implications for nutritional interventions. Addiction. 2012;107(3):635–41.
37. McIlwraith F, Betts KS, Jenkinson R, Hickey S, Burns L, Alati R. Is low BMI associated with specific drug use among injecting drug users? Subst Use Misuse. 2014;49(4):374–82.
38. Mysels DJ, Sullivan MA. The relationship between opioid and sugar intake: review of evidence and clinical applications. J Opioid Manag. 2010;6(6):445–52.
39. Pereska Z, Bozinovska C, Dimitrovski C, Cakalarovski K, Chibishev A, Zdravkovska M, Babulovska A, Janicevic D. Heroin dependence duration influences the metabolic parameters: mechanisms and consequences of impaired insulin sensitivity in hepatitis C virus seronegative heroin dependents. J Addict Med. 2012;6(4):304–10. https://doi.org/10.1097/ADM.0b013e31826bd76c.
40. Levine AS, Grace M, Billington CJ. The effect of centrally administered naloxone on deprivation and drug-induced feeding. Pharmacol Biochem Behav. 1990;36(2):409–12.
41. Peles E, Schreiber S, Sason A, Adelson M. Risk factors for weight gain during methadone maintenance treatment. Subst Abus. 2016;37(4):613–8.
42. Hu T, Yang Z, Li MD. Pharmacological effects and regulatory mechanisms of tobacco smoking effects on food intake and weight control. J Neuroimmune Pharmacol. 2018;13:453.
43. Chawla N, Charan D, Kumar S, Pattanayak RD. Pica associated with initiation of atypical antipsychotic drugs: Report of two cases. Psychiatry Clin Neurosci. 2016;70(8):363–4.
44. Huang JH, Shiah IS, Lee WK, Tzang RF, Chang KJ. Olanzapine-associated pica in a schizophrenia patient. Psychiatry Clin Neurosci. 2010;64(4):444.
45. Chawla N, Mandal P, Chatterjee B, Dhawan A. Tramadol-associated pica. Psychiatry Clin Neurosci. 2019;73(1):43.
46. Nzwalo H, Ferreira L, Peralta R, Bentes C. Sleep-related eating disorder secondary to zolpidem. BMJ Case Rep. 2013:2013.
47. Müller TD, Clemmensen C, Finan B, DiMarchi RD, Tschöp MH. Anti-obesity therapy: from rainbow pills to polyagonists. Pharmacol Rev. 2018;70(4):712–46.

Disordered Eating Behaviors in Other Psychiatric Disorders

Anna Rita Atti, Maurizio Speciani, and Diana De Ronchi

9.1 Disordered Eating in Schizophrenia

In the fifth edition of the *Diagnostic and Statistical Manual of Mental Disorders* (DSM-5) [1], disordered eating is not explicitly listed in the criteria for the diagnosis of schizophrenia. However, "a lack of interest in eating or food refusal" is reported in the "Associated Features Supporting Diagnosis." Even though disorganized eating behaviors did not formally make the list, the relationship between peculiarities in nutritional patterns and psychoses has long been observed and highlighted. Emil Kraepelin, in his book *Dementia Praecox and Paraphrenia* [2], recalls how the "taking of food" may fluctuate "from complete refusal to the greatest voracity," while Eugen Bleuler, in his *Textbook of Psychiatry* [3], highlighted a tendency of schizophrenics "to swallow all kinds of things."

Disordered eating behaviors may result from thought content alterations and perceptual disturbances, as a direct consequence of the most specific symptoms of the disease. In our professional experience, it's not uncommon that delusions may focus on food and eating, especially when persecutory delusions or delusions of poisoning characterize the clinical picture. In-depth analyses of disordered eating in schizophrenia have been collected in a case series by Yum and colleagues [4], highlighting the aforementioned effects of delusions on nutritional patterns with great detail. However, a growing body of evidence has been steadily growing in the last few decades, emphasizing how disordered eating behaviors do not only stem from delusions and hallucinations, painting a more complex clinical picture.

A. R. Atti (✉) · M. Speciani · D. De Ronchi
Department of Biomedical and Neuromotor Science, University of Bologna, Bologna, Italy
e-mail: annarita.atti@unibo.it; maurizio.speciani@studio.unibo.it; diana.deronchi@unibo.it

© Springer Nature Switzerland AG 2022
E. Manzato et al. (eds.), *Hidden and Lesser-known Disordered Eating Behaviors in Medical and Psychiatric Conditions*,
https://doi.org/10.1007/978-3-030-81174-7_9

For example, in 1999, Brown and colleagues [5] found, in a community sample of 102 schizophrenics, a predilection for a diet higher in fat and lower in fiber when compared to the general population, even after controlling for social class. Another study [6], less than a decade later, found a comparable dietary pattern in a sample of 30 hospitalized patients. However, in a 2003 paper, Strassnig and colleagues [7] did not find significant differences in terms of types of preferred foods in schizophrenics, but they found that they ate significantly more calories than their healthy counterparts. Furthermore, in 2013, Palmese and colleagues identified a higher rate of night eating in obese individuals with a diagnosis of schizophrenia or schizoaffective disorder compared to the general population [8]. As results from multiple studies on the matter were often conflicting, and the methodology varied considerably, an initial review of the evidence was published by Strassnig and colleagues in 2005 [9], which did not find a peculiar dietary pattern in schizophrenics. Eight years later, a much needed systematic review taking into consideration the most recently published evidence was published by Dipasquale and colleagues [10]. They highlighted a number of critical issues in the recollection of eating patterns, which sometimes were analyzed through short questionnaires and in a few cases even without any standardized assessment. They found that patients were more likely to consume less fiber and fruit, while their intake of saturated fats was higher and sometimes that consumption of monounsaturated and polyunsaturated fatty acids was lower. Some studies also found a higher total calorie intake, while a few did not report any significant difference compared to controls. They found that some studies identified factors which correlated with dietary patterns. Gender differences were found to be sometimes positively and sometimes negatively correlated to a healthier diet. Stress, through cortisol secretion and the balance of hypothalamic–pituitary–adrenal axis, was investigated, but no conclusion could be drawn. Dietary patterns as a consequence of pharmacological treatment were also investigated, but they were far from conclusive: olanzapine treatment was found to be associated in one study with increased consumption of sweet food and in another one with increased calorie intake. Treatment with clozapine was found to be associated with increased consumption of fats and proteins along with decreased fiber and carbohydrates in one study, compared to risperidone, although both seemed to be associated with higher fat intake compared to clinical recommendations. However, a number of studies did not find statistical differences in macronutrients or caloric intake, and a few did not even find any effect on diet from antipsychotic treatment.

In 2019, a systematic review and meta-analysis by Teasdale and colleagues [11], which focused on both bipolar disorder and schizophrenia, found an association between psychoses and a higher calorie intake, particularly because of decreased intakes of fruit and vegetables and increased intakes of convenience foods and sugar-sweetened drinks. They also attempted to discern and discriminate the effects of antipsychotic medication on dietary patterns but considered the available evidence to be insufficiently detailed in order to reach conclusions.

Stemming from the expanding knowledge of eating symptomatology in schizophrenia, a number of hypotheses have been proposed to better understand the link between eating disorders and psychoses, as described by Seeman in a recent publication [12]. The seven hypotheses are described as follows:

1. Eating disorders and schizophrenia are entirely separate diseases which may co-occur.
2. Starvation in eating disorders or in psychoses can cause the other disease.
3. Control of food (in eating disorders or in psychoses) provides a sense of achievement which may help to ward off the primary disease.
4. Eating disorders are, because of body image distortions, essentially psychotic disorders.
5. Eating symptoms are prodromes of an impending psychosis, and psychotic symptoms can be harbingers of a developing eating disorder.
6. Antipsychotics can lead to weight gain, therefore inducing an eating disorder, or conversely, antidepressants can trigger psychosis.
7. Psychotic symptoms are severity markers in eating disorders, while food refusal is a severity marker in psychosis.

Although the quality of evidence did not allow to recognize a more substantiated hypothesis than the others, nor to detect any causal relationship between eating disorders and psychoses, as recognized by the author, it may be useful to keep in mind these hypotheses when treating a schizophrenic patient with manifest symptoms of disordered eating. In a recent study by Zhang and colleagues, another link between psychosis and disordered eating was found in a large-scale familiar study. A family member of a patient with an eating disorder was found to be at a higher risk of developing schizophrenia, and schizophrenia was also found to be a risk factor for the development of an eating disorder in other family members. This bidirectional relationship, found to be relevant in a study involving millions of subjects, may suggest that the alterations in eating behaviors which are found in psychoses may constitute subthreshold manifestations of formally diagnosed eating disorders [13].

From a neurobiological point of view, evidence regarding dysregulation of dopaminergic, cholinergic, and opioid pathways involved in eating modulation in schizophrenia is emerging [14, 15] and may further clarify the development of disordered eating and could, in the future, provide alternative means to better control the symptoms.

9.2   Disordered Eating in Bipolar Disorders

In DSM-5 [1], disordered eating is not part of the criteria for the diagnosis of bipolar disorder. Evidence linking disordered eating and bipolar disorder is not as abundant as there is for other psychiatric disorders such as psychoses, although in the last few years several papers highlighting a correlation between eating symptoms and bipolar disorders have been published.

In 2005, a review of the evidence by McElroy and colleagues [16] emphasized that bipolar disorders and eating disorders share specific clinical features, as patients experiencing mood episodes—whether they are manic, hypomanic, or depressive—often manifest a disruption of their usual eating patterns; more specifically, they identified common characteristics between bipolar and eating disorders: alterations of the mood (such as behavioral activation, lability, and cyclicity) as symptoms of eating disorders, eating and weight dysregulation as symptoms of bipolar disorders, and impulsivity and compulsivity as symptoms of both. Furthermore, they highlighted how the diseases appear to share a common course since they both typically begin in adolescence or early adulthood, they both may be characterized by phasic or cyclic patterns, and both may share some similarities in the way they respond— or in the way they do not—to pharmacological drugs. Thus, the authors proposed three distinct models to understand these similarities: the first, where eating disorders and bipolar disorders co-occur by chance, even though at significant frequency; the second, where they overlap because they share similar pathophysiological disruptions regarding mood dysregulation, disordered eating, body weight, and impulse control; and a third, wherein they co-occur because they are pathophysiological related, but they are ultimately separate disorders. Hence, even though the evidence available at the time did not allow the authors to favor one model compared to the others, the reviewed literature strongly suggested that bipolar and eating disorders are related.

Clinical studies also investigated which characteristics appear to be more closely associated with disordered eating and bipolar disorders. A relationship between bipolar disorder and binge eating disorder was highlighted in a paper by Ramacciotti and colleagues [17] which found a disproportionately higher frequency of eating disorders (bulimia nervosa and binge eating disorder) in their sample of 51 bipolar patients. In particular, they found that binge eating episodes developed at the same time or following the onset of bipolar disorder. Therefore, they suggested a model wherein binge eating develops as a means of regulating mood with food, but could also be due to psychopharmacological side effects. In 2007, a paper by Kilbourne and colleagues [18] found significant differences in eating patterns in bipolar patients compared to controls. Specifically, bipolar patients were more likely to have suboptimal eating patterns, such as eating fewer than two meals per day, and they were more likely to eat alone most of the time. Furthermore, they reported having difficulties cooking or obtaining food, a difference that remained significant even after adjusting for socio-demographic and clinical factors. The authors hypothesized that these differences could be due to depressive and manic episodes and their behavioral consequences on food intake. However, in consideration of the results by Ramacciotti and colleagues as previously described, it may also be hypothesized that a lower frequency of meals in a day could, in some cases, be due to compensatory restriction of calories after a disproportionate calorie intake in a single meal, such as after a binge eating episode.

More recently, in 2015, a study by Bernstein and colleagues [19] further investigated the link between obesity and bipolar disorder on a sample of 37 female patients. They found that restraint was correlated with healthily eating, while perceived hunger and disinhibition were directly correlated with a higher BMI. Accordingly, Martin and colleagues [20] found a higher prevalence of binge eating and emotional eating in a population of 82 bipolar patients; emotional dysregulation and impulsivity were significantly correlated with maladaptive nutritional behaviors. Boulanger and colleagues [21] also found emotional dysregulation and impulsivity to be correlated to binge eating behaviors in bipolar patients. Additionally, higher levels of anxiety were also found to be significantly associated with binge eating behaviors.

The binge eating behavior "phenotype" in bipolar disorder and its characteristics were thoroughly investigated by McElroy and colleagues [22] in a 2016 paper. Bipolar patients with an eating disorder diagnosis and who manifested binge eating behaviors were found, compared to non-binge eating/non-eating disordered bipolar patients, to manifest significantly higher levels of eating psychopathology, mood instability, suicidality, and comorbidity (especially for anxiety disorders); they also had a higher BMI, a higher prevalence of obesity, and a higher medical illness burden. Bipolar patients who manifested binge eating behaviors but did not fulfill the criteria for an eating disorder diagnosis, in terms of clinical characteristics, more closely resembled those who did not have any eating symptomatology than those with an eating disorder comorbidity.

Not only binge eating behaviors are more frequently comorbid in bipolar patients; evidence suggests night eating syndrome could be more prevalent as well in this population. In an assessment of 80 bipolar patients and 40 healthy controls, Melo and colleagues [23] found that night eating syndrome has a higher prevalence in bipolar patients compared to controls (8.8% in their sample, against none in the control group); this subpopulation also expressed more anxiety, worse functioning, and impaired sleeping.

A review of the available evidence regarding bipolar disorder and disordered eating from McDonald and colleagues [24] has been recently published. In accordance with many of the studies previously described in this chapter, they found a higher prevalence of eating disorders in bipolar patients, especially binge eating symptomatology, while restrictive symptoms were not as prevalent. Subgroups of bipolar patients with eating symptomatology were also expressing heightened rates of mood instability, alcohol abuse, and suicidality.

In conclusion, bipolar disorder appears to be significantly correlated with eating symptomatology, particularly binge eating symptomatology; emotional dysregulation, mood instability, and other clinical characteristics appear to be associated with a bipolar-eating disordered comorbid phenotype.

9.3 Disordered Eating in Depressive Disorders

In DSM-5 [1], eating symptomatology is reported among the criteria for the diagnosis of depressive disorders such as major depressive disorder, persistent depressive disorder (dysthymia), and premenstrual dysphoric disorder. Both overeating and lack of appetite have been recognized as symptoms of depressive illnesses for a long time and have been part of the criteria for the diagnosis of major depressive episode since DSM-III [25].

Eating symptomatology is deemed a possible risk factor for depressive disorders, and depressive disorders are also considered a risk factor for eating disorders [26–28]. Evidence suggests that disordered eating—even in the absence of a categorical diagnosis of eating disorder—may be more frequent in mood disorders, as highlighted in a 2011 study from Touchette and colleagues [29]. They found subclinical eating symptomatology to be significantly associated with a mood disorder diagnosis in a sample of adolescent girls. Specifically, they found subclinical bulimia nervosa and subclinical binge eating disorder to be significantly correlated to a diagnosis of major depression or dysthymia compared to controls. Criterion A3 in major depression (weight/appetite gain or loss when not dieting) and criterion B1 in dysthymia appear to be the most closely associated criteria with eating symptomatology in their sample.

It is still unclear whether any specific eating pattern is an effect or a risk factor for depressive disorders, and a review of the available evidence from Quirk and colleagues [30] found methodological difficulties and conflicting results and thus could not evaluate significant associations on the matter. Further studies are needed to systematically review new evidence which may have emerged in the last few years.

Although eating symptomatology is widely accepted as one of the many phenomena which characterize depressive illnesses, less is known about its neurobiological basis. In the last few years, a number of studies investigated possible factors which may play a role in a biochemical imbalance resulting in disordered eating symptomatology. One of the most recent developments regarding the biological link between eating and mental health involves the so-called gut-brain axis, a bidirectional network between neurobiological alterations and the microbiome population. A paper from Valles-Colomer and colleagues [31] published in *Nature Microbiology* in early 2019 highlighted the strong relationship between specific populations of bacteria in the microbiome and depression. Additionally, chronic inflammation seems to be also involved in the pathophysiology of depression and dysbiosis [32]. Since the microbiota is affected by eating patterns and evidence suggests that both depression risk and its course could be influenced by food [33], the microbiota seems to play a role in this bidirectional relationship and may be a factor implicated in the maintenance of the disease. Further studies are needed to better understand whether disordered eating symptomatology in depression also has a role in the maintenance of the disease, perhaps through alterations in the microbiota and immune equilibrium.

9.4 Disordered Eating in Anxiety Disorders

In the most recent edition of the DSM [1], there is no specific mention of eating symptomatology as a specific criterion in the Anxiety Disorders chapter. However, a number of studies throughout the years highlighted the significant comorbidity which characterizes anxiety disorders (which, until DSM-5, included OCD) and eating symptomatology.

Even when neither eating disorders nor anxiety disorders are categorically diagnosed, anxiety seems to influence eating behavior. In 1987, a paper from Herman and colleagues [34] found that anxiety could either diminish or augment hunger depending on usual and previous food intake in an otherwise healthy population of college students. When people who were hungry felt anxious, their feeling of hunger became more intense, and when people who were not hungry felt anxious, their feeling of hunger decreased significantly. In more recent years, a lot of papers found significantly high rates of comorbidity between categorically diagnosed eating disorders and anxiety disorders. For example, a review by Swinbourne and Touyz [35] found that, although it seems clear that anxiety disorders and eating disorders more frequently co-occur compared to the general population, inconsistent findings from previous studies did not clarify whether eating symptomatology emerged as a consequence of anxiety disorders or if they are fully distinct diseases sharing similar contributing factors or features. In some cases, an anxiety disorder was reported to have emerged earlier than eating symptomatology. Therefore, even though the available evidence was far from conclusive, anxiety symptomatology could be deemed a contributing factor to the development of eating struggles. Accordingly, population studies also found a higher prevalence of disordered eating behaviors in a population of more than 20,000 women [36]. More specifically, they found disordered eating to be significantly associated with social phobia in women over 25 years old, with agoraphobia in women between the ages of 15 and 44, and with panic disorder in women of all age groups. Since a previous study by Hinrichsen and colleagues [37] found social phobia to be associated with bulimia nervosa, the authors hypothesized that the significant association they found between disordered eating with social phobia in women over 25 years old could be due to the fact that the shift from restrictive type, which may precede bulimia nervosa, already happened in their sample and thus was not highlighted by their methodology. It appears anxiety influences eating behavior in less frequently investigated age groups for eating disorders as well; it was found to be significantly correlated with both emotional eating and uncontrolled eating in a population of women from 40 to 65 years old in a recent study by Janjetic and colleagues [38]. Perfectionism has been suggested as the mediator between social phobia and bulimic symptomatology [39]. Social anxiety was not only correlated with bulimia nervosa but with binge eating as well; Ostrovsky and colleagues [40] investigated disordered eating in an overweight and obese population and found a significant association between social anxiety, binge eating symptomatology, and emotional eating. Disordered eating and anxiety seem to share a bidirectional relationship in which both influence each other, as highlighted in a paper by Puccio and colleagues [41].

A paper by Thornton and colleagues in 2011 investigated the relationship between generalized anxiety disorder and anorexia nervosa [42]. They hypothesize that a number of behavioral strategies, such as exercise or fasting, which happen more frequently in this population, may be due to their diminishing effects on anxiety; it could be because of such practices that their lowest BMI was lower than individuals with anorexia nervosa only; they therefore deemed this comorbid population as high risk.

Regarding subclinical eating disturbances in anxiety disorders, Touchette and colleagues [29] found separation anxiety disorder to be significantly correlated with subclinical anorexia nervosa-restricting type and generalized anxiety disorder to be significantly associated with subclinical bulimia nervosa and subclinical binge eating disorder, in a sample of 833 adolescent girls. It is, however, still unclear how these subclinical syndromes may evolve in time.

A specific phobia phenotype (SPOV: specific phobia of vomiting) was investigated by Veale and colleagues [43] in a sample of 94 patients. They were divided in those who restricted food for fear of vomiting and those who did not. The whole population was found to manifest eating disturbances, as they frequently smelled and checked food for expiry dates and freshness, and the restricting subtype cooked food for significantly longer than most would consider necessary.

In conclusion, anxiety disorders and disordered eating appear to more frequently co-occur. Social anxiety appears to be the most common anxiety disorder comorbid with eating symptomatology and seems to more frequently correlate with bulimic and binge eating tendencies. The role of generalized anxiety disorder in the development of categorically diagnosed eating disorder is still unclear. Further studies are needed to better clarify the relationship between specific anxiety disorders and disordered eating.

9.5 Disordered Eating in Obsessive-Compulsive Disorders

In the last edition of the DSM, there is no specific mention of eating symptomatology in the obsessive-compulsive disorders criteria. It is known that OCD and disordered eating may co-occur [35, 44]. It is still unclear whether eating disorders occur more frequently in OCD patients compared to anxiety disorders [45]. A number of features appear to predict eating symptomatology in obsessive-compulsive disordered patients. Obsessions for symmetry and compulsions for ordering and arranging were found to be more common in eating disordered OCD patients, compared to OCD patients alone in a small sample of female patients, in a study from Matsunaga and colleagues [46]. Accordingly, in a population of 141 college students, Roberts [47] found "ordering and arranging" to be the most significant predictor of disordered eating. Furthermore, in a study from Humphreys and colleagues [48], disordered eating significantly correlated with OC symptoms and ordering/cleaning compulsions. In a recent review of the available literature, Bozzini and colleagues found a correlation between OCD symptoms, anxiety, and higher eating behavior inflexibility [49]. Hoarding was not found to be predictive nor significantly correlated with eating symptomatology [47, 48]. Additionally, OC symptoms were found to correlate positively with eating disorder severity in a paper by Jiménez-Murcia and colleagues [50].

From a dimensional point of view, perfectionism and neuroticism have been found to be significantly correlated with eating disorder symptomatology [44]. Accordingly, obsessive-compulsiveness, obsessive personality traits, and perfectionism were found to be accurate predictors of eating disorder severity [50]. Additionally, a recent paper by Froreich and colleagues [51] investigated and compared measures of control dimensions with OC symptoms in a community sample; they found ineffectiveness and fear of losing control as the most significant predictors of eating disordered symptomatology.

In conclusion, the available evidence on OCD and disordered eating appears to support an underlying relationship between the diseases, as they seem to influence each other. While it is still unclear how frequently they co-occur, many dimensional characteristics of OC symptomatology seem to predict eating symptoms in OCD patients. Further studies are needed to better understand eating behaviors and patterns of OCD patients.

9.6 Disordered Eating in Dissociative Disorders

Eating symptomatology is not included in criteria for the diagnosis of dissociative disorders in DSM-5 [1]. Dissociative symptoms happen to be common in a number of psychiatric diagnoses [52]. However, a relationship between disordered eating and dissociative symptoms has long been shown in scientific publications. Rosen and Petty [53] found significant correlations between measures of dissociation (measured by Dissociative Experiences Scale, DES, and Perceptual Alteration Scale, PAS) and disordered eating in a community sample; the cognitive dimension was not significantly correlated with the severity and intensity of eating symptoms, suggesting disordered eating in presence of dissociative tendencies to be related to modifications of affect and feelings of loss of control, rather than to a byproduct of an alteration of cognitive components. More specifically, Everill and colleagues [54] found a significant association between dissociation (measured by DES) and binge tendencies in a non-clinical community sample and between dissociation and frequency of binge eating episodes in a clinical sample of eating disordered patients. Accordingly, Engelberg and colleagues [55] found dissociation to be elevated prior to binge episodes in a clinical sample of bulimic patients; negative affect was found to be significantly elevated prior to binge episodes as well. Fuller-Tyszkiewicz and Mussap [56] actually found that dissociation was significantly correlated with binge eating and more specifically with somatoform dissociation as a mediator of binge episodes. It has been hypothesized that binge eating episodes may be a way to decrease negative affect, while the lack of awareness could allow patients to prevent the development of feelings of despair and guilt following the episode. Another hypothesis is that both binge eating episodes and dissociative episodes work synergistically as a way to diminish both negative affect and self-awareness [57]. The nature and role of this relationship are still unclear. Recent evidence appears to confirm the significant association between negative affect and dissociation, and since negative affect appears to diminish after a binge eating episode, regardless of dissociation, it has been hypothesized that both dissociation and binge eating may function as independent factors regulating negative affect [58]. Furthermore, a relationship between traumatic experiences—which could mediate long-term negative affect, dissociation, and binge eating—has long been recognized in scientific literature [59]. Accordingly, somatoform dissociation and childhood traumatic experiences have been found to accurately predict the severity of binge eating symptoms [60].

In conclusion, binge eating symptoms appear to be significantly correlated to dissociative symptoms, especially somatoform dissociation, and may perform similar functions on mood, working jointly in order to decrease negative emotions. Further studies are needed in order to better understand how frequently disordered eating co-occurs in categorically diagnosed dissociative disorders.

9.7 Disordered Eating in Sleep-Wake Disorders

Sleep disturbances have long been known to correlate with disordered eating patterns. Sleep loss, stress, and eating patterns appear to be interlinked through neuroendocrinological pathways which promote weight gain [61]. Even in community samples, in the absence of a categorically diagnosed disorder, the association between eating symptomatology and sleep disturbances appears conspicuous. Bos and colleagues found that bulimic behaviors, as measured by EAT-40 scores, correlated with difficulties in sleeping, especially insomnia [62]. Tromp and colleagues also found a correlation between scores in eating disorder scales and sleep disorder scales in a community sample [63]. The association between poor sleep and disordered eating was also found in a community sample of children between the ages of 5 and 12, in which shorter sleep duration and poor sleep continuity were found to promote eating behaviors which could lead to overeating and weight gain and could raise obesity risk [64].

It has been hypothesized that the neuroendocrinological basis of the bidirectional relationship between sleep and hunger lies in the balance of ghrelin (orexigenic hormone) and leptin (anorexigenic hormone) [65]. Sleep loss has been significantly correlated with a dysregulation of these hormones, more specifically with decreased leptin levels and higher ghrelin levels in a sleep-deprived sample [66]. In obstructive sleep apnea syndrome, a clinical syndrome frequently associated with obesity and disturbances in sleep, an alteration of the equilibrium of leptin and ghrelin was also found by Ulukavak Ciftci and colleagues [67]. Another hypothesis on the link between the two disturbances is related to the effects of orexins, peptides also known as hypocretins which have been found to mediate both sleep-related and hunger-related effects, and to be involved in the pathophysiology of narcolepsy [68]. Accordingly, narcoleptic patients have been found to be more overweight and to manifest significantly more severe bulimic symptomatology than controls [69, 70]. Furthermore, psychopharmaceutical effects of drugs used to treat sleeping disorders may have a role in the development of eating disordered symptomatology. Zolpidem appears to have an effect on eating behaviors, since a direct relationship between disordered eating symptoms and zolpidem has been reported in the literature [71–73].

In conclusion, eating behavior and sleep behavior appear to be correlated. A number of neurobiological pathways have been hypothesized to be involved. Further studies are needed to better discern the effects of disturbed sleeping from contributing and confounding factors and to better understand the relationship between psychopharmaceutical drugs for sleeping and consequential disturbed eating behaviors.

9.8 Disordered Eating in Personality Disorders

Personality traits are implicated in the onset, in the phenotypic expression, and in the maintenance of EDs: common personality features observed along the ED spectrum are perfectionism, obsessive-compulsiveness, neuroticism, negative emotionality, harm avoidance, low self-directedness, low cooperativeness, and avoidant traits. It is also well acknowledged that AN patients demonstrate high constraint and persistence and low novelty seeking, while BN patients are characterized by high impulsivity, sensation seeking, and novelty seeking [74]. In a systematic literature revision published in 2005, the estimated personality disorder (PD) rates among individuals with AN and BN range from 0 to 58%, although self-report instruments are deemed to greatly overestimate PD prevalence [74]. More recently, network analyses have been increasingly applied to psychiatric populations to understand the relationships among symptoms. A network analysis published in 2018 [75] performed on 2068 adult patients with mixed ED assessed by the Symptom Check-List 90 (SCL-90), the Eating Disorder Inventory (EDI), and the Tridimensional Personality Questionnaire (TPQ) demonstrated the relevance of interpersonal sensitivity and ineffectiveness among all EDs but not in patients with AN, thus excluding that personality had a central role in the network of symptoms of AN [76].

A network analysis on self-report data from 753 adults (81.5% women), of whom 109 reported a lifetime ED diagnosis, investigated several transdiagnostic variables including insecure attachment, rejection sensitivity, emotion dysregulation, a theory of mind, and emotion recognition. Findings demonstrated that comorbidity between borderline personality disorder (BPD) and ED symptoms was only partially conceptualized through the transdiagnostic variables. The centrality indices from the network analysis indicated that emotion dysregulation and abandonment were the most central elements in the network. Conversely, the theory of mind and emotion recognition had very few connections with the other transdiagnostic variables in the network [77].

The idea that personality disorders could not be diagnosed before the age of 18 has been recently overcome by studies published in the last decade that revealed that personality disorders can be observed in children and adolescents. Given the high prevalence and incidence of EDs during adolescence, several recent studies have investigated this issue.

Adolescents with EDs differed from the non-ED group according to traits related to negative affectivity, detachment, and conscientiousness. The presence of AN moderated the relationship between an ED and personality traits; anorexia itself was more strongly associated with conscientious traits compared to other EDs [78]. Girls ($n = 73$) aged 11–18 presenting for mental health treatment at an outpatient psychiatry clinic in a large metropolitan hospital were evaluated by means of the Diagnostic Interview for Borderline Personality Disorder-Revised, Borderline Personality Questionnaire, and Short Screen for Eating Disorders. Girls with borderline personality disorder had significantly more disordered eating behavior compared to controls. Of the nine facets of BPD, eight were highly correlated with disordered eating, suggesting important shared variance between the constructs of

BPD and disordered eating; rejection sensitivity significantly mediated the relationship between BPD symptoms and disordered eating [79].

Relevant differences between personality profiles associated with AN and BN might occur also during adolescence as demonstrated in a study on 104 patients with AN and BN that employed an instrument specifically suitable for adolescents the Millon Adolescent Clinical Inventory (MACI). The personality profiles that differ significantly in both AN and BN were submissive, egotistic, unruly, forceful, conforming, oppositional, self-demeaning, and borderline. The most frequent profiles in AN were conforming (33.33%), egotistic (22.72%), and dramatizing (18.18%), while in the case of BN, those profiles were unruly (18.42%), submissive (18.42%), and borderline (15.78%). The author concluded that tailored therapeutic interventions for this specific population would be important [80].

9.9 Conclusions

To conclude, although physiological factors play an important role in human eating, eating behavior is also influenced by a variety of psychological factors and personality traits. Research from laboratory settings suggests that the only factor that triggers eating in unrestrained eaters is hunger. Conversely, restrained eaters overeat after experiencing anxiety or positive or negative moods, but not hunger. Understanding the triggers of eating in everyday life in patients affected by psychiatric disorders is crucial for the implementation of interventions to promote healthy eating and to prevent disordered eating among them.

References

1. American Psychiatric Association, editor. Diagnostic and statistical manual of mental disorders: DSM-5. 5th ed. Washington, D.C: American Psychiatric Association; 2013.
2. Emil Kraepelin Dementia praecox and paraphrenia; 1919, pp. 87. Chicago Medical Co.
3. Eugen B. Textbook of psychiatry. New York: Macmillan Co; 1924. p. 149. [original published 1911]. The Macmillan Company.
4. Yum SY, Caracci G, Hwang MY. Schizophrenia and eating disorders. Psychiatr Clin. 2009;32:809–19.
5. Brown S, Birtwistle J, Roe L, Thompson C. The unhealthy lifestyle of people with schizophrenia. Psychol Med. 1999;29:697–701.
6. Amani R. Is dietary pattern of schizophrenia patients different from healthy subjects? BMC Psychiatry. 2007;7(15)
7. Strassnig M, Brar JS, Ganguli R. Nutritional assessment of patients with schizophrenia: a preliminary study. Schizophr Bull. 2003;29:393–7.
8. Palmese LB, Ratliff JC, Reutenauer EL, Tonizzo KM, Grilo CM, Tek C. Prevalence of night eating in obese individuals with schizophrenia and schizoaffective disorder. Compr Psychiatry. 2013;54:276–81.
9. Strassnig M, Brar JS, Ganguli R. Dietary intake of patients with schizophrenia. Psychiatry (Edgmont). 2005;2:31–5.
10. Dipasquale S, Pariante CM, Dazzan P, Aguglia E, McGuire P, Mondelli V. The dietary pattern of patients with schizophrenia: a systematic review. J Psychiatr Res. 2013;47:197–207.

11. Teasdale SB, Ward PB, Samaras K, Firth J, Stubbs B, Tripodi E, Burrows TL. Dietary intake of people with severe mental illness: systematic review and meta-analysis. Br J Psychiatry. 2019;214:251–9.
12. Seeman MV. Eating disorders and psychosis: seven hypotheses. World J Psychiatry. 2014;4:112–9.
13. Zhang R, Larsen JT, Kuja-Halkola R, Thornton L, Yao S, Larsson H, Lichtenstein P, Petersen LV, Bulik CM, Bergen SE. Familial co-aggregation of schizophrenia and eating disorders in Sweden and Denmark. Mol Psychiatry. 2020; https://doi.org/10.1038/s41380-020-0749-x.
14. Elman I, Borsook D, Lukas SE. Food intake and reward mechanisms in patients with schizophrenia: implications for metabolic disturbances and treatment with second-generation antipsychotic agents. Neuropsychopharmacology. 2006;31:2091–120.
15. Avena NM, Bocarsly ME. Dysregulation of brain reward systems in eating disorders: neurochemical information from animal models of binge eating, bulimia nervosa, and anorexia nervosa. Neuropharmacology. 2012;63:87–96.
16. McElroy SL, Kotwal R, Keck PE, Akiskal HS. Comorbidity of bipolar and eating disorders: distinct or related disorders with shared dysregulations? J Affect Disord. 2005;86:107–27.
17. Ramacciotti CE, Paoli RA, Marcacci G, Piccinni A, Burgalassi A, Dell'Osso L, Garfinkel PE. Relationship between bipolar illness and binge-eating disorders. Psychiatry Res. 2005;135:165–70.
18. Kilbourne AM, Rofey DL, McCarthy JF, Post EP, Welsh D, Blow FC. Nutrition and exercise behavior among patients with bipolar disorder. Bipolar Disord. 2007;9:443–52.
19. Bernstein EE, Nierenberg AA, Deckersbach T, Sylvia LG. Eating behavior and obesity in bipolar disorder. Aust N Z J Psychiatry. 2015;49:566–72.
20. Martin K, Woo J, Timmins V, Collins J, Islam A, Newton D, Goldstein BI. Binge eating and emotional eating behaviors among adolescents and young adults with bipolar disorder. J Affect Disord. 2016;195:88–95.
21. Boulanger H, Tebeka S, Girod C, Lloret-Linares C, Meheust J, Scott J, Guillaume S, Courtet P, Bellivier F, Delavest M. Binge eating behaviours in bipolar disorders. J Affect Disord. 2018;225:482–8.
22. McElroy SL, Crow S, Blom TJ, et al. Clinical features of bipolar spectrum with binge eating behaviour. J Affect Disord. 2016;201:95–8.
23. Melo MCA, de Oliveira Ribeiro M, de Araújo CFC, de Mesquita LMF, de Bruin PFC, de Bruin VMS. Night eating in bipolar disorder. Sleep Med. 2018;48:49–52.
24. McDonald CE, Rossell SL, Phillipou A. The comorbidity of eating disorders in bipolar disorder and associated clinical correlates characterised by emotion dysregulation and impulsivity: a systematic review. J Affect Disord. 2019;259:228–43.
25. American Psychiatric Association, American Psychiatric Association, DSM-III Task Force. Diagnostic and statistical manual of mental disorders: DSM-3. Washington, DC: American Psychiatric Association; 1980.
26. Stice E. Risk and maintenance factors for eating pathology: a meta-analytic review. Psychol Bull. 2002;128:825–48.
27. Jacobi C, Hayward C, de Zwaan M, Kraemer HC, Agras WS. Coming to terms with risk factors for eating disorders: application of risk terminology and suggestions for a general taxonomy. Psychol Bull. 2004;130:19–65.
28. Puccio F, Fuller-Tyszkiewicz M, Ong D, Krug I. A systematic review and meta-analysis on the longitudinal relationship between eating pathology and depression. Int J Eat Disord. 2016;49:439–54.
29. Touchette E, Henegar A, Godart NT, Pryor L, Falissard B, Tremblay RE, Côté SM. Subclinical eating disorders and their comorbidity with mood and anxiety disorders in adolescent girls. Psychiatry Res. 2011;185:185–92.
30. Quirk SE, Williams LJ, O'Neil A, Pasco JA, Jacka FN, Housden S, Berk M, Brennan SL. The association between diet quality, dietary patterns and depression in adults: a systematic review. BMC Psychiatry. 2013;13:175.

31. Valles-Colomer M, Falony G, Darzi Y, et al. The neuroactive potential of the human gut microbiota in quality of life and depression. Nat Microbiol. 2019;4:623–32.
32. Koopman M, El Aidy S, MIDtrauma Consortium. Depressed gut? The microbiota-diet-inflammation trialogue in depression. Curr Opin Psychiatry. 2017;30:369–77.
33. Lang UE, Beglinger C, Schweinfurth N, Walter M, Borgwardt S. Nutritional aspects of depression. Cell Physiol Biochem. 2015;37:1029–43.
34. Herman CP, Polivy J, Lank CN, Heatherton TF. Anxiety, hunger, and eating behavior. J Abnorm Psychol. 1987;96:264–9.
35. Swinbourne JM, Touyz SW. The co-morbidity of eating disorders and anxiety disorders: a review. Eur Eat Disord Rev. 2007;15:253–74.
36. Gadalla T, Piran N. Psychiatric comorbidity in women with disordered eating behavior: a national study. Women Health. 2008;48:467–84.
37. Hinrichsen H, Wright F, Waller G, Meyer C. Social anxiety and coping strategies in the eating disorders. Eat Behav. 2003;4:117–26.
38. Janjetic MA, Rossi ML, Acquavía C, Denevi J, Marcolini C, Torresani ME. Association between anxiety level, eating behavior, and nutritional status in adult women. J Am Coll Nutr. 2019:1–6.
39. Menatti AR, Weeks JW, Levinson CA, McGowan MM. Exploring the relationship between social anxiety and bulimic symptoms: mediational effects of perfectionism among females. Cogn Ther Res. 2013;37:914–22.
40. Ostrovsky NW, Swencionis C, Wylie-Rosett J, Isasi CR. Social anxiety and disordered overeating: an association among overweight and obese individuals. Eat Behav. 2013;14:145–8.
41. Puccio F, Fuller-Tyszkiewicz M, Youssef G, Mitchell S, Byrne M, Allen N, Krug I. Longitudinal bi-directional effects of disordered eating, depression and anxiety. Eur Eat Disord Rev. 2017;25:351–8.
42. Thornton LM, Dellava JE, Root TL, Lichtenstein P, Bulik CM. Anorexia nervosa and generalized anxiety disorder: further explorations of the relation between anxiety and body mass index. J Anxiety Disord. 2011;25:727–30.
43. Veale D, Costa A, Murphy P, Ellison N. Abnormal eating behaviour in people with a specific phobia of vomiting (emetophobia). Eur Eat Disord Rev. 2012;20:414–8.
44. Pollack LO, Forbush KT. Why do eating disorders and obsessive compulsive disorder co-occur? Eat Behav. 2013;14:211–5.
45. Tyagi H, Patel R, Rughooputh F, Abrahams H, Watson AJ, Drummond L. Comparative prevalence of eating disorders in obsessive-compulsive disorder and other anxiety disorders. Psychiatry J. 2015;2015:186,927.
46. Matsunaga H, Miyata A, Iwasaki Y, Matsui T, Fujimoto K, Kiriike N. A comparison of clinical features among Japanese eating-disordered women with obsessive-compulsive disorder. Compr Psychiatry. 1999;40:337–42.
47. Roberts M. Disordered eating and obsessive-compulsive symptoms in a subclinical student population. N Z J Psychol. 2006;35(45)
48. Humphreys JD, Clopton JR, Reich DA. Disordered eating behavior and obsessive compulsive symptoms in college students: cognitive and affective similarities. Eat Disord. 2007;15:247–59.
49. Bozzini AB, Malzyner G, Maximino P, Machado RHV, Ramos C de C, Ribeiro L, Fisberg M. Should pediatricians investigate the symptoms of obsessive-compulsive disorder in children with feeding difficulties? Rev Paul Pediatr. 2019;37:104–9.
50. Jiménez-Murcia S, Fernández-Aranda F, Raich RM, Alonso P, Krug I, Jaurrieta N, Alvarez-Moya E, Labad J, Menchón JM, Vallejo J. Obsessive-compulsive and eating disorders: comparison of clinical and personality features. Psychiatry Clin Neurosci. 2007;61:385–91.
51. Froreich FV, Vartanian LR, Grisham JR, Touyz SW. Dimensions of control and their relation to disordered eating behaviours and obsessive-compulsive symptoms. J Eat Disord. 2016;4(14)
52. Matsui Y, Naito K, Matsuishi K, Kato H, Maeda K, Tanaka K. Assessment of dissociation symptoms in patients with mental disorders by the Dissociation Questionnaire (DIS-Q). Kobe J Med Sci. 2011;56:E263–9.
53. Rosen EF, Petty LC. Dissociative states and disordered eating. Am J Clin Hypn. 1994;36:266–75.

54. Everill J, Waller G, Macdonald W. Dissociation in bulimic and non-eating-disordered women. Int J Eat Disord. 1995;17:127–34.
55. Engelberg MJ, Steiger H, Gauvin L, Wonderlich SA. Binge antecedents in bulimic syndromes: an examination of dissociation and negative affect. Int J Eat Disord. 2007;40:531–6.
56. Fuller-Tyszkiewicz M, Mussap AJ. The relationship between dissociation and binge eating. J Trauma Dissociation. 2008;9:445–62.
57. La Mela C, Maglietta M, Castellini G, Amoroso L, Lucarelli S. Dissociation in eating disorders: relationship between dissociative experiences and binge-eating episodes. Compr Psychiatry. 2010;51:393–400.
58. Mason TB, Lavender JM, Wonderlich SA, Steiger H, Cao L, Engel SG, Mitchell JE, Crosby RD. Comfortably numb: the role of momentary dissociation in the experience of negative affect around binge eating. J Nerv Ment Dis. 2017;205:335–9.
59. Vanderlinden J, Vandereycken W, van Dyck R, Vertommen H. Dissociative experiences and trauma in eating disorders. Int J Eat Disord. 1993;13:187–93.
60. Palmisano GL, Innamorati M, Susca G, Traetta D, Sarracino D, Vanderlinden J. Childhood traumatic experiences and dissociative phenomena in eating disorders: level and association with the severity of binge eating symptoms. J Trauma Dissociation. 2018;19:88–107.
61. Hirotsu C, Tufik S, Andersen ML. Interactions between sleep, stress, and metabolism: From physiological to pathological conditions. Sleep Sci. 2015;8:143–52.
62. Bos SC, Soares MJ, Marques M, Maia B, Pereira AT, Nogueira V, Valente J, Macedo A. Disordered eating behaviors and sleep disturbances. Eat Behav. 2013;14:192–8.
63. Tromp MD, Donners AA, Garssen J, Verster JC. Sleep, eating disorder symptoms, and daytime functioning. Nat Sci Sleep. 2016;8:35–40.
64. Burt J, Dube L, Thibault L, Gruber R. Sleep and eating in childhood: a potential behavioral mechanism underlying the relationship between poor sleep and obesity. Sleep Med. 2014;15:71–5.
65. Aspen V, Weisman H, Vannucci A, Nafiz N, Gredysa D, Kass AE, Trockel M, Jacobi C, Wilfley DE, Taylor CB. Psychiatric co-morbidity in women presenting across the continuum of disordered eating. Eat Behav. 2014;15:686–93.
66. Spiegel K, Tasali E, Penev P, Van Cauter E. Brief communication: sleep curtailment in healthy young men is associated with decreased leptin levels, elevated ghrelin levels, and increased hunger and appetite. Ann Intern Med. 2004;141:846–50.
67. Ulukavak Ciftci T, Kokturk O, Bukan N, Bilgihan A. Leptin and ghrelin levels in patients with obstructive sleep apnea syndrome. Respiration. 2005;72:395–401.
68. Stahl SM. Stahl's essential psychopharmacology: neuroscientific basis and practical application. 4th ed. Cambridge; New York: Cambridge University Press; 2013.
69. Chabas D, Foulon C, Gonzalez J, Nasr M, Lyon-Caen O, Willer J-C, Derenne J-P, Arnulf I. Eating disorder and metabolism in narcoleptic patients. Sleep. 2007;30:1267–73.
70. Palaia V, Poli F, Pizza F, et al. Narcolepsy with cataplexy associated with nocturnal compulsive behaviors: a case-control study. Sleep. 2011;34:1365–71.
71. Najjar M. Zolpidem and amnestic sleep related eating disorder. J Clin Sleep Med. 2007;3:637–8.
72. Kim HK, Kwon JT, Baek J, Park DS, Yang KI. Zolpidem-induced compulsive evening eating behavior. Clin Neuropharmacol. 2013;36:173–4.
73. Park Y-M, Shin H-W. Zolpidem induced sleep-related eating and complex behaviors in a patient with obstructive sleep apnea and restless legs syndrome. Clin Psychopharmacol Neurosci. 2016;14:299–301.
74. Cassin SE, von Ranson KM. Personality and eating disorders: a decade in review. Clin Psychol Rev. 2005;25:895–916.
75. Solmi M, Collantoni E, Meneguzzo P, Degortes D, Tenconi E, Favaro A. Network analysis of specific psychopathology and psychiatric symptoms in patients with eating disorders. Int J Eat Disord. 2018;51:680–92.
76. Solmi M, Collantoni E, Meneguzzo P, Tenconi E, Favaro A. Network analysis of specific psychopathology and psychiatric symptoms in patients with anorexia nervosa. Eur Eat Disord Rev. 2019;27:24–33.

77. De Paoli T, Fuller-Tyszkiewicz M, Huang C, Krug I. A network analysis of borderline personality disorder symptoms and disordered eating. J Clin Psychol. 2020; https://doi.org/10.1002/jclp.22916.
78. Dufresne L, Bussières E-L, Bédard A, Gingras N, Blanchette-Sarrasin A, Bégin C. Personality traits in adolescents with eating disorder: a meta-analytic review. Int J Eat Disord. 2019; https://doi.org/10.1002/eat.23183.
79. Al-Salom P, Boylan K. Borderline personality disorder and disordered eating behaviour: the mediating role of rejection sensitivity. J Can Acad Child Adolesc Psychiatry. 2019;28:72–81.
80. Barajas Iglesias B, Jáuregui Lobera I, Laporta Herrero I, Santed Germán MÁ. Eating disorders during the adolescence: personality characteristics associated with anorexia and bulimia nervosa. Nutr Hosp. 2017;34:1178–84.

Avoidant/Restrictive Food Intake Disorder (ARFID) in Adults

10

Patrizia Todisco

10.1 Introduction

The avoidant/restrictive food intake disorder (ARFID) is a newly recognized category belonging to the feeding and eating disorder (FED) diagnosis according to the 5th edition of the American Psychiatric Association's *Diagnostic and Statistical Manual of Mental Disorders* (DSM-5) [1] published in 2013 and in the 11th revision of the World Health Organization's *International Statistical Classification of Diseases and Related Health Problems* published in 2019 [2]. This disorder was introduced to recognize and expand what previously defined as a feeding disorder of infancy and early childhood and to improve the clinical utility by adding greater detail to and widening the diagnostic criteria to be applicable across the lifespan [1]. ARFID is an agnostic diagnosis as to etiology and, in fact, describes patients who avoid or are disinterested in food for a variety of reasons, but not due to a wish to lose weight or to body image disturbance, that result in functional impairments (also in social life), nutritional deficiencies, and/or weight loss, as well as medical complications of malnutrition [1]. Since its recent definition, studies on the prevalence, diagnosis, treatment, and outcome are lacking, above all in adult populations. In this chapter, we summarize the literature available at present on ARFID in adulthood.

P. Todisco (✉)
Eating Disorders Unit, Casa Di Cura Villa Margherita, Arcugnano (VI), Italy
e-mail: patrizia.todisco1964@gmail.com

© Springer Nature Switzerland AG 2022
E. Manzato et al. (eds.), *Hidden and Lesser-known Disordered Eating Behaviors in Medical and Psychiatric Conditions*,
https://doi.org/10.1007/978-3-030-81174-7_10

10.2 Assessment

10.2.1 Diagnostic Criteria According to DSM-5 and Differential Diagnosis

ARFID is characterized by persistent avoidant or restrictive eating resulting in one (or more) of the following (criterion A): significant weight loss or failure to achieve expected weight gain (criterion A1), nutritional deficiency such as anemia (criterion A2), dependence on enteral feeding or oral nutritional supplements (criterion A3), and interference with psychosocial functioning (criterion A4). The psychosocial impairment can take the form of depression or social anxiety, otherwise the inability to eat outside the home at restaurants, school, or friend's houses with a sense of social isolation and impossibility to sustain relationships [3].

DSM-5 describes three core ARFID presentations: (1) apparent lack of interest in eating or food; (2) avoidance based on the sensory characteristics of food; and (3) fear of aversive consequences associated with food intake [1]. Individuals with the lack of interest profile typically endorse a lack of hunger or premature fullness, otherwise distractibility or hyperarousal before/during mealtime leading them to forget to eat or consume small volumes of food. The sensory sensitivity profile is characterized by food avoidance due to sensory properties of food (e.g., texture, taste, or appearance) and for some individuals is the experience of intense, detailed perceptions of food qualities such that subtle differences in a saltine cracker can taste distinctively or be found to be aversive if it is not the preferred brand [4]. This restriction manifests behaviorally as "picky" eating [1] that has been defined as an aversion to, and usually refusal to eat, a wide variety of commonly accepted foods, even after sampling them. Food neophobia, a general refusal to try unfamiliar foods, is a distinct though commonly co-occurring phenomenon [1]. Finally, patients with fear of aversive consequences profile exhibit food avoidance or restriction usually following a traumatic event related to eating (e.g., choking, vomiting).

The restricted food intake results in either macronutrient or micronutrient insufficiency and is not due to body image disturbance as in anorexia nervosa (AN) (criterion C) or another mental or physical health disorder (criterion D) [5]. When a medical or a psychiatric disorder is present, the diagnosis of ARFID is justified when all diagnostic criteria are met and when the eating disturbance requires specific treatment [1, 6]. The eating disturbance should not be included in the context of poor socioeconomic resources (e.g., food insecurity) or religious or cultural observations (e.g., Ramadan) (criterion B) [1].

The previous diagnosis of feeding disorder of infancy and early childhood defined feeding disturbances whose onset was prior to 6 years of age and resulted in lack of weight gain or growth, while ARFID hasn't an age of onset criterion and captures a more extensive spectrum of cases including food avoidance/restriction at different developmental periods and accepts a broader range of impairment. Thus, the diagnostic space covered by ARFID is broad [6], and the extension from a disorder of childhood to a disorder that may occur throughout lifespan was a notable departure in conceptualization. This integration reflects a wish to adopt a life course approach to psychopathology by emphasizing the continuity between child, adolescent, and adult manifestations of the same disorders, rather than treating psychiatric disorders in the pediatric population as a separate entity [5]. For some authors, ARFID possesses characteristics relevant to both feeding and eating disorders and may represent the missing link between these differing types of disorders [7].

ARFID in adulthood is also conceptualized as a disorder that previously may have been diagnosed as an anxiety disorder, a specific phobia to a type of food or swallowing [5].

To improve ARFID identification, in 2018, a small multidisciplinary pool of international experts in feeding and eating disorder clinical practice and research convened, as the Radcliffe ARFID workgroup, to consider operationalization of DSM-5 ARFID diagnostic criteria to guide research in this disorder [8]. They proposed to eliminate criteria A1–A3 clarifying that A4 (the interference with psychosocial functioning) would satisfy criterion A [8]. Some studies in children-adolescents support this suggestion [9, 10].

An important factor that distinguishes ARFID from other restrictive eating disorders, such as AN, is that in ARFID there are no undue influence of body shape and weight on self-evaluation, no fear of gaining weight, and no disturbance in the way one's body weight or shape is experienced (criterion B). In clinical settings, it may be difficult to differentiate people with ARFID from those with anorexia nervosa who may minimize or deny the extent of weight/shape over-valuation. The same difficulty may be found in cultures with different expression of distress around body image and/or where mental illness is more commonly expressed through somatization rather than psychological reactions [5]. Moreover, ARFID shares similar presentations with the so-called non-fat phobic anorexia nervosa (NFP-AN) in some cases and appears to precede AN in a substantial minority (12%) of patients with ARFID [7]. Differential diagnosis between NFP-AN and ARFID can be challenging, and explicit endorsements do not necessarily match internal beliefs [11]. The individuals with so-called NFP-AN often endorse low appetite or gastrointestinal distress as rationales for food restriction [12, 13], blurring the distinction between ARFID and AN [14]. Thus, it is sometimes unclear whether individuals who present with NFP-AN are minimizing or denying underlying shape and weight concerns, have alternate rationales for food restriction, or actually have ARFID [14]. An interesting study [11], supporting this doubt, demonstrated that adolescent and young females with NFP-AN have implicit beliefs that may not match their explicitly expressed beliefs toward dieting.

A systematic scoping review [5] evaluated the diagnostic validity of ARFID based on Feighner criteria [15]. According to this review [5], we can consider satisfied the first Feighner criterion (the description of a clearly distinguishable clinical picture) because a predominant clinical presentation emerges from the literature and specific epidemiological features can be identified, despite the heterogeneity of clinical descriptions. Literature supports also the fourth Feighner criterion (the category demonstrated a typical course over time) even though research is not exhaustive [5]. As many other psychiatric disorders, ARFID does not fulfill the second and fifth criteria—the identification of biomarkers or comparable psychological tests (or effective treatments) and of patterns of heritability—but Strand and colleagues [5] suggest that it is not to be excluded that the diagnosis is clinically applicable. The distinction from other diseases (the third Feighner criterion) seems more difficult: the differences between ARFID and AN are sufficiently clear, apart from NFP-AN, because the two disorders differ conceptually and there is evidence to support separate epidemiological characteristics [5]. The problems arise in applying the ARFID diagnostic criteria in situations where there are comorbid psychiatric or medical conditions that may cause restrictive eating and food avoidance or selectivity [e.g., autism spectrum disorder [ASD], anxiety disorders, obsessive-compulsive disorder, attention-deficit/hyperactivity disorder, affective disorders, gastrointestinal disease, metabolic disorders, etc.] [5]. Whereas such comorbidity is of course not always difficult to integrate with an ARFID diagnosis, evidence points to recurrent conceptual bewilderment that makes the ARFID category unnecessarily obscure.

Some authors [5] proposed to modify the current diagnostic criteria to overcome their weakness emphasizing the three-dimensional clinical picture that is currently only hinted at in the DSM-5 diagnostic criteria. There is emerging evidence to support such a model. Thomas and co-workers [16] introduced a hypothetical three-dimensional model whereby "a given individual's ARFID presentation can be plotted as a single point along a three-dimensional space, meaning that the three prototypic presentations vary in severity and are not mutually exclusive." Even though further research is needed, clustering ARFID patients into specific clinical subtypes allows clinicians and researchers to consider and conceptualize different treatment regimens that may be better suited to patients in the context of subtype-specific presentations and etiologies [5].

As suggested in DSM-5, a combination of neurobiological factors and developmental stressors may engender traditional eating disorder psychopathology in subjects with ARFID. This disorder may (1) share endophenotypes with symptoms of other EDs, simultaneously increasing risk for all forms of disordered eating, and/or (2) ARFID symptoms themselves or accommodation to ARFID symptoms may precipitate additional eating pathology [9].

Even though screening and identification of possible ARFID should be made by any healthcare professional [8], because affected patients often present to settings other than mental health clinics, assessment has to be multidimensional because medical, nutritional, and psychological-psychiatric aspects have to be investigated as for every ED. A medical professional (e.g., primary care physician, nurse practitioner) is recommended to complete the medical and nutritional assessment of avoidant/restrictive eating. Such evaluation should include a physical assessment to ascertain eating history, acute and potential long-term medical and nutritional complications of avoidant/restrictive eating such as sequelae of low weight (e.g., hypogonadism and bone loss) or obesity, as well as malnutrition (e.g., insufficient vitamin and mineral consumption), which can occur in individuals with ARFID across the weight spectrum. Medical assessment should also explore the presence of underlying systemic or gastrointestinal disorders which may contribute to the onset or persistence of ARFID, such as celiac disease, peptic or allergic gastrointestinal disease (including eosinophilic esophagitis), Crohn's disease, and functional gastrointestinal disorders including constipation and irritable bowel syndrome. Nutritional/dietary assessment should determine the adequacy of dietary diversity and caloric needs. A mental health clinician (e.g., psychologist, psychiatrist, social worker) should complete the diagnostic interviews and assessment of psychosocial impairment and functioning with special attention to anxiety, avoidance learning, and cognitive features such as rigidity or detail orientation that may be transdiagnostic across psychiatric or neurodevelopmental disorders and impact ARFID maintenance and outcomes. Some diagnostic tools are available and will be described later, but their psychometric features have to be fully assessed. Additional opinion and input from specialists may be needed for more complex ARFID presentations (such as gastrointestinal pathology, autoimmune disease/atopy, swallowing difficulties, respiratory compromise of undiagnosed etiology, difficulty with self-care tasks or self-regulation). In addition, mealtime observations are also acknowledged as forming a useful component of assessment to measure bites consumed, food selected, facial expressions, and more.

10.2.2 Diagnostic Tools

A number of diagnostic rating scales have been developed and have shown promising results in terms of sensitivity and specificity and may contribute to ED assessment. However, little is known about how ARFID patients differ from patients with other EDs on these instruments. There are few measures (self-report questionnaires or structured interview) of the specific psychopathology of ARFID because it is a relatively new diagnosis.

The "ARFID symptom checklist" was developed to identify picky eaters experiencing weight loss, nutritional deficiencies, nutritional supplement dependence, or psychosocial impairment [4]. Its ability to identify a group reporting significant comorbidity and impairment, and distinctive eating behaviors, supports its usefulness as a screening instrument for ARFID but is not commonly used.

A new self-report screening tool for adults is the "Nine Item ARFID Screen" (NIAS) [17] that yields dimensional symptom ratings rather than diagnoses. The NIAS [17] is a brief multidimensional and reliable instrument to measure ARFID-associated eating behaviors. Exploratory and confirmatory factor analyses provided evidence for three factors. The NIAS subscales demonstrated high internal consistency, test-retest reliability, invariant item loadings between two samples, and convergent/discriminant validity with other measures of picky eating, appetite, fear of negative consequences, and psychopathology. The scales were also correlated with measures of ARFID-like symptoms (e.g., low BMI, low fruit/vegetable variety and intake, and eating-related psychosocial interference/distress), although the picky eating, appetite, and fear scales had distinct independent relationships with these constructs [17].

Published structured interviews to diagnose ARFID are: (a) the Eating Disorder Assessment for DSM-5 (EDA-5) [18], used to confer ARFID, pica, and rumination disorder (RD) diagnoses, although its diagnostic properties have not been evaluated for these groups; and (b) the Structured Clinical Interview for DSM-5 (SCID-5) [19] which can also be employed to diagnose ARFID but does not evaluate constructs relating to pica or RD.

There are also preliminary reports on the new ARFID module of the Eating Disorder Examination [20].

The first specific structured clinical interview to assess ARFID across the lifespan is the "Pica, ARFID, and Rumination Disorder Interview" (PARDI) [21]. The PARDI includes items assessing the level of endorsement and overall severity of common ARFID features organized into profiles (i.e., sensory sensitivity, lack of interest in eating, and fear of aversive consequences) to facilitate treatment planning and algorithms for diagnosing ARFID, pica, and RD. This interview is available in four versions, one of which is suitable for young people and adults (14 years and up). On average, the PARDI takes 39 min to complete, appears acceptable to respondents, and has demonstrated adequate reliability and validity (individuals with ARFID scored significantly higher than healthy controls on ARFID severity and ARFID profiles) in an initial sample [21], while larger-scale validation studies are underway.

It will be crucial to develop and refine psychometric measures that help us to distinguish among ARFID presentations, as well as other ED diagnoses across different ages [17].

10.2.3 Epidemiology

There are consistent findings regarding epidemiological features such as age and gender patterns that distinguish ARFID from other eating disorders in childhood-adolescence, but there is a lack of evidence on how common and how much troubling ARFID is among adults.

Nevertheless, we can affirm that the gender difference between ARFID and AN found in children-adolescents is less pronounced in adult samples [22] and in patients requiring acute medical hospitalization [23]. One study [24] reported that only 4 of 45 malnourished adult patients were categorized as having ARFID. A retrospective chart review was conducted in a cohort of patients, aged 15–40 years, who sought treatment for an eating disorder at Kyoto University Hospital between 1990 and 2005 [22] and between 1990 and 1997 [25]. Respectively, 95 (9.2%) of 1029 [22] and 27 (11.0%) out of the 245 [25] adult patients with a feeding and eating disorder met the criteria for ARFID; contrary to previous studies in pediatric patients [26], all adult patients with ARFID were women. Other results of those retrospective researches in ARFID patients were the following: most of them had restrictive eating related to emotional problems; some patients had multiple gastrointestinal complaints as contributing factors for restrictive eating; no patients reported food avoidance related to sensory characteristics or functional dysphagia or exhibited binge eating or purging behaviors or excessive exercise; and a few patients had enteral feeding. Moreover, the ARFID group had a significantly shorter duration of illness, lower rates of hospital admission history, and less severe eating disorder pathology and psychopathology and reported significantly better outcome results than the AN group [22, 25]. Hay and colleagues [27] conducted two sequential population-based surveys in Australia including individuals aged over 15 years who were interviewed in 2014 ($n = 2732$) and 2015 ($n = 3005$). The 2014 and 2015 3-month prevalence of ARFID were 0.3% (95% CI 0.1–0.5) and 0.3% (95% CI 0.2–0.6). Mental health-related quality of life was particularly poor for those with ARFID who also had lower role performance. These prevalence estimates were similar to those of other specified EDs (AN 0.4%–0.5%; BN 1.1%–1.2%) and lower than those for other specified feeding or eating disorder (3.2%) and unspecified feeding or eating disorder (10.4%) [27]. An online eating disorder screening to adults in the USA [28] found that 86.3% of the whole sample ($n = 71362$) had a possible clinical or subclinical ED; in particular, 4.5% ($n = 2923$) of the sample screened as ARFID and rates of current treatment were lowest for people in this category (1.1%) [28]. A retrospective review of charts from 410 consecutive referrals (ages 18–90 years; 73.0% female) to a tertiary care center for neurogastroenterology examination [29] identified 26 cases (6.3%) who met the full criteria for ARFID and 71 cases (17.3%) who had clinically significant avoidant or restrictive eating behaviors with insufficient information for a definitive diagnosis of ARFID. Of patients with ARFID symptoms, 92.8% (90 out of 97) cited fear of gastrointestinal symptoms as motivation for their avoidant or restrictive eating [29]. A series of binary logistic regressions showed that the likelihood of having ARFID symptoms increased significantly in patients with eating- or weight-related complaints (odds ratio [OR], 5.09; 95% CI, 2.54–10.21); with dyspepsia, nausea, or vomiting (OR, 3.59; 95% CI, 2.04–6.32); with abdominal pain (OR, 4.72; 95% CI, 1.87–11.81); or with more than one diagnosis of a gastrointestinal disorder (OR, 1.63; 95% CI, 1.26–2.10) [29]. A recent study [30] had similar findings. The authors assessed adult patients presenting with symptoms of gastroparesis and characterized 39.9% as meeting conservative self-report cut-off for ARFID symptoms, with 23.3% patients having documented psychosocial/medical impairment. In addition, gastroparesis symptom severity was moderately and significantly associated with greater ARFID symptom severity ($b = 0.45$, $P < 0.001$), but neither positive gastric emptying scintigraphy nor other FED symptoms [30]. Thus, gastroparesis/dyspepsia symptoms may mimic but also hide ARFID diagnosis, and clinicians have to keep it in mind [30].

10.3 Clinical Characteristics

10.3.1 Presentations, Comorbidities, and Severity

ARFID is very heterogeneous, and the clinical presentations are unified by the avoidant/restrictive eating patterns, but the rationales for restriction and medical sequelae differ: low weight or failure to gain weight is common but it is possible normal weight or even overweight or obesity. This demonstrates the variety and complexity of its underlying pathophysiology [31]. Some individuals may remain in healthy weight range via the use of tube feeding or energy-dense supplements, while others, reliant on carbohydrates or energy-dense processed foods, bear excess weight. While individuals with AN often limit food intake to low-calorie options, those with ARFID favor a calorie-dense diet high in processed foods, carbohydrates, and added sugars and low in vegetables and protein [31, 32]. Harshman and coworkers [32] collected and analyzed 4-day food record data for 52 participants with full or subthreshold ARFID and 52 healthy controls (HCs) (9–22 years). Participants with full or subthreshold ARFID did not report any fruit or vegetable category in their top five most commonly reported food categories, whereas these food groups occupied three of the top five groups for HCs. Vegetable, protein, and vitamin K and B12 intakes were significantly lower, while intakes of added sugars and total carbohydrates were significantly higher in full or subthreshold ARFID compared to HCs [32].

The food avoidance/restriction can lead to medical and mental health consequences that further exacerbated symptoms (e.g., diabetes, cardiovascular disease, fatigue, poor self-esteem, family mealtime conflict, peer social isolation, and difficulties with relationships and work). In an Australian epidemiological study [27], individuals with ARFID (aged 24–60 years) had lower mental health-related quality of life and more days of being unable to function due to emotional or physical health problems than people without EDs [27]. Similarly, in an online study, adults with symptoms of ARFID self-reported greater internalizing distress than those without ARFID and comparable levels of distress to individuals with symptoms of other EDs [4].

Clinically significant picky eating (PE), also referred to as "selective" or "selective/neophobic" eating, can lead to a diagnosis of avoidant/restrictive food intake disorder [1, 7, 10, 16, 33, 34]. Adult PE has received increased attention due to its important association with adult ARFID [35]. Picky eaters with ARFID symptoms can be differentiated from picky eaters without these symptoms on the basis of three eating behaviors (stronger endorsement of food neophobia, inflexible eating behaviors, and eating from a very narrow range of foods) and by their higher endorsement of internalizing distress, OCD symptoms, and eating-related quality of life impairment [36]. Retrospective reports of greater parental pressure to eat, higher disgust sensitivity, lower PE age of onset, and experiencing an aversive food event were associated with general adult PE behavior [36]. However, additional research is needed to understand the extent to which parental pressure is a reaction to or perhaps compounds the development of problematic eating behavior [36]. Results also indicated parental encouragement of healthy eating may be a protective factor and that men endorsed higher levels of adult PE.

PE is one of the three patterns of restrictive eating that have been linked to ARFID symptoms both in nonclinical samples [17] and in treatment-seeking patients diagnosed with ARFID [10, 33]. The other two ARFID presentations involve restrictive eating due to apparent lack of appetite or interest in eating and restrictive eating due to fear of aversive consequences from eating, such as choking and vomiting. Although the ARFID presentations show significant overlap in both nonclinical and diagnosed samples [17, 21, 33], there is also evidence that they are phenomenologically and statistically distinct from each other. Therefore, it is likely that each presentation has its own etiological and maintenance mechanisms linked to severity of restrictive eating and likelihood of experiencing ARFID symptoms. As reported before, Thomas and colleagues [16] proposed a conceptual three-dimensional neurobiological model of ARFID (consistent with the National Institute of Mental Health's Research Domain Criteria [RDoC] approach) wherein the three core presentations occur along a continuum of severity and are not mutually exclusive [16]. According to this dimensional model, the three ARFID profiles share similarities with other DSM-5 diagnoses: the sensory sensitivity profile shares similarities with ASD; the fear of aversive consequences profile shares similarities with anxiety disorders; and the lack of interest profile shares similarities with major depressive disorder. Similar to the sensory sensitivity profile of ARFID, selective eating (e.g., unwillingness to try new foods, avoiding certain food groups) is common among children with ASD [37] and may be related to sensory processing deficits in the areas of taste or smell [38, 39]. Reilly and colleagues [33] reported that the prevalence of ASD in young individuals with the "selective eating" presentation of ARFID was approximately 5%. Similar to the fear of aversive consequences profile of ARFID, those with anxiety disorders may display heightened distress in the presence of anxiety-provoking or feared stimuli, typically resulting in avoidance. Indeed, Norris and co-workers [40] found that individuals with the ARFID "aversive" profile had a 70% prevalence of anxiety disorders, and Zickgraf and colleagues [10] found that 77% of those exhibiting the fear profile had a comorbid anxiety disorder. Given that the fear of aversive consequences presentation of ARFID can lead to rapid weight loss and require urgent action due to acute food refusal, patients report significant psychological and medical symptoms [9]. A recent study suggested that increased disgust might partially explain the association between anxiety and food avoidance [41]. Moreover, lack of appetite is common in major depressive disorder (MDD) and may be due to decreases in experiences of pleasure or reward associated with food consumption. Thomas and colleagues [16, 42] proposed also neurobiological underpinnings for each of the three presentations:

1. The ARFID subdomain, presenting as lack of interest in food, might be associated with differences in activation of appetite-regulating centers in the brain.
2. The selective eating subdomain might be related to oversensitivity in taste perception [43].
3. The fear of aversive consequences subdomain might be linked to hyperactivation of fear processing brain circuitry.

At present, different studies in adolescents [34, 44, 45] support the hypothesis by Thomas and colleagues [16, 42]. ARFID subgroups exhibit differences on various clinical (e.g., degree of medical morbidity) and demographic variables, suggesting that distinct etiological and maintenance factors may be associated with different restrictive eating patterns. A better understanding of diagnostic differences among

ARFID subtypes will most benefit from ongoing dialogue between clinicians and researchers [46] and will contribute to a greater comprehension of the factors associated with risk for, etiology of, and maintenance of restrictive eating behaviors not characterized by weight or shape concerns [10]. Research in a wider variety of settings and clinical populations should help clarify the relative prevalence of different ARFID presentations and the degree to which they overlap with one another and with other forms of disordered eating. In fact, ARFID symptoms exist independent of symptoms of other EDs and are characterized by several distinct eating behaviors and associated with distress and impairment at levels comparable to symptoms of anorexia and bulimia [4]. Becker and colleagues [9] demonstrated, although in an age-heterogeneous sample (mean age 22.2 ± 11.88 years; range 10–78), that the addition of psychosocial impairment as a criterion sufficient for an ARFID diagnosis altered the presentation of ARFID in expected ways such that, without the requirement for insufficient energy intake or presence of nutritional deficiencies, the ARFID sample was, on average, within a normal weight range [9]. In the same sample, compared to AN subjects, ARFID individuals had an earlier age of disorder onset; presented for treatment at a younger age; scored lower on measures of eating pathology, depression, anxiety, and clinical impairment; but scored similar on restrictive eating and scored higher on food neophobia. Also as expected, a higher proportion of those with ARFID were males compared with the proportion of males with AN [9]. Previously Nakai and collaborators [25], in a retrospective chart review study, found that the ARFID group had a significantly shorter duration of illness, lower rates of admission history, less severe psychopathology, and significantly better outcome results than the AN group and was composed by women [25]. It's worth to notice that there is a percentage of patients that meet the criteria initially for ARFID and crossover to AN or appear with overlapping presentations [26, 45]. The majority of patients reclassified as having AN initially presented with feeding specific concerns most consistent with the ARFID aversive subtype and commonly reported worries relating to general health as opposed to weight or shape at the time of assessment [47].

Because ARFID diagnosis is relatively new, the information about specific medical complications are limited. When patients with eating problems, that cannot be explained by their medical condition and the severity may exceed that expected for a given condition and/or may persist beyond the usual resolution period, present in treatment settings it's possible that such eating difficulties are attributable to a combination of medical and psychiatric factors, and can be diagnosed as ARFID. In ARFID, it is reasonable to examine dietary idiosyncrasies and consider specific complications of nutritional deficiencies [48]. Recently, some authors [31] compared in a sample of female, aged 10–22 years, low-weight individuals affected by ARFID with AN patients and healthy controls in order to assess the differences in medical complications and endocrine alterations. Medical comorbidities and endocrine features overlapped in ARFID and AN even though there were also key differences, suggesting that low-weight ARFID should be treated as intensively as AN but they have distinct pathophysiology [31]. Medical and psychiatric comorbidities were greater in low-weight ARFID versus HC, but disease onset was earlier in

ARFID than in AN and so may have earlier and more prolonged developmental exposure to negative consequences of undernutrition [31]. While low-weight ARFID and AN had higher rates of anxiety and depression than HC, only AN reported a higher prevalence of obsessive-compulsive disorder consistent with the ritualistic behavior observed clinically in AN [31]. Use of psychiatric medications did not differ between ARFID and AN. However, ARFID reported greater use of appetite-stimulating antihistamines, not typically prescribed for AN, highlighting the divergent perceived pathophysiology of low weight among clinicians. ARFID and AN had more gastrointestinal (GI) symptoms than HC, which may be a cause or consequence of undernutrition [31]. Both reported low blood pressure (BP), but only AN had lower systolic BP versus HC. Those with AN reported a higher prevalence of bradycardia and had lower heart rate on exam than ARFID, which might reflect more acute weight loss in AN. Asthma was more common in ARFID than AN or HC, and both ARFID and AN reported greater frequency of food or drug allergies than HC. The data by Aulinas and colleagues [31] suggest that immunological mechanisms may be involved in the pathogenesis and/or maintenance of ARFID. The finding of atopy in ARFID also raises the question of undiagnosed immune-mediated disorders contributing to symptoms. Despite similar low weight and leptin levels in ARFID and AN, the same authors observed a greater waist-to-hip ratio (marker of visceral fat) in ARFID [31] that may reflect dietary differences (a calorie-dense diet in ARFID [32] versus a low-calorie diet in AN) or may simply indicate differences in developmental stage because the waist-to-hip ratio no longer differed after controlling for age [31]. The authors observed also distinct medical and endocrine alterations in ARFID compared to AN, such as a lower number of menses missed in the preceding 9 months, higher total T3 levels, and lower total T4/total T3 ratio; these differences persisted after adjusting for age and might reflect differences in pathophysiology, acuity of weight fluctuations, and/or nutritional composition of food consumed [31].

Another research on medical complications [49] found that the 18% of ARFID men (18–63 years) had bone mineral density (BMD) Z-scores at spine and hip <-2 at ≥ 1 site. They resulted at significant risk of low BMD above all at the spine level, but have preserved estimated hip strength and a body mass index (BMI) of 15.3 ± 1.5 near to that of AN male patients (14.7 ± 1.8).

It was suggested that [9] items that could be relevant in considering ARFID severity could include number of foods consumed in each of the five basic food groups, how frequently the exact same meals are repeated, avoidance of trying new foods and important social eating opportunities, fears related to eating (choking, vomiting, allergic reactions, GI distress), and the need for major family accommodation of aberrant eating behaviors [21, 42]. Finally, the Radcliffe ARFID workgroup [8] achieved a consensus proposal for ARFID recovery that included having a diet that is adequate in volume and variety associated with the following: (a) eating foods from all the major food groups (fruits or vegetables, grains, protein foods, and dairy) regularly (e.g., having all food groups represented several days [e.g., 2, 3] per week); (b) weight no longer in the under-weight range (based on individualized clinical assessment) and height growth and physical development (e.g., maturation) resumed; (c) no nutritional deficiencies; (d) no more than one nutritional supplement drink per day; and (e) no longer avoiding, requiring major accommodation, or experiencing significant distress in social eating situations.

10.4 Treatment

Evidence-based treatment of ARFID is in its infancy, and there is no evidence-based psychological treatment suitable for all forms of ARFID at this time. The current evidence base for ARFID treatment relies primarily on case reports, case series, and retrospective chart reviews, with scarce randomized controlled trials in young children. Studies in adults are lacking, and it's under research if the treatments used for other EDs could be applicable and useful also for ARFID.

In fact, for all EDs (including ARFID), the main treatment as delineated in the current national and international guidelines is a form of psycho-behavioral therapy that can most usually be provided on an outpatient basis [50].

Fewer case reports related to adults with chronic ARFID exist [51, 52] and focus on comorbid physical illnesses (i.e., gastroesophageal reflux disease, supraventricular tachycardia, Crohn's disease), while treatment of a chronic course of ARFID in adults has yet to be documented [53].

ARFID treatments for children/adolescents recently described in the literature include family-based treatment and parent training, cognitive-behavioral (CBT) approaches, hospital-based refeeding including tube feeding, family-centered partial hospitalization, and adjunctive pharmacotherapy [42]. For adults, we can assume that some of the treatments used for children/adolescents will work the same. In ED, evidence-based therapies delivered by an eating disorders-informed clinician are considered most efficacious and are preferred by patients, and this approach may also be more cost-effective and reduce hospitalizations [50]. The presence of specific complications of nutritional deficiencies in ARFID supports the need for diet diversification as part of therapeutic interventions to reduce risk for nutrient insufficiencies and related complications [32]. People with more severe symptoms and so nutritionally compromised or who are not improving with less restrictive care may be treated in a partial (day) or full hospital specialist program [50] to reach medical stabilization [54]. Treatment should be adapted depending on the severity of the nutritional problem and tailored to account for the behavioral, organic, oral-motor, and dietary concerns often present and may involve hospitalization with multidisciplinary care (nutritional therapist, physician, dietitian, psychologist, psychiatrist, speech-language pathology/occupational therapist, etc.). Some findings [55] suggest that patients with ARFID who exhibit an acute onset of severe food restriction can be successfully treated in the same partial-hospital program as patients with other ED, with comparable improvements in weight and psychopathology over a shorter time period [55]. In the absence of published criteria for admission and refeeding protocols for ARFID patients, it seems that providers rely on established AN criteria for hospital admission (e.g., bradycardia, orthostatic hypotension, electrolyte abnormalities, and low weight) and also adopt AN refeeding protocols. Solid food and nasogastric tube (NGT) feeds are most commonly used for nutritional rehabilitation, but the variability in the treatment approaches to the inpatient medical stabilization of patients with ARFID highlights the evidence gap regarding optimal treatment of this disorder, and probably no single treatment works best for all ARFID patients. Katzman and co-workers [56] advise to consider cautiously the use of NGT feedings due to the oral sensitivities inherent in many individuals with ARFID and the potential psychological consequences like iatrogenic conditioned food aversions.

Given the lack of empirical data on the treatment strategies of ARFID, best practice treatment guidelines have not yet been developed, which potentially increases the risk of prolonged resource-intensive hospital stays for complex cases [26]. As for others ED also for ARFID multidisciplinary team is likely important to the effectiveness of treatment [54], but not all individuals with ARFID would require it. The Radcliffe ARFID workgroup [8] stated that patients generally require a minimum of a primary care practitioner to monitor physical health. The need for multidisciplinary involvement decreases at older ages and with lower levels of severity and medical complexity; in these conditions, patients may manage treatment with a single practitioner whose expertise is most relevant to the case. Furthermore, experts noted that ARFID is phenotypically heterogeneous and patients' needs might differ depending on what factors are thought to be driving the distress and eating disturbances, and these variable presentations may in turn call for variable interventions, only some of which would be multidisciplinary. Significant themes were identified [8] across existing psychosocial interventions including (1) psychoeducation about ARFID, nutrition, and principles of exposure and habituation; (2) caregiver or family involvement for support and to reinforce change; (3) exposure therapy involving both in- and out-of-session work [57]; and (4) structured mealtimes. Other commonly implemented strategies included use of reinforcements to promote behavior change, sensory and self-regulation treatments (for ARFID who avoid food to avoid internal sensations) [58], management of anxiety and other comorbidities, pharmacotherapy, tube weaning, and other medical interventions, as needed. Given that community-based expertise in ARFID is limited, it was considered a strength that these competencies can be scaffolded based on existing expertise (e.g., with other EDs, anxiety disorders, etc.) and clinicians work to advance time-limited and outcome-guided interventions and to improve access to care and treatment efficacy.

Identifying mechanisms contributing to food avoidance is essential to develop effective interventions because the treatment can focus on drivers. Harris and collaborators [41] suggested that increased disgust, probably tied to formation of taste aversions, might partially explain the association between anxiety and food avoidance. Exploring fully the function of disgust among individuals with selective eating in the context of ARFID could aid in delineating more specific etiological models as well as formulation of more tailored, effective treatment strategies. Conceptual deconstruction techniques [59], secondary appraisals of one's ability to cope with disgust [60], counter-conditioning methods (wherein disgust-eliciting stimuli are paired with rewarding stimuli or with safety signals) [61, 62], and pilot testing techniques that focus on targeting evaluative associations may be helpful [63].

A novel form of outpatient cognitive-behavioral therapy specific for ARFID (CBT-AR) is one treatment currently under study. CBT-AR is appropriate for children, adolescents, and adults ages 10 years and more [42]. The CBT-AR model posits that biological vulnerabilities including sensory sensitivity, anxiety, and/or low appetite, with or without a negative experience with eating, contribute to negative feelings and predictions about eating, which lead to food avoidance or restriction. Avoidant/restrictive eating has a series of physical and psychosocial consequences that maintain the maladaptive cycle. Regardless of whether the patient has one, two, or all three primary presentations, CBT-AR challenges the avoidant-restrictive eating head-on in order to interrupt and correct the maintaining mechanisms [42]. The symptoms that unify all clinical presentations are food avoidance and restriction which are the primary targets of treatment that is flexible to overcome different presentations. To address heterogeneity in age at presentation, CBT-AR can be applied in either a family-supported or individual format. To address heterogeneity in maintaining mechanisms, CBT-AR always proceeds through four stages, but Stage 3 features three optional modules that the therapist can implement depending on the primary maintaining mechanism(s) of the individual patient. Lastly, to address heterogeneity in weight status and clinical complexity, the treatment spans 20–30 sessions in length, affording additional time for patients who have significant weight to gain or must address multiple maintaining mechanisms. Regardless of the version of the treatment employed, all forms of CBT-AR include important common features such as a structured session format, at-home practice assignments, common therapeutic goals, and consistent therapist stance [42].

At present, there are neither evidence-based treatment approaches nor medications for ARFID. Most of clinicians prescribed selective serotonin reuptake inhibitors [54] and atypical antipsychotics [54]. One medication of interest seems to be mirtazapine because it promotes appetite and weight gain, decreases nausea and vomiting, improves gastric emptying [64], is an effective treatment for depression and anxiety symptoms in adults, and is generally well tolerated [64]. Among atypical antipsychotics, a case report in adolescents and children [65] showed that low-dose olanzapine, when used as an adjunct to other treatment modalities, may facilitate eating, weight gain, and the reduction of anxious, depressive, and cognitive symptoms in ARFID patients [65], but its use in adults has to be demonstrated. A systematic review of cyproheptadine concluded that it had some benefits for avoidant-restrictive food intake disorder [66].

10.5 Conclusions

ARFID is a recently defined ED, and it's poorly recognized above all among adult for insufficient knowledge of characterization and epidemiology and lack of established assessment, screening tools, and treatment protocols. For the same reasons, there is also an ongoing widespread inconsistent use of terminology. Treatment will commonly include psychological interventions, nutritional advice or intervention, and medical monitoring or intervention. Some individuals with ARFID may present with extreme low weight, resulting in similar complications to people with anorexia nervosa. Others may present with longstanding serious nutritional compromise, impairing physical development and functioning. In many cases, it will be neither realistic nor necessarily desirable to achieve an eating pattern without any avoidance or restriction. A more appropriate aim may be to minimize physical or nutritional risk through behavioral change and/or to help the individuals learn to manage their own anxiety about trying new foods or extending their dietary intake.

Although the lifespan approach of DSM-5 is commendable, there is an urgent need for research on ARFID in adult populations and also on how established treatment models for eating disorders can be modified to accommodate for the specific features of ARFID [46]. The existent findings highlight the importance of ARFID-specific screening instruments and a thorough initial assessment as well as challenges associated with present diagnostic criteria of restrictive eating disorders. Researchers must develop a unified approach to the study of ARFID subtypes drawing from populations across the lifespan and in varied settings in order to best understand if this approach has merit and how to best meet the needs of all ARFID patients. Many subjects with ARFID have complex presentations that often require specialized treatment; it will be important that clinicians be educated about ARFID, have knowledge of the diagnostic characteristics of the illness, and have an understanding of how a patient's needs should be managed. Currently, there are no prospective studies that have reported outcomes on interventions that have targeted patients with ARFID across the lifespan. As these evidence-based treatments become available, it will be crucial to apply treatments that optimize outcomes in hopes of minimizing morbidity associated with the illness [26].

References

1. American Psychiatric Association. Diagnostic and Statistical Manual of Mental Disorders (5th edn) (DSM-5). Washington DC: American Psychiatric Association; 2013.
2. World Health Organization. International statistical classification of diseases and related health problems, 11th revision (ICD-11). Geneva: World Health Organization; 2019.
3. Menzel J. Avoidant/restrictive food intake disorder: assessment and treatment. In: Anderson LK, Murray ST, Kaye WH, editors. Clinical handbook of complex and atypical eating disorders. New York: Oxford University Press Print Publication; 2017. p. 149–68.
4. Zickgraf HF, Franklin ME, Rozin P. Adult picky eaters with symptoms of avoidant/restrictive food intake disorder: comparable distress and comorbidity but different eating behaviors compared to those with disordered eating symptoms. J Eat Disord. 2016;4(26) https://doi.org/10.1186/s40337-016-0110-6.
5. Strand M, von Hausswolff-Juhlin Y, Welch E. A systematic scoping review of diagnostic validity in avoidant/restrictive food intake disorder. Int J Eat Disord. 2019;52(4):331–60. https://doi.org/10.1002/eat.22962.
6. Zucker N. Avoidant/Restrictive Food Intake Disorder (ARFID). In: Wade T, editor. Encyclopedia of feeding and eating disorders. Singapore: Springer Science+Business Media; 2016. p. 1–4.

7. Kennedy GA, Wick MR, Keel PK. Eating disorders in children: is avoidant-restrictive food intake disorder a feeding disorder or an eating disorder and what are the implications for treatment? F1000Res. 2018;7(88) https://doi.org/10.12688/f1000research.13110.1.
8. Eddy KT, Harshman SG, Becker KR, et al. Radcliffe ARFID Workgroup: Toward operationalization of research diagnostic criteria and directions for the field. Int J Eat Disord. 2019;52(4):361–6. https://doi.org/10.1002/eat.23042.
9. Becker KR, Breithaupt L, Lawson EA, Eddy KT, Thomas JJ. Co-occurrence of avoidant/restrictive food intake disorder and traditional eating psychopathology. J Am Acad Child Adolesc Psychiatry. 2020;59(2):209–12. https://doi.org/10.1016/j.jaac.2019.09.037.
10. Zickgraf HF, Lane-Loney S, Essayli JH, Ornstein RM. Further support for diagnostically meaningful ARFID symptom presentations in an adolescent medicine partial hospitalization program. Int J Eat Disord. 2019;52(4):402–9. https://doi.org/10.1002/eat.23016.
11. Izquierdo A, Plessow F, Becker KR, Mancuso CJ, Slattery M, Murray HB, Hartmann AS, Misra M, Lawson EA, Eddy KT, Thomas JJ. Implicit attitudes toward dieting and thinness distinguish fat-phobic and non-fat-phobic anorexia nervosa from avoidant/restrictive food intake disorder in adolescents. Int J Eat Disord. 2019;52(4):419–27. https://doi.org/10.1002/eat.22981.
12. Becker AE, Thomas JJ, Pike KM. Should non-fat-phobic anorexia nervosa be included in DSM-V? Int J Eat Disord. 2009;42(7):620–35. https://doi.org/10.1002/eat.20727.
13. Lee S, Ng KL, Kwok KP, Thomas JJ, Becker AE. Gastrointestinal dysfunction in Chinese patients with fat-phobic and nonfat-phobic anorexia nervosa. Transcult Psychiatry. 2012;49(5):678–95. https://doi.org/10.1177/1363461512459487.
14. Thomas JJ, Hartmann AS, Killgore WD. Non-fat-phobic eating disorders: why we need to investigate implicit associations and neural correlates. Int J Eat Disord. 2013;46(5):416–9. https://doi.org/10.1002/eat.22098.
15. Feighner JP, Robins E, Guze SB, Woodruff RA Jr, Winokur G, Munoz R. Diagnostic criteria for use in psychiatric research. Arch Gen Psychiatry. 1972;26(1):57–63. https://doi.org/10.1001/archpsyc.1972.01750190059011.
16. Thomas JJ, Lawson EA, Micali N, Misra M, Deckersbach T, Eddy KT. Avoidant/restrictive food intake disorder: a three-dimensional model of neurobiology with implications for etiology and treatment. Curr Psychiatry Rep. 2017;19(8):54. https://doi.org/10.1007/s11920-017-0795-5.
17. Zickgraf HF, Ellis JM. Initial validation of the Nine Item Avoidant/Restrictive Food Intake disorder screen (NIAS): a measure of three restrictive eating patterns. Appetite. 2018;123:32–42. https://doi.org/10.1016/j.appet.2017.11.111.
18. Sysko R, Glasofer DR, Hildebrandt T, Klimek P, Mitchell JE, Berg KC, Peterson CB, Wonderlich SA, Walsh BT. The eating disorder assessment for DSM-5 (EDA-5): development and validation of a structured interview for feeding and eating disorders. Int J Eat Disord. 2015;48(5):452–63. https://doi.org/10.1002/eat.22388.
19. First MB, Williams JBW, Karg RS, Spitzer RL. User's guide for the structured clinical interview for DSM-5 disorders, clinical version (SCID-5-CV). Arlington, VA: American Psychiatric Association; 2015.
20. Schmidt R, Kirsten T, Hiemisch A, Kiess W, Hilbert A. Interview-based assessment of avoidant/restrictive food intake disorder (ARFID): a pilot study evaluating an ARFID module for the eating disorder examination. Int J Eat Disord. 2019;52(4):388–97. https://doi.org/10.1002/eat.23063.
21. Bryant-Waugh R, Micali N, Cooke L, Lawson EA, Eddy KT, Thomas JJ. Development of the Pica, ARFID, and rumination disorder interview, a multi-informant, semi-structured interview of feeding disorders across the lifespan: a pilot study for ages 10-22. Int J Eat Disord. 2019;52(4):378–87. https://doi.org/10.1002/eat.22958.
22. Nakai Y, Nin K, Noma S, Teramukai S, Wonderlich SA. Characteristics of avoidant/restrictive food intake disorder in a cohort of adult patients. Eur Eat Disord Rev. 2016;24(6):528–30. https://doi.org/10.1002/erv.2476.

23. Strandjord SE, Sieke EH, Richmond M, Rome ES. Avoidant/restrictive food intake disorder: illness and hospital course in patients hospitalized for nutritional insufficiency. J Adolesc Health. 2015;57(6):673–8. https://doi.org/10.1016/j.jadohealth.2015.08.003.
24. Tanaka S, Yoshida K, Katayama H, Kohmura K, Kawano N, Imaeda M, Kato S, Ando M, Aleksic B, Nishioka K, Ozaki N. Association of beck depression inventory score and temperament and character inventory-125 in patients with eating disorders and severe malnutrition. J Eat Disord. 2015;3(36) https://doi.org/10.1186/s40337-015-0077-8.
25. Nakai Y, Nin K, Noma S, et al. Clinical presentation and outcome of avoidant/restrictive food intake disorder in a Japanese sample. Eat Behav. 2017;24:49–53. https://doi.org/10.1016/j.eatbeh.2016.12.004.
26. Norris ML, Spettigue WJ, Katzman DK. Update on eating disorders: current perspectives on avoidant/restrictive food intake disorder in children and youth. Neuropsychiatr Dis Treat. 2016;12:213–8. https://doi.org/10.2147/NDT.S82538.
27. Hay P, Mitchison D, Collado AEL, González-Chica DA, Stocks N, Touyz S. Burden and health-related quality of life of eating disorders, including Avoidant/Restrictive Food Intake Disorder (ARFID), in the Australian population. J Eat Disord. 2017;5(21). https://doi.org/10.1186/s40337-017-0149-z.
28. Fitzsimmons-Craft EE, Balantekin KN, Graham AK, Smolar L, Park D, Mysko C, Funk B, Taylor CB, Wilfley DE. Results of disseminating an online screen for eating disorders across the U.S.: Reach, respondent characteristics, and unmet treatment need. Int J Eat Disord. 2019;52(6):721–9. https://doi.org/10.1002/eat.23043.
29. Murray HB, Bailey AP, Keshishian AC, Silvernale CJ, Staller K, Eddy KT, Thomas JJ, Kuo B. Prevalence and characteristics of avoidant/restrictive food intake disorder in adult neurogastroenterology patients. Clin Gastroenterol Hepatol. 2020;18(9):1995–2002.e1. https://doi.org/10.1016/j.cgh.2019.10.030.
30. Burton Murray H, Jehangir A, Silvernale CJ, Kuo B, Parkman HP. Avoidant/restrictive food intake disorder symptoms are frequent in patients presenting for symptoms of gastroparesis. Neurogastroenterol Motil. 2020:e13931. https://doi.org/10.1111/nmo.13931.
31. Aulinas A, Marengi DA, Galbiati F, Asanza E, Slattery M, Mancuso CJ, Wons O, Micali N, Bern E, Eddy KT, Thomas JJ, Misra M, Lawson EA. Medical comorbidities and endocrine dysfunction in low-weight females with avoidant/restrictive food intake disorder compared to anorexia nervosa and healthy controls. Int J Eat Disord. 2020;53(4):631–6. https://doi.org/10.1002/eat.23261.
32. Harshman SG, Wons O, Rogers MS, Izquierdo AM, Holmes TM, Pulumo RL, Asanza E, Eddy KT, Misra M, Micali N, Lawson EA, Thomas JJA. Diet high in processed foods, total carbohydrates and added sugars, and low in vegetables and protein is characteristic of youth with avoidant/restrictive food intake disorder. Nutrients. 2019;11(9):2013. https://doi.org/10.3390/nu11092013.
33. Reilly EE, Brown TA, Gray EK, Kaye WH, Menzel JE. Exploring the cooccurrence of behavioural phenotypes for avoidant/restrictive food intake disorder in a partial hospitalization sample. Eur Eat Disord Rev. 2019;27(4):429–35. https://doi.org/10.1002/erv.2670.
34. Zickgraf HF, Murray HB, Kratz HE, Franklin ME. Characteristics of outpatients diagnosed with the selective/neophobic presentation of avoidant/restrictive food intake disorder. Int J Eat Disord. 2019;52(4):367–77. https://doi.org/10.1002/eat.23013.
35. Wildes JE, Zucker NL, Marcus MD. Picky eating in adults: results of a web-based survey. Int J Eat Disord. 2012;45(4):575–82. https://doi.org/10.1002/eat.20975.
36. Ellis JM, Galloway AT, Webb RM, Martz DM, Farrow CV. Recollections of pressure to eat during childhood, but not picky eating, predict young adult eating behavior. Appetite. 2016;97:58–63. https://doi.org/10.1016/j.appet.2015.11.020.
37. Nadon G, Feldman DE, Dunn W, Gisel E. Association of sensory processing and eating problems in children with autism spectrum disorders. Autism Res Treat. 2011;2011:541926. https://doi.org/10.1155/2011/541926.

38. Tomchek SD, Dunn W. Sensory processing in children with and without autism: a comparative study using the short sensory profile. Am J Occup Ther. 2007;61(2):190–200. https://doi.org/10.5014/ajot.61.2.190.
39. Wiggins LD, Robins DL, Bakeman R, Adamson LB. Brief report: sensory abnormalities as distinguishing symptoms of autism spectrum disorders in young children. J Autism Dev Disord. 2009;39(7):1087–91. https://doi.org/10.1007/s10803-009-0711-x.
40. Norris ML, Robinson A, Obeid N, Harrison M, Spettigue W, Henderson K. Exploring avoidant/restrictive food intake disorder in eating disordered patients: a descriptive study. Int J Eat Disord. 2014;47(5):495–9. https://doi.org/10.1002/eat.22217.
41. Harris AA, Romer AL, Hanna EK, Keeling LA, LaBar KS, Sinnott-Armstrong W, Strauman TJ, Wagner HR, Marcus MD, Zucker NL. The central role of disgust in disorders of food avoidance. Int J Eat Disord. 2019;52(5):543–53. https://doi.org/10.1002/eat.23047.
42. Thomas JJ, Eddy KT. Cognitive-behavioral therapy for avoidant/restrictive food intake disorder: children, adolescents, and adults. Cambridge: Cambridge University Press; 2018.
43. Kauer J, Pelchat ML, Rozin P, Zickgraf HF. Adult picky eating. Phenomenology, taste sensitivity, and psychological correlates. Appetite. 2015;90:219–28. https://doi.org/10.1016/j.appet.2015.03.001.
44. Norris ML, Spettigue W, Hammond NG, Katzman DK, Zucker N, Yelle K, Santos A, Gray M, Obeid N. Building evidence for the use of descriptive subtypes in youth with avoidant restrictive food intake disorder. Int J Eat Disord. 2018;51(2):170–3. https://doi.org/10.1002/eat.22814.
45. Duncombe Lowe K, Barnes TL, Martell C, Keery H, Eckhardt S, Peterson CB, Lesser J, Le Grange D. Youth with avoidant/restrictive food intake disorder: examining differences by age, weight status, and symptom duration. Nutrients. 2019;11(8):1955. https://doi.org/10.3390/nu11081955.
46. Sharp WG, Stubbs KH. Avoidant/restrictive food intake disorder: a diagnosis at the intersection of feeding and eating disorders necessitating subtype differentiation. Int J Eat Disord. 2019;52(4):398–401. https://doi.org/10.1002/eat.22987.
47. Norris ML, Santos A, Obeid N, Hammond NG, Valois DD, Isserlin L, Spettigue W. Characteristics and clinical trajectories of patients meeting criteria for avoidant/restrictive food intake disorder that are subsequently reclassified as anorexia nervosa. Eur Eat Disord Rev. 2020;28(1):26–33. https://doi.org/10.1002/erv.2710.
48. Wassenaar E, O'Melia AM, Mehler PS. A causality dilemma: ARFID, malnutrition, psychosis, and hypomagnesemia. Int J Eat Disord. 2018;51(9):1113–6. https://doi.org/10.1002/eat.22939.
49. Schorr M, Drabkin A, Rothman MS, Meenaghan E, Lashen GT, Mascolo M, Watters A, Holmes TM, Santoso K, Yu EW, Misra M, Eddy KT, Klibanski A, Mehler P, Miller KK. Bone mineral density and estimated hip strength in men with anorexia nervosa, atypical anorexia nervosa and avoidant/restrictive food intake disorder. Clin Endocrinol (Oxf). 2019;90(6):789–97. https://doi.org/10.1111/cen.13960.
50. Hay P. Current approach to eating disorders: a clinical update. Intern Med J. 2020;50(1):24–9. https://doi.org/10.1111/imj.14691.
51. King LA, Urbach JR, Stewart KE. Illness anxiety and avoidant/restrictive food intake disorder: Cognitive-behavioral conceptualization and treatment. Eat Behav. 2015;19:106–9. https://doi.org/10.1016/j.eatbeh.2015.05.010.
52. Tsai K, Singh D, Pinkhasov A. Pudendal nerve entrapment leading to avoidant/restrictive food intake disorder (ARFID): a case report. Int J Eat Disord. 2017;50(1):84–7. https://doi.org/10.1002/eat.22601.
53. Steen E, Wade TD. Treatment of co-occurring food avoidance and alcohol use disorder in an adult: Possible avoidant restrictive food intake disorder? Int J Eat Disord. 2018;51:373–7. https://doi.org/10.1002/eat.22832.
54. Guss CE, Richmond TK, Forman S. A survey of physician practices on the inpatient medical stabilization of patients with avoidant/restrictive food intake disorder. J Eat Disord. 2018;6(22) https://doi.org/10.1186/s40337-018-0212-4.

55. Ornstein RM, Essayli JH, Nicely TA, Masciulli E, Lane-Loney S. Treatment of avoidant/restrictive food intake disorder in a cohort of young patients in a partial hospitalization program for eating disorders. Int J Eat Disord. 2017;50(9):1067–74. https://doi.org/10.1002/eat.22737.
56. Katzman DK, Norris ML, Zucker N. Avoidant restrictive food intake disorder: First do no harm. Int J Eat Disord. 2019;52(4):459–61. https://doi.org/10.1002/eat.23021.
57. Dumont E, Jansen A, Kroes D, de Haan E, Mulkens S. A new cognitive behavior therapy for adolescents with avoidant/restrictive food intake disorder in a day treatment setting: a clinical case series. Int J Eat Disord. 2019;52(4):447–58. https://doi.org/10.1002/eat.23053.
58. Zucker NL, LaVia MC, Craske MG, Foukal M, Harris AA, Datta N, Savereide E, Maslow GR. Feeling and body investigators (FBI): ARFID division-An acceptance-based interoceptive exposure treatment for children with ARFID. Int J Eat Disord. 2019;52(4):466–72. https://doi.org/10.1002/eat.22996.
59. Rozin P, Fallon AE. A perspective on disgust. Psychol Rev. 1987;94(1):23–41.
60. Teachman BA. Pathological disgust: In the thoughts, not the eye, of the beholder. Anxiety Stress Coping. 2006;19(4):335–51.
61. Bosman RC, Borg C, de Jong PJ. Optimising extinction of conditioned disgust. PLoS One. 2016;11(2):e0148626.
62. Engelhard IM, Leer A, Lange E, Olatunji BO. Shaking that icky feeling: effects of extinction and counterconditioning on disgust-related evaluative learning. Behav Ther. 2014;45(5):708–19. https://doi.org/10.1016/j.beth.2014.04.003.
63. Menzel JE, Reilly EE, Luo TJ, Kaye WH. Conceptualizing the role of disgust in avoidant/restrictive food intake disorder: Implications for the etiology and treatment of selective eating. Int J Eat Disord. 2019;52(4):462–5. https://doi.org/10.1002/eat.23006.
64. Gray E, Chen T, Menzel J, Schwartz T, Kaye WH. Mirtazapine and weight gain in avoidant and restrictive food intake disorder. J Am Acad Child Adolesc Psychiatry. 2018;57(4):288–9. https://doi.org/10.1016/j.jaac.2018.01.011.
65. Brewerton TD, D'Agostino M. Adjunctive use of olanzapine in the treatment of avoidant restrictive food intake disorder in children and adolescents in an eating disorders program. J Child Adolesc Psychopharmacol. 2017;27(10):920–2. https://doi.org/10.1089/cap.2017.0133.
66. Harrison ME, Norris ML, Robinson A, Spettigue W, Morrissey M, Isserlin L. Use of cyproheptadine to stimulate appetite and body weight gain: a systematic review. Appetite. 2019;137:62–72. https://doi.org/10.1016/j.appet.2019.02.012.

Drunkorexia

11

Crystal D. Oberle

11.1 Epidemiology: Characteristics, Prevalence, and Determinants

Drunkorexia is a term that first appeared in various media outlets in 2008 [1, 2] to describe a pattern of behavior whereby some individuals engage in compensatory diet-related behaviors when consuming alcohol. These behaviors include restricting behaviors, such as skipping meals or cutting back on calories or fat intake, as well as purging behaviors such as excessive exercising, vomiting, or laxative use. Performing such behaviors prior to alcohol consumption inherently enhances the effects of alcohol on the body and substantially raises the health and behavioral risks associated with drinking [3–9]. Although some researchers have proposed alternative labels such as food and alcohol disturbance (FAD) [10] and alcoholimia [11], drunkorexia is the term most often used in the literature and will be used throughout the remainder of this chapter.

Regarding prevalence rates of this behavior pattern, the researchers of many studies have assessed drunkorexia with a single item asking people how often they restrict their food, calories, or fat intake on days that they plan to consume alcohol, and people who indicate that they do so at least some of the time (i.e., not a "never" response) are considered "restrictors" who exhibit drunkorexia behavior. Using this method, these studies have found prevalence rates ranging from 12% to 39% in college student samples [6–8, 12–18]. In studies that use more comprehensive assessment measures with multiple items asking about various restricting and purging behaviors done before, during, and after consuming alcohol, researchers have found greater prevalence rates ranging from 54% to 58% in college student samples [3, 19, 20].

C. D. Oberle (✉)
Texas State University, San Marcos, TX, USA
e-mail: oberle@txstate.edu

© Springer Nature Switzerland AG 2022
E. Manzato et al. (eds.), *Hidden and Lesser-known Disordered Eating Behaviors in Medical and Psychiatric Conditions*,
https://doi.org/10.1007/978-3-030-81174-7_11

Research reveals two primary reasons given for drunkorexia behaviors: avoiding weight gain (i.e., restricting and purging behaviors for the purpose of offsetting the calories of the alcohol consumed) and experiencing enhanced alcohol effects (i.e., restricting and purging behaviors for the purposes of getting drunk faster and becoming more drunk with less alcohol) [6, 7, 12–14]. The first reason concerning the avoidance of weight gain is supported by research showing that drunkorexia behaviors are associated with greater levels of disordered eating [7, 21], including body dissatisfaction [5, 19, 22–25], drive for thinness [5, 17, 18, 24, 25], fasting [17], binge eating [4], and bulimia symptoms [4, 5, 8, 18, 25, 26]. Likewise, the second reason concerning the enhancement of alcohol effects is supported by research showing that drunkorexia behaviors are associated with greater levels of alcohol consumption [3–6, 9, 13, 15, 16, 20, 21, 24, 25]; binge drinking episodes [9, 12, 13, 16–19, 25, 26]; alcohol-related problems such as getting into a fight, memory loss, unprotected sex, and sexual victimization [3–9, 24]; and illicit drug use [16, 20].

The aforementioned research relates to the phenomenon of comorbidity between eating disorders and alcohol use disorders [27, 28] and leads to the question of whether extreme drunkorexia behaviors comprise an eating disorder, an alcohol disorder, or both. Based partly on the finding that disordered eating is a slightly better predictor than disordered alcohol consumption in women [4], some researchers [11] propose that drunkorexia should be included as a subcategory of other specified feeding and eating disorders (OSFED) in the *Diagnostic and Statistical Manual of Mental Disorders, Fifth Edition* (DSM-5) [29]. As another proposal, other researchers [10] suggest that drunkorexia be considered as an application of the transdiagnostic model of eating disorders [30]. Accordingly, in people with extreme drunkorexia, poor emotion regulation in the presence of negative life stressors will increase the desire to binge drink (and to quickly and more effectively experience the effects of alcohol). Yet, their overemphasis on weight and shape will lead to caloric restriction and purging compensatory behaviors to offset the effects of alcohol's calories and to avoid potential weight gain from both upcoming and recently completed binge drinking episodes. Although both proposals involve officially categorizing drunkorexia as an eating disorder, both also recognize the dual presence of both disordered eating and substance use that make drunkorexia unique from other disorders.

11.2 Demographic Differences and Other Correlates

Research findings regarding potential demographic differences in drunkorexia behaviors have been mixed. For instance, although some studies found women to exhibit greater drunkorexia behaviors than men [3, 12, 14, 15], other research reveals no significant gender differences [5, 13, 16–18, 24–26, 31]. Additionally, although two studies found greater drunkorexia behaviors among college freshmen [6, 15], other studies failed to find any significant age effects [5, 17, 31, 32]. Meta-analyses, weighted based on study quality, would be useful in better determining behavioral differences based on gender and age. In addition, future research should further explore potential interactions. Regarding gender, for example, some research suggests that while women may be more likely than men to engage in compensatory behaviors for the purpose of avoiding weight gain, women and men do not differ in doing these behaviors for the purpose of experiencing enhanced alcohol effects [6, 32]. As to demographic variables with consistent findings, Hispanic and non-Hispanic Caucasians tend to exhibit greater drunkorexia behaviors than African Americans [6, 15, 20], and drunkorexia behaviors have been shown to be unrelated to body mass index [13, 18, 32]. Regarding the latter finding, however, it is important to note that important clinical research on severe and extreme cases of drunkorexia is missing from the literature at this time.

Some studies have already explored how drunkorexia is potentially related to various personality, emotion, and mental health variables. Regarding personality, two studies found that drunkorexia behaviors are associated with greater sensation seeking tendencies [22, 23], which is consistent with the desire to experience enhanced alcohol effects. Regarding emotion and mental health, several studies found that drunkorexia behaviors are associated with emotion dysregulation, including limited access to emotion regulation strategies, impulse control difficulties, and difficulties in recognizing and responding to emotional states [17, 32]. Such emotion dysregulation may lead to poor coping strategies such as binge drinking to dull the negative affect or disordered restricting and purging dietary behaviors as an attempt to gain control. Either way, the emotional conflict has been shown to lead to lower levels of self-esteem [32] and greater levels of anxiety and depression [7].

11.3 Proposed Diagnostic Criteria

The negative impacts of both eating disorders and alcohol use disorders have been clearly demonstrated elsewhere. Here, we introduce a possible disorder that encompasses aspects of both, which could be even more debilitating. Moreover, severe restriction of food prior to alcohol consumption enhances the alcohol's effects and leads to even greater alcohol-related health and behavioral risks including sexual victimization and alcohol-related accidents that could be fatal [3–9]. Although much more research is needed prior to establishing drunkorexia as a formal disorder in the DSM-5, the following diagnostic criteria have tentatively been proposed [11]: the co-occurrence of high-risk drinking and diet-related compensatory behaviors for at least three consecutive months, self-evaluation being unduly influenced by body weight/shape (like both anorexia and bulimia), and the person experiencing significant distress and impairment. The severity of the drunkorexia may be mild (1–3 episodes per month), moderate (4–7 episodes per month), severe (8–14 episodes per month), or extreme (14 or more episodes per month). These proposed criteria could help guide future research in the field, allowing researchers to gain better insight into whether drunkorexia is indeed a disorder that is unique from other eating and substance use disorders.

References

1. Kershaw S. Starving themselves, cocktail in hand, New York Times; 2008. https://www.nytimes.com/2008/03/02/fashion/02drunk.html
2. CBS News. Drunkorexia: health dangers for women. CBS News; 2008. https://www.cbsnews.com/news/drunkorexia-health-danger-for-women/
3. Choquette EM, Ordaz DL, Melioli T, Delage B, Chabrol H, Rodgers R, Thompson JK. Food and alcohol disturbance (FAD) in the US and France: nationality and gender effects and relations to drive for thinness and alcohol use. Eat Behav. 2018;31:113–9. https://doi.org/10.1016/j.eatbeh.2018.09.002.
4. Hunt TK, Forbush KTI. "drunkorexia" an eating disorder, substance use disorder, or both? Eat Behav. 2016;22:40–5. https://doi.org/10.1016/j.eatbeh.2016.03.034.
5. Pinna F, Milia P, Mereu A, di Santa Sofia SL, Puddu L, Fatteri F, et al. Validation of the Italian version of the compensatory eating and behaviors in response to alcohol consumption scale (CEBRACS). Eat Behav. 2015;19:120–6. https://doi.org/10.1016/j.eatbeh.2015.08.004.
6. Giles SM, Champion H, Sutfin EL, McCoy TP, Wagoner K. Calorie restriction on drinking days: an examination of drinking consequences among college students. J Am Coll Health. 2009;57:603–9. https://doi.org/10.3200/JACH.57.6.603-610.
7. Roosen KM, Mills JS. Exploring the motives and mental health correlates of intentional food restriction prior to alcohol use in university students. J Health Psychol. 2015;20:875–86. https://doi.org/10.1177/1359105315573436.
8. Ward RM, Galante M. Development and initial validation of the Drunkorexia Motives and Behaviors scales. Eat Behav. 2015;18:66–70. https://doi.org/10.1016/j.eatbeh.2015.04.003.
9. Ward RM, Oswald BB, Galante M. Prescription stimulant misuse, alcohol abuse, and disordered eating among college students. J Alcohol Drug Educ. 2015;60:59–80.
10. Choquette EM, Rancourt D, Kevin Thompson J. From fad to fad: a theoretical formulation and proposed name change for "drunkorexia" to food and alcohol disturbance. Int J Eat Disord. 2018;51:831–4. https://doi.org/10.1002/eat.22926.
11. Thompson-Memmer C, Glassman T, Diehr A. Drunkorexia: a new term and diagnostic criteria. J Am Coll Health. 2019;67:620–6. https://doi.org/10.1080/07448481.2018.1500470.
12. Bryant JB, Darkes J, Rahal C. College students' compensatory eating and behaviors in response to alcohol consumption. J Am Coll Health. 2012;60:350–6. https://doi.org/10.1080/07448481.2011.630702.
13. Burke SC, Cremeens J, Vail-Smith K, Woolsey C. Drunkorexia: calorie restriction prior to alcohol consumption among college freshman. J Alcohol Drug Educ. 2010;54:17–34.
14. Peralta RL. Alcohol use and the fear of weight gain in college: reconciling two social norms. Gend Issues. 2002;20:0–42. https://doi.org/10.1007/s12147-002-0021-5.
15. Eisenberg MH, Fitz CC. "Drunkorexia": exploring the who and why of a disturbing trend in college students' eating and drinking behaviors. J Am Coll Health. 2014;62:570–7. https://doi.org/10.1080/07448481.2014.947991.
16. Lupi M, Martinotti G, Di Giannantonio M. Drunkorexia: an emerging trend in young adults. Eat Weight Disord. 2017;22:619–22. https://doi.org/10.1007/s40519-017-0429-2.
17. Pompili S, Laghi F. Drunkorexia among adolescents: the role of motivations and emotion regulation. Eat Behav. 2018;29:1–7. https://doi.org/10.1016/j.eatbeh.2018.01.001.
18. Pompili S, Laghi F. Drunkorexia: disordered eating behaviors and risky alcohol consumption among adolescents. J Health Psychol. 2018:1–11. https://doi.org/10.1177/1359105318791229.
19. Knight A, Castelnuovo G, Pietrabissa G, Manzoni GM, Simpson S. Drunkorexia: an empirical investigation among Australian female university students. Aust Psychol. 2017;52:414–23. https://doi.org/10.1111/ap.12212.
20. Peralta RL, Schnellinger RP, Wade JM, Barr PB, Carter JR. The association between Food and Alcohol Disturbance (FAD), race, and ethnic identity belonging. Eat Weight Disord. 2019;24:705–14. https://doi.org/10.1007/s40519-019-00718-4.

21. Gorrell S, Walker DC, Anderson DA, Boswell JF. Gender differences in relations between alcohol-related compensatory behavior and eating pathology. Eat Weight Disord. 2018;24:715–21. https://doi.org/10.1007/s40519-018-0545-7.
22. Griffin BL, Vogt KS. Drunkorexia: is it really "just" a university lifestyle choice? Eat Weight Disord. 2020; https://doi.org/10.1007/s40519-020-01051-x.
23. Hill EM, Lego JE. Examining the role of body esteem and sensation seeking in drunkorexia behaviors. Eat Weight Disord. 2019; https://doi.org/10.1007/s40519-019-00784-8.
24. Simons RM, Hansen JM, Simons JS, Hovrud L, Hahn AM. Drunkorexia: normative behavior or gateway to alcohol and eating pathology? Addict Behav. 2021;112:1–8. https://doi.org/10.1016/j.addbeh.2020.106577.
25. Rahal CJ, Bryant JB, Darkes J, Menzel JE, Thompson JK. Development and validation of the Compensatory Eating and Behaviors in Response to Alcohol Consumption Scale (CEBRACS). Eat Behav. 2012;13:83–7. https://doi.org/10.1016/j.eatbeh.2011.11.001.
26. Ward RM, Galante M, Trivedi R, Kahrs J. An examination of drunkorexia, Greek affiliation, and alcohol consumption. J Alcohol Drug Educ. 2015;59:48–66.
27. Gadalla T, Piran N. Co-occurrence of eating disorders and alcohol use disorders in women: a meta analysis. Arch Womens Ment Health. 2007;10:133–40. https://doi.org/10.1007/s00737-007-0184-x.
28. Harrop EN, Marlatt GA. The comorbidity of substance use disorders and eating disorders in women: prevalence, etiology, and treatment. Addict Behav. 2010;35:392–8. https://doi.org/10.1016/j.addbeh.2009.12.016.
29. American Psychiatric Association. Diagnostic and statistical manual of mental disorders. 5th ed. Washington, DC: American Psychiatric Association; 2013.
30. Fairburn CG. Cognitive behavior therapy and eating disorders. New York: Guilford Press; 2008.
31. Hill EM, Martin JD, Lego JE. College students' engagement in drunkorexia: examining the role of sociocultural attitudes toward appearance, narcissism, and Greek affiliation. Curr Psychol. 2019; https://doi.org/10.1007/s12144-019-00382-y.
32. Laghi F, Pompili S, Bianchi D, Lonigro A, Baiocco R. Psychological characteristics and eating attitudes in adolescents with drunkorexia behavior: an exploratory study. Eat Weight Disord. 2019; https://doi.org/10.1007/s40519-019-00675-y.

Eating Disorders and Bariatric Surgery

Donatella Ballardini, Livia Pozzi, Elena Dapporto, and Elena Tomba

12.1 Introduction

Recently, an increasing proportion of patients with severe obesity undergo bariatric surgery. This intervention is recommended in subjects with a body mass index (BMI) of 40 kg/m^2 and over or 35 kg/m^2 in the presence of one or more associated medical comorbidities. This treatment option relates to the fact that non-surgical therapies, including drug treatment, dietary treatment and lifestyle interventions, produce modest and short-term benefits in patients with severe obesity [1, 2].

Bariatric treatment produces significant weight loss and the improvement or resolution of the associated medical comorbidities, along with significant physical, psychological and social functioning improvements [3, 4]. Despite this, the results of weight loss present an important variability, even with the most effective bariatric surgery modalities [5]. Indeed, a significant proportion of patients who are undergoing bariatric surgery does not achieve the expected weight loss or regains weight in the following decade after surgery [6]. The Toronto Bariatric Surgery Psychosocial (Bari-PSYCH) cohort study [7] assessed patients who underwent Roux-en-Y gastric bypass, showing a significant weight reduction in the first post-operative year, while, between the second and third post-operative years, a significant weight regain was observed. Two years after surgery, 21.9% of patients had regained more than

---

D. Ballardini (✉) · L. Pozzi · E. Dapporto
Centro Gruber, Diagnosis and Treatment Outpatient Centre of Eating and Weight Disorders, Anxiety and Psychosomatic Disorders, Via Santo Stefano, 10, Bologna, Italy
e-mail: segreteria@centrogruber.org; donatella.ballardini@centrogruber.org; livia.pozzi@centrogruber.org; elena.dapporto@centrogruber.org

E. Tomba
Department of Psychology, University of Bologna, Bologna, Italy
e-mail: elena.tomba@unibo.it

10% of total weight loss (TWL) in the first year, 11.5% had regained more than 15% of TWL, and 4.9% of patients had regained more than 25% of TWL [7].

Many studies show that post-operative eating disorders and problematic eating behaviours may represent a major obstacle to achieve and maintain the weight loss in patients undergoing bariatric surgery. Therefore, the outcomes of bariatric intervention, although often significant, are not universal: between 20% and 30% [8] of patients have suboptimal weight loss experience or significant weight regain within the first post-operative years. Also, patients undergoing bariatric surgery present both short-term and long-term malnutrition risks [9]. All these outcomes probably involve both physiological processes and behavioural and psychological factors. Evidence suggests that pre-operative psychosocial status and psychological functioning may contribute to suboptimal weight loss, nutritional deficits or post-operative psychosocial distress. Several studies suggest that the presence of pre-operative psychopathology is associated with suboptimal weight loss, post-operative complications and limited positive psychosocial outcomes [8].

12.2 Eating Disorders and Problematic Eating Behaviours

Within the first post-operative year, a decline in eating psychopathology is generally associated with bariatric surgery. Eating disorders are frequently observed in patients awaiting bariatric surgery which in turn tend to improve after surgery. More specifically, within the first year after surgery, the episodes of objective binge eating episodes tend to disappear [7, 10]. However, many studies advise that the relapse of dysfunctional eating behaviours could occur beyond this initial year [10, 11]. After bariatric surgery, the weight regaining risk would remain for life. Behavioural factors could play a modulating role: an increase in dietary impulses, severe decrease in post-operative psychological well-being, problems related to alcohol or drug use seemed to be predictors of significant weight regain in a study where a group of patients with extreme obesity underwent Roux-en-Y gastric bypass. Therefore, involvement of patients by encouraging the use of self-monitoring strategies plays a protective role in weight regain [12].

Bariatric surgery creates anatomical and physiological modifications that could impact on patients' capacity to introduce large amounts of food. However, the development of eating disorders and the onset of problematic eating behaviours have been reported in the literature [13, 14]. Post-operative anatomical and physiological alterations can impact significantly on patients' diet and eating behaviour. Patients may develop new forms of dysfunctional eating behaviour such as loss of control over eating. These binge episodes, characterized by a feeling of loss of control perceived by the patient followed by negative emotional experiences and guilt, could be objective, but also subjective, which means that they occur in the absence of large amounts of consumed food [15]. The prevalence rates of binge eating disorder (BED) [16] in candidates for bariatric surgery range from 2% to 53%, with variations related to the method used during the investigation (clinical interview or self-report questionnaires) [17]. After depression syndrome, BED is the second most widespread psychiatric comorbidity in candidates for bariatric intervention population [18], while post-operative BED prevalence rates (DSM-5 criteria) appear low, ranging from 0% to 10.3% [19]. Prevalence rates of subjective experiences of loss of control over eating range from 6% to 64% [20]. In a 12-month follow-up study, BED, night eating syndrome (NES) [16] and uncontrolled food consumption reduced after surgery, while patients with pre-operative BED changed their eating patterns, switching to eat meals smaller in volume, but increased in frequency [21].

Pre-operative BED seems to attenuate weight loss. However, in another study (Chao et al. 2016) [22] conducted 24 months after bariatric surgery, surgically treated BED patients lost 18.6% of their initial weight compared to 23.9% of patients without BED ($p = 0.049$). The authors thus recommend that patients with this condition, as well as other eating disorders, receive specific psychological support.

After bariatric surgery, patients may experience unplanned and frequent consumption of small amounts of high-calorie foods, which circumvent the action mechanism of bariatric surgery [23, 24]. The most frequent clinical conditions of such problematic eating behaviours are described below.

Grazing is defined as the repetitive consumption of small and/or modest amounts of unplanned food not related to hunger. The term "repetitive" has been defined as eating more than twice in a limited period during the day (e.g. morning, evening or during the day) without prolonged intervals between food episodes. It is possible to differentiate between *compulsive grazing*, in which there is a loss of control present in every episode, and *non-compulsive grazing*, in which the act of eating occurs repeatedly in a distracted and unconscious manner. Since small meal consumption is a recommended therapeutic indication, because of the limited gastric capacity, an adequate assessment of food patterns is therefore essential in order to recognize if the food choice and consumption are controlled and if patients recognize hunger and satiety stimuli appropriately [23]. The prevalence of grazing in pre-operative patients is estimated at 26.4% [25], whereas in post-operative patients, it is estimated at 46.6% [26].

Picking or *nibbling* indicates the consumption of small amounts of food between meals, carried out in a repetitive and unconscious way. Very often, the patient is not able to reconstruct precisely the manner and amount of food ingested at the beginning of the episode and/or during the episodes; the feature of control loss is absent.

Another aspect of differentiation between *picking* and *grazing* is identified by the fact that in both subtypes of *grazing*, patients are able to reconstruct the situation or the way in which the episodes begin; moreover, the period of time in which the episodes occur is not always marked by planned meals [23].

Grazing or *picking* or *nibbling* eating behaviours are maladaptive phenomena, common in the post-bariatric population, probably exacerbated by prescriptive eating patterns in patients with premorbid altered eating difficulties. All these problematic eating behaviours occur more frequently after surgery with prevalence rates as high as 47.1% [24]; a correlation with poor weight loss has also been reported [27].

There is a lack of data on the prevalence of bulimia nervosa (BN) preceding bariatric surgery, perhaps because of the denial or minimization of symptoms for reasons of admissibility to surgery [23]. Using DSM-5 criteria, 343 patients who were candidates for bariatric surgery have been evaluated (Williams et al. 2017), and the 7.6% met the criteria for BN. In the entire sample, the most frequent compensatory behaviour was fasting (20.4%), followed by excessive physical exercise (11.7%), use of laxatives (5.6%) and self-induced vomiting (1.8%) [28]. The presence of BN after bariatric surgery is rare, and BN rates are little known. In the postoperative phase, patients may experience spontaneous or induced vomiting, which may occur in response to the consumption of poorly tolerated foods, too rapid meal or insufficient chewing, or, sometimes, may be a useful tool to alleviate symptoms of excessive gastric replenishment. Often, surgeons themselves advise or encourage the patient to relieve these unpleasant physical symptoms through self-induced vomiting. In patients who have significant weight and body image concerns, vomiting may become a strategy for a faster body weight loss. Therefore, a careful assessment about the reason and the expected outcome of the vomiting is necessary in order to understand whether it is considered as compensatory behaviour or not [24]. Another post-operative common clinical syndrome that can be used as a compensatory measure is *dumping* syndrome. Since this phenomenon may occur as a result of a high consumption of sweets and/or large amounts of food causing strong diarrhoea, it is important to assess whether patients experience such feature as a possible loss of control with compensation mechanism. The use of other compensation mechanisms such as the abuse of laxatives and diuretics following bariatric surgery seems to be rare [29].

There are numerous case reports of patients undergoing bariatric surgery who develop symptoms attributable to anorexia nervosa (AN) symptomatology: significant weight loss, excessive fear of weight gain, major dietary restrictions and disorders of weight and body image [30].

It is frequent that medical teams in charge of post-surgical follow-up encourage the patients to limit the volume of meals, to strictly adhere to dietary programmes, to weigh the food, to break the food into small pieces and to avoid specific foods for better food management. These recommendations can be overindulged by patients up to developing eating behaviours and typical rituals of people suffering from AN.

Other eating behaviours that should be considered in bariatric and post-bariatric population are *emotional eating, craving* and *sweet eating*.

Emotional eating, that is, eating in response to emotional distress and stress, is present in 38–59% of surgical candidates [31] and has been linked to other behaviours such as binge eating [32]. Such food consumption associated with emotional states seems to improve after bariatric surgery [33], but data in the literature on this behaviour are limited since there are mostly short-term follow-up studies in which the use of validated measures is not always available. *Craving* is an eating behaviour that leads to the consumption of food or a specific food, as a result of intense physiological or psychological impulses other than physiological hunger. *Craving* phenomena are more frequent in candidates for bariatric surgery compared to normal-weight patients and are present in most post-bariatric patients. Guthrie H et al. (2014) [34] found that only about 10% of post-operative patients do not report craving.

Sweet eating is generally characterized by excessive intake of high-calorie sweet foods, but its definition varies from one study to another, making difficult to compare data among studies. The lack of a shared definition in the literature may also explain the discordant results on the effect that *sweet eating* has on weight in post-bariatric patients [23].

Finally, a recent study by Lydecker and colleagues (2019) [35] evaluates the behaviour of secretive eating, loss of control (LOC) and psychopathology related to eating disorders through the Eating Disorder Examination-Bariatric Surgery Version (EDEBSV) in 168 adults who experience LOC following bariatric surgery (6 months later). As a result, 37% of patients report behaviour of secretive eating, of which 54% meet the criteria for BED and 25% report subthreshold symptoms of BED. Symptoms of eating disorders (frequency of LOC episodes, overall severity, dietary restriction, overestimation of body weight/body shape and dissatisfaction with the body) were higher among patients with secretive eating behaviour, while weight-related variables (BMI and % of TWL) were not significantly associated with secretive eating.

The lack of significant differences for weight variables suggests that secretive eating may be more related to body dissatisfaction than to weight loss after surgery [35].

Another eating disorder that should be mentioned in this section is night eating syndrome (NES), which is included in DSM-5 (APA 2013) [16] as one of "other specified feeding and eating disorders". NES is clinically defined by the presence of evening hyperphagia, nocturnal ingestion, morning anorexia and sleep problems. It seems to be associated with a higher risk of psychopathology, mood disorders, anxiety and sleep problems [36].

There are inconsistent data on NES prevalence in post-operative patients, while pre-operative prevalence is up to 17.7% [37]. Little is known about the impact of bariatric surgery on this syndrome. Some authors argue that since this disorder involves a shift in the circadian pattern of eating that disrupts sleep, it may continue after bariatric surgery. Moreover, it does not consist in the objective ingestion of large amounts of food. According to some studies, the symptoms of NES seem to decrease after bariatric surgery. To date, there is no evidence that pre-operative NES has a negative impact on weight loss after surgery [38].

12.3 Body Perception and Body Misperception in Obese Patients

The success of bariatric surgery is defined by the occurrence of a rapid and intensive weight loss, which typically improves body image. However, changes in body image are quite complex, and such a physical change is not always associated with a self-image adjustment. In fact, several studies report that many patients may continue to internally perceive themselves as being fat, configuring a phenomenon called "mind-body lag" or "allocentric lock". Faccio and colleagues (2016) [39] observed that although patients are satisfied in terms of weight loss outcomes, after the bariatric intervention, they show considerable difficulties in adapting their identity to the new body; even after a year, patients tend to think and behave as obese people. The impact of the external world on body image, cognitive, emotional and behavioural changes that occur in relation to body image and coping mechanisms to mitigate the undesirable changes of body image (e.g. the development of excess skin) should be assessed [40].

Neuroscience data underscore that the amygdala seems to play a crucial role in processing allocentric sensory input to long-term memory structures. The social stigma related to being obese may be associated with negative emotions that are stored in the amygdala and repeatedly rise in bariatric surgery patients' brain, even once the body condition has changed [41, 42].

In the same study, Perdue et al. (2018) [41] assessed 40 female patients between 18 and 30 months post-operative bariatric surgery, investigating whether evolving self-view, health locus of control, tendency towards alexithymic thoughts and health quality of life may present significant relationships. The "Evolving Self-View After Bariatric Surgery" (ESV) is a specific measure created to identify patient's orientation as "obese" or "ex-obese" person. Despite weight loss, the majority of women identified themselves in the "obese" category ($n = 28$, 70%) compared to the women in the sample who defined themselves in the "ex-obese" category ($n = 12$, 30%). Such results seem to confirm the multifactorial nature of obesity, characterized by biological, environmental and psychological components. Obese identity seems associated with greater difficulties in describing feelings and a tendency to feel less energetic, less calm and less happy. Therefore, it seems important not only to define pre-operative psychological issues that can influence post-operative conditions but also to provide psychological support to facilitate greater adaptation in the post-operative phase.

If therefore the maintenance of an obese "self-identity" could affect the quality of life and satisfaction with the results of slimming, patients undergoing bariatric surgery may present dissatisfaction with body image also related to overestimation of body weight or shape. Weight or shape overvaluation is a concept that occurs when self-assessment or self-esteem is based mainly and/or excessively on one's own weight or body shape [43]. This is recognized as a fundamental and central cognitive feature of many eating disorders [16, 44]. In BED, overestimation of the body image is not a diagnostic criterion, but when present it has been associated with greater level of psychopathology and severity [45–47] and is a predictor of worse treatment outcomes [48]. Unfortunately, little is known regarding overvaluation among individuals who undergo bariatric surgery and those with post-operative eating disorders. Ivezaj et al. (2019) [49] recently published a study on the role of weight or body shape overestimation in post-bariatric surgery patients with loss of control (LOC) eating. In particular, the frequency of body overvaluation and the association between overvaluation and clinical patterns were examined. Weight and clinical patterns in patients with or without clinical levels of overevaluation of body and shape following bariatric surgery were also compared. The study was conducted in a sample of 145 adults after 6 months of sleeve gastrectomy, and all participants had experienced regular LOC episodes. Half of the patients reported clinical levels of body and weight overestimation which was also found to be associated with greater eating disorder psychopathology, depression symptomatology and disability/poorer functioning. Future research is needed to examine the prognostic significance of overestimating body weight and shape before or after a bariatric operation in individuals with or without an eating disorder.

The assessment of problems in weight and shape in post-operative bariatric patients represents a complex clinical process. The fear of weight gain in this population is realistic. Clinicians encourage these patients to monitor weight and control those factors that may promote weight gain. Weight loss is often accompanied by important aesthetic and functional side effects that can cause high body dissatisfaction and disappointment with the expected weight and shape improvement. Conventional body satisfaction assessment may not capture the complex nuances of body dissatisfaction in a population marked by specific changes in body shape.

12.4 Case Report

This section presents an illustrative clinical case of a patient with a severe eating disorder who underwent gastric banding (GB) at the age of 20 years (pre-operative BMI: 38 kg/m^2). This case brings up noteworthy clinical features for further discussion and reflection.

A 27-year-old woman, normal weight (BMI: 22 kg/m^2), arrived at a specialized outpatient treatment clinic for feeding and eating disorders, referred by her general practitioner.

She referred to suffer of bulimia nervosa and to be afraid of being affected for many years during which for a long time she attributed her symptomatology to the GB. She had recourse to vomit after more abundant meals than her post-operative diet indicated. She could not tolerate that sense of stuffing and declared to vomit for this reason. Later on, she began using vomiting also to manage objective binge eating episodes. The patient reported a complete "loss of control" of her symptoms, feeling like in a tunnel and looking for an adequate treatment to recover.

Specialized multidisciplinary assessment including medical and nutritional assessment, integrated to psychiatric, psychological and psychotherapeutic assessment, was conducted. Figure 12.1 describes the model of the structured multidisciplinary diagnostic-therapeutic process which integrates medical and nutritional therapy with psychiatric, psychological and CBT-based psychotherapeutic therapy [50].

The following psychometric instruments to support, respectively, psychiatric diagnoses and eating disorder-related psychopathology and general psychopathology severity were used: Structured Clinical Interview for DSM-5, Clinical Version (SCID-5-CV) and SCID-5 Personality Disorders (SCID-5-PD) [51], Eating Disorder Inventory-3 [52], Eating Attitude Test [53] and Three-Factor Eating Questionnaire [54].

Figure 12.2 provides a graphic representation of the patient's complex anamnesis.

Specialized Multidisciplinary Outpatient Treatment for Eating Disorders

Medical and Nutritional Sector →
- **Management of Medical Issues**
- **Psychoterapies** (Cognitive Therapies CT's, Cognitive Behavioral Therapy CBT, Schema-Focused Therapy SFT, Trauma Therapy, Motivational Therapy MET) ← **Psychiatric, Psychological and Psychotherapeutic Sector**
- **Psycho-Nutritional Rehabilitation in CBT** (Basic and enlarged for comorbidity)
- **Psycho-Education** ←
- **Psychiatric Therapy** ←
- **Family Counseling and Therapy** ←
- Group Psychotherapies (Clinical Assertiveness Training ATP, Clinical Emotional Communication Therapy EMO, Group CBT) ←
- Biofeedback ←
- Body Therapy (Mindfulness, **Relaxation Training**)
- **Coordination with other medical specialists** (gynaecologist, cardiologist etc.)
- **Collaboration with family doctor and with territorial services**

Fig. 12.1 The model of the structured multidisciplinary diagnostic-therapeutic process. The model integrates medical and nutritional therapy with psychiatric, psychological and CBT-based psychotherapeutic therapy. Patient's treatment plan is **underlined** in the figure

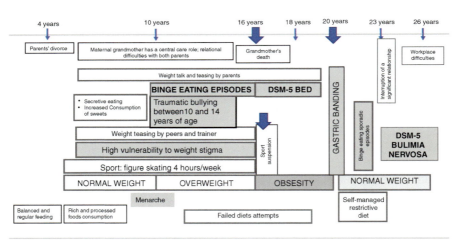

Fig. 12.2 A graphic representation of the patient's complex anamnesis

It was given a diagnosis of BN (DSM-5) [16] with at least three binge eating episodes per day, both subjective and objective, followed by self-induced vomiting. The patient reported an eating pattern characterized by several small meals between episodes of loss of control. This symptomatology worsened in the last year, and its onset occurred about 3 years after a restrictive eating pattern period. After GB intervention, the patient managed to follow a strict diet, with rare episodes of loss of control followed by vomiting. The patient complained about gastro-oesophageal reflux associated with a retro-sternal burning and pharyngitis. Sleep is very disturbed with two or three awakenings per night. The menstrual cycle is regular. The patient's blood test showed critical clinical concerns, such as a serious microcytic hypochromic anaemia (Hb 8.0 g/dL, VN 12.0–16.0) associated with iron, folic acid and vitamin B_{12}, vitamin D deficiency and a slight rise in transaminases; electrolyte, inflammatory and coagulation parameters were in normal ranges; kidney function is not impaired. Cardiological evaluation described a satisfactory hemodynamic compensation in a condition of healthy cardiovascular system, except for moderate bradycardia and hypotension. Instead, significant alterations occurred in the oesophagus and stomach, gastric sac extensive dilatation above the bandage, class B reflux esophagitis [55] and hyperaemia of the gastric wall; the search for *Helicobacter pylori* resulted negative. The gastroenterologist indicated gastric banding removal, initially refused by the patient because of the fear of gaining weight without it.

It should be noted that it was not possible to refer to the medical record of the GB operation since it was carried out in a private hospital of a different region. Pre-operation assessment consisted only in two interviews (with surgeon and psychologist). During the assessment, the patient omitted to declare her frequent binge eating episodes fearing that she would be refused for the surgery. Since at age of 16 years, the patient presented binge eating episodes, without conduct of elimination or compensatory methods; the symptomatology pattern described by the patient could fulfil a retrospective diagnosis of BED (DSM-5 criteria) [16]. Moreover, the patient did not attend the follow-up visits after the surgical operation. She managed to control her diet for a few years even though she had sporadic binges (no more than 1 episode per month) which were always followed by vomiting. Three years before, after the interruption of a romantic relationship, the binge episodes intensified in frequency and became planned, and the vomiting became self-induced. The patient started perceiving a significant body dissatisfaction and reported "I am still an obese person as before the bariatric surgery". She has never been motivated for entering in specialized ED clinical programme treatment; only recently she asked her family doctor help for a specialized treatment support.

Clinical and psychometric assessment highlighted the following psychopathological features: body dissatisfaction, drive for thinness, bulimia and worry about food, low self-esteem, poor psychological well-being (in particular impairment in autonomy, environmental mastery, personal growth, positive relations with others, purpose in life, self-acceptance) and high social insecurity. In addition to the symptoms of the eating disorders, the clinical evaluation made by the psychotherapist pointed out previous traumatic experiences related to bullying and the sudden death of the grandmother (the main caregiver in her childhood). Her childhood was characterized by parental emotional neglect, lack of attention and insecure attachment—mainly related to the aspects of physical as well as emotional care—feeling of loneliness and guilt linked to the extremely conflictual parental divorce. Affective instability, difficulty in emotional identification, constant feeling of emptiness and high fear of being abandoned and obsessions related to food and body shape were present at the time of taking charge. Moreover, interpersonal relationship

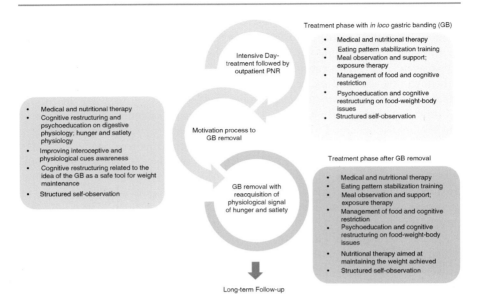

Fig. 12.3 Psycho-nutritional rehabilitation (PNR) treatment

difficulties seemed to be characterized by personal insecurity, vulnerability to the judgment of others and isolation.

The treatment consisted of a psychotherapeutic therapy, integrated with a psycho-nutritional rehabilitation. The psychotherapeutic treatment, cognitive and cognitive-behavioural orientated, had the following objectives: establishing and maintaining a therapeutic alliance; managing and decreasing the severity of ED symptomatology (in particular, binges and vomiting episodes); promoting adaptive relational and communicative skills; interventions oriented to the internal processing of the traumatic experiences; and promoting mentalization functions. Psycho-nutritional treatment included, in its first treatment phase, in loco GB; consequently, a motivation phase was oriented to the GB removal (removed after 5 months). Then, treatment was oriented to support nutritional problems and any worries and phobias that emerged after GB removal. Figure 12.3 presents in detail the psycho-nutritional rehabilitation process.

After a 2-year follow-up, the patient maintained remission from the eating disorder and a BMI of 22.5 kg/m^2.

The patient provided consent for this case report.

12.5 Discussion

The clinical detection of any eating disorder and problematic eating behaviours in patients who are candidates for bariatric surgery, as well as their possible maintenance or exacerbation following surgery, is little investigated. Moreover, such lack of data is perhaps underestimated [24]. The clinical case presented offers several clinical insights here discussed in detail.

First of all, conducting a clinical evaluation to determine whether surgery is safe and appropriate is crucial. This assessment should include an adequate period of time during which the patient should be observed, and it should be repeated before surgery, especially when a candidate has been on a waiting list for a long time. The assessment should be structured and performed by an experienced multidisciplinary team composed of physician, dietician, surgeon, psychologist and psychiatrist [56]. Medical history, physical examination and laboratory investigations, mental health assessment and interviews to determine the patient's motivation for bariatric surgery should be included. Also, it is important that patient understands the procedures, the possible complications and post-operative therapeutic needs. This must be assessed in order to improve the shared decision-making as well as determine whether the patient has the necessary and appropriate social support. Psychosocial analysis is needed to evaluate the environmental, cultural, economic and working conditions that may support or hinder the patient's compliance with the post-operative programme.

A critical element during this clinical evaluation relates to the clinicians' skills to understand when patients minimize eating psychopathology and other psychopathological symptoms in order to receive authorization to proceed to surgery (as our patient reported). Ambwani et al. (2013) [57] studied the prevalence of such "socially desirable response style" measured using two scales on socially desirable response styles, in particular Marlowe-Crowne's Social Desirability Scale (MCSD) and the Inventory Positive Impression Management (PAI-PIM). Among the participants (N=359), 33–40% of them scored higher than the cut-off score established for the Inventory Positive Impression Management; 62–67% scored one standard deviation above the normative average on Marlowe-Crowne's Social Desirability Scale. Therefore, such data support that many bariatric surgery candidates present a response style associated with lower reporting on psychological problems which in turn may interfere with an accurate assessment of the patient's functioning. These patient attitudes should be evaluated not as a desire to "lie", but rather as a "symptom" of the patient's own suffering from which the diagnostic responsibility of the bariatric team clinicians derives.

Psychological and psychiatric eligibility criteria for bariatric intervention should be further explored. Psychopathology can compromise a patient's ability to manage not only the surgery but the complex and demanding post-surgical phase, in both the short and long term. Patients with a higher degree of obesity present also a higher rate of mental illness, addiction disorders and sexual abuse [58] and have a higher likelihood of suffering from depressive disorders. Therefore, studies suggest that patients should be screened for depressive disorders, with particular attention to suicidal ideation, mania, anxiety disorders, psychosis, substance use and abuse, history of sexual abuse, family history of mental health problems and any previous psychiatric treatment experiences.

To date, there are no clear and shared guidelines for the psychological evaluation [56], procedures, techniques, timing and duration of the bariatric patient assessment. For this reason, it is necessary to keep the clinical behaviour more protective for the patient. As already reported, eating disorders are frequent in patients who are candidates for bariatric surgery, so their screening is necessary. BN, BED and NES are all clinically relevant clinical disorders and syndromes that should be considered when defining eligibility for surgery. The presence of BN should represent an absolute contraindication for surgery; whereas BED is not contraindicated, it should be carefully examined (e.g. the presence of emotional triggers for eating and the medical history). In the presented case, the onset of BED pattern developed subsequently a history of childhood eating disorders characterized by loss of food control, childhood obesity, stigmatization and weight teasing in the early adolescence and severe grief in adolescence. Clinicians must consider the possibility that bariatric intervention may favour the development of an eating disorder or a switch towards another form of eating disorder. In the case of our patient, the urge to thinness, high body dissatisfaction, loss of food control since childhood and failed dietary attempts may all be considered as predisposing factors to BN.

Post-bariatric therapeutic indications (e.g. dietary restriction, use of laxatives for the constipation, vomiting to manage gastric discomfort) can exacerbate eating behaviours and pathologic practices in order to control weight fluctuations. This, in association with the presence of *emotional eating*, LOC eating and an increase in impulsive behaviours in response to emotions and negative experiences, would further explain the development of an ED or a relapse [59, 60].

Many authors evaluated the frequency and behavioural characteristics associated with a form of post-operative binge eating disorder that could be defined as "bariatric binge eating disorder". This condition fulfils all criteria for DSM-5 binge eating disorder, except for the requirement of an unusually large amount of food, consumed during loss of control eating [15, 37, 60].

Another important debate relates to bariatric surgery in children, adolescents and young adults. In the developmental phase, eating disorders are generally common; in particular, for eligible patients for bariatric surgery, such disorders are present in a substantial percentage, almost 25% [61]. Adolescence is a complex period characterized by biological, psychological and social development changes, and bariatric surgery in adolescents may be therefore associated with potentially different outcomes from those considered for adults. Bariatric surgery for adolescents and young people involves medical and ethical dilemmas that are certainly superior than those in adults. Systematic reviews identified significant health benefits [61], but long-term data are still scarce in particular regarding both nutritional and psychological complications and social and life outcomes [62].

Mackey (2018) evaluated the rates of psychiatric diagnoses in a clinical population of adolescents undergoing bariatric surgery; in particular, 71% of adolescents qualified for a psychiatric disorder (anxiety, 26%; depression, 42%; ADHD, 22%; eating disorders, 8%). The presence or absence or number of diagnoses before surgery was not associated with weight loss outcomes after surgery [63].

Adolescents with loss of control (LOC) over eating seem to gain greater advantages from surgical treatment, precisely because of the possibility to recover an adequate dimension of social life in a relatively short time. In adolescence, the shape and body image represent a pivotal factor in the acceptance by peers, and therefore the opportunity to reduce the risk of depressive syndrome, isolation, suicidal ideation and chronic eating disorders may constitute a noteworthy treatment option [64].

Recently, Goldschmidt et al. (2018) studied LOC over eating in a group of patients ($n = 234$) aged 13–19 years. The emerged results underscored that although pre-surgical LOC over eating was not related to relative weight loss after surgery, post-operative LOC over eating may adversely affect long-term weight outcomes. LOC over eating episodes decreased in the first 6 months post-surgery, but increased thereafter. Therefore, targeting such behavioural feature may justify further empirical and clinical attention, suggesting the need for longer follow-up studies [65].

12.6 Conclusions

Bariatric surgery currently represents one of the most important and innovative therapeutic strategies for people affected by severe obesity. Bariatric approach can drastically reduce cardiovascular risk and mortality in obese patients, promoting weight loss and several metabolic and weight-related improvements, both in adults and in paediatric-age patients. Despite this, further researches are still needed to establish clinical evaluation criteria for patients eligible for the intervention and the post-bariatric management. Particular attention must be paid to the psychopathology, to paediatric-age patients and young adults. It should also be highlighted that most of the studies presents short and limited follow-up periods; moreover, a notable rate of patients abandon post-bariatric follow-up: as a result, a possible limitation of significance may occur.

In consequence, an adequate post-surgical nutritional rehabilitation is needed, as well as a psychological and psychiatric re-assessment, specifically indicated for patients affected by eating disorders and depressive syndromes in order to start a specific therapeutic programme.

Specific diagnostic-therapeutic programme should be structured for the post-bariatric patient, referring to pre-bariatric assessment, post-surgery monitoring which considers metabolic aspects and weight issues, as well as mental health and quality of life issues.

Finally, to provide post-surgery improvements, it is important to entrust the bariatric patient management to an experienced multidisciplinary team which should include, in addition to the surgical team, professionals as psychiatrists, psychotherapists, physicians and dietitians (specifically trained for the ED identification). The post-bariatric patient needs not only specific nutritional support (essential for malnutrition prevention) but also a long-term multidisciplinary support, in order to avoid dysfunctional behaviours consequent to cognitive and dietary restriction, needed after the intervention. So, it would be desirable to organize a long-term nutritional counselling, associated with an accurate assessment of eating behaviours, in all bariatric patients, in order to early identify the possible development of ED patterns or subthreshold EDs and problematic eating behaviours.

References

1. National Institute for Health and Clinical Excellence. Obesity: identification, assessment and management; 2014. Nice.org.uk/guidance/cg189
2. National Institute for Health and Clinical Excellence. Surgery for obese adults; 2019. http://pathways.nice.org.uk/pathways/obesity
3. Buchwald H, Avidor Y, Braunwald E, Jensen MD, Pories W, Fahrbach K, Schoelles K. Bariatric surgery: a systematic review and meta-analysis. JAMA. 2004;292(14):1724–37.
4. Thomson L, Sheehan KA, Meaney C, Wnuk S, Hawa R, Sockalingam S. Prospective study of psychiatric illness as a predictor of weight loss and health related quality of life one year after bariatric surgery. J Psychosom Res. 2016;86:7–12.
5. Carlin AM, Zeni TM, English WJ, Hawasli AA, Genaw JA, Krause KR, Schram JL, Kole KL, Finks JF, Birkmeyer JD, Share D. The comparative effectiveness of sleeve gastrectomy, gastric bypass, and adjustable gastric banding procedures for the treatment of morbid obesity. Ann Surg. 2013;257(5):791–7.
6. Sjöström L, Lindroos AK, Peltonen M, Torgerson J, Bouchard C, Carlsson B, Dahlgren S, Larsson B, Narbro K, Sjöström CD, Sullivan M. Lifestyle, diabetes, and cardiovascular risk factors 10 years after bariatric surgery. N Engl J Med. 2004;351(26):2683–93.
7. Nasirzadeh Y, Kantarovich K, Wnuk S, Okrainec A, Cassin SE, Hawa R, Sockalingam S. Binge eating, loss of control over eating, emotional eating, and night eating after bariatric surgery: results from the Toronto Bari-PSYCH Cohort Study. Obes Surg. 2018;28(7):2032–9.
8. Sarwer DB, Allison KC, Wadden TA, Ashare R, Spitzer JC, McCuen-Wurst C, LaGrotte C, Williams NN, Edwards M, Tewksbury C, Wu J. Psychopathology, disordered eating, and impulsivity as predictors of outcomes of bariatric surgery. Surg Obes Relat Dis. 2019;
9. Torres AJ, Rubio MA. The endocrine society's clinical practice guideline on endocrine and nutritional management of the post-bariatric surgery patient: commentary from a European perspective. Eur J Endocrinol. 2011;165(2):171–6.
10. Devlin MJ, King WC, Kalarchian MA, White GE, Marcus MD, Garcia L, Yanovski SZ, Mitchell JE. Eating pathology and experience and weight loss in a prospective study of bariatric surgery patients: 3-year follow-up. Int J Eat Disord. 2016;49(12):1058–67.
11. Courcoulas AP, Christian NJ, Belle SH, Berk PD, Flum DR, Garcia L, Horlick M, Kalarchian MA, King WC, Mitchell JE, Patterson EJ. Weight change and health outcomes at 3 years after bariatric surgery among individuals with severe obesity. JAMA. 2013;310(22):2416–25.
12. Courcoulas AP, King WC, Belle SH, Berk P, Flum DR, Garcia L, Gourash W, Horlick M, Mitchell JE, Pomp A, Pories WJ. Seven-year weight trajectories and health outcomes in the Longitudinal Assessment of Bariatric Surgery (LABS) study. JAMA Surg. 2018;153(5):427–34.
13. Marino JM, Ertelt TW, Lancaster K, Steffen K, Peterson L, de Zwaan M, Mitchell JE. The emergence of eating pathology after bariatric surgery: a rare outcome with important clinical implications. Int J Eat Disord. 2012;45(2):179–84.
14. Conceição E, Orcutt M, Mitchell J, Engel S, LaHaise K, Jorgensen M, Woodbury K, Hass N, Garcia L, Wonderlich S. Eating disorders after bariatric surgery: a case series. Int J Eat Disord. 2013;46(3):274–9.
15. Meany G, Conceição E, Mitchell JE. Binge eating, binge eating disorder and loss of control eating: effects on weight outcomes after bariatric surgery. Eur Eat Disord Rev. 2014;22(2):87–91.
16. American Psychiatric Association. Diagnostic and statistical manual of mental disorders—5th Edition. BCM Med. 2013;17:133–7.
17. Tess BH, Maximiniano-Ferreira L, Pajecki D, Wang YP. Bariatric surgery and binge eating disorder: should surgeons care about it? A literature review of prevalence and assessment tools. Arq Gastroenterol. 2019;56(1):55–60.
18. Dawes AJ, Maggard-Gibbons M, Maher AR, Booth MJ, Miake-Lye I, Beroes JM, Shekelle PG. Mental health conditions among patients seeking and undergoing bariatric surgery: a meta-analysis. JAMA. 2016;315(2):150–63.

19. de Zwaan M, Hilbert A, Swan-Kremeier L, Simonich H, Lancaster K, Howell LM, Monson T, Crosby RD, Mitchell JE. Comprehensive interview assessment of eating behavior 18–35 months after gastric bypass surgery for morbid obesity. Surg Obes Relat Dis. 2010;6(1):79–85.
20. Niego SH, Kofman MD, Weiss JJ, Geliebter A. Binge eating in the bariatric surgery population: a review of the literature. Int J Eat Disord. 2007;40(4):349–59.
21. Colles SL, Dixon JB, O'Brien PE. Night eating syndrome and nocturnal snacking: association with obesity, binge eating and psychological distress. Int J Obes (Lond). 2007;31(11):1722–30.
22. Chao AM, Wadden TA, Faulconbridge LF, Sarwer DB, Webb VL, Shaw JA, Thomas JG, Hopkins CM, Bakizada ZM, Alamuddin N, Williams NN. Binge-eating disorder and the outcome of bariatric surgery in a prospective, observational study: Two-year results. Obesity. 2016;24(11):2327–33.
23. Conceição EM, Utzinger LM, Pisetsky EM. Eating disorders and problematic eating behaviours before and after bariatric surgery: characterization, assessment and association with treatment outcomes. Eur Eat Disord Rev. 2015;23(6):417–25.
24. Conceição E, Mitchell JE, Vaz AR, Bastos AP, Ramalho S, Silva C, Cao L, Brandão I, Machado PP. The presence of maladaptive eating behaviors after bariatric surgery in a cross sectional study: importance of picking or nibbling on weight regain. Eat Behav. 2014;15(4):558–62.
25. Colles SL, Dixon JB, O'Brien PE. Grazing and loss of control related to eating: two high-risk factors following bariatric surgery. Obesity. 2008;16(3):615–22.
26. Kofman MD, Lent MR, Swencionis C. Maladaptive eating patterns, quality of life, and weight outcomes following gastric bypass: results of an Internet survey. Obesity. 2010;18(10):1938–43.
27. Conceição EM, Mitchell JE, Engel SG, Machado PP, Lancaster K, Wonderlich SA. What is "grazing"? Reviewing its definition, frequency, clinical characteristics, and impact on bariatric surgery outcomes, and proposing a standardized definition. Surg Obes Relat Dis. 2014;10(5):973–82.
28. Williams GA, Hawkins MA, Duncan J, Rummell CM, Perkins S, Crowther JH. Maladaptive eating behavior assessment among bariatric surgery candidates: evaluation of the Eating Disorder Diagnostic Scale. Surg Obes Relat Dis. 2017;13(7):1183–8.
29. Conceição E, Teixeira F, Rodrigues T, de Lourdes M, Bastos AP, Vaz A, Ramalho S. Problematic eating behaviors after bariatric surgery: a national study with a Portuguese sample. Acta Med Port. 2018;31(11):633–40.
30. Marino JM, Ertelt TW, Lancaster K, Steffen K, Peterson L, de Zwaan M, Mitchell JE. The emergence of eating pathology after bariatric surgery: a rare outcome with important clinical implications. Focus. 2014;12(4):470–5.
31. Opolski M, Chur-Hansen A, Wittert G. The eating-related behaviours, disorders and expectations of candidates for bariatric surgery. Clin Obes. 2015;5(4):165–97.
32. Fischer S, Chen E, Katterman S, Roerhig M, Bochierri-Ricciardi L, Munoz D, Dymek-Valentine M, Alverdy J, Le Grange D. Emotional eating in a morbidly obese bariatric surgery-seeking population. Obes Surg. 2007;17(6):778–84.
33. Castellini G, Godini L, Amedei SG, Faravelli C, Lucchese M, Ricca V. Psychological effects and outcome predictors of three bariatric surgery interventions: a 1-year follow-up study. Eat Weight Disord. 2014;19(2):217–24.
34. Guthrie H, Tetley D, Hill AJ. Quasi-prospective, real-life monitoring of food craving post-bariatric surgery: comparison with overweight and normal weight women. Clin Obes. 2014;4(3):136–42.
35. Lydecker JA, Ivezaj V, Grilo CM. Secretive eating and binge eating following bariatric surgery. Int J Eat Disord. 2019;
36. McCuen-Wurst C, Ruggieri M, Allison KC. Disordered eating and obesity: associations between binge eating-disorder, night-eating syndrome, and weight-related co-morbidities. Ann N Y Acad Sci. 2018;1411(1):96.
37. Mitchell JE, King WC, Courcoulas A, Dakin G, Elder K, Engel S, Flum D, Kalarchian M, Khandelwal S, Pender J, Pories W. Eating behavior and eating disorders in adults before bariatric surgery. Int J Eat Disord. 2015;48(2):215–22.

38. de Zwaan M, Marschollek M, Allison KC. The night eating syndrome (NES) in bariatric surgery patients. Eur Eat Disord Rev. 2015;23(6):426–34.
39. Faccio E, Nardin A, Cipolletta S. Becoming ex-obese: narrations about identity changes before and after the experience of the bariatric surgery. J Clin Nurs. 2016;25(11–12):1713–20.
40. Lyons K, Meisner BA, Sockalingam S, Cassin SE. Body image after bariatric surgery: a qualitative study. Bariatric Surg Pract Patient Care. 2014;9(1):41–9.
41. Perdue TO, Schreier A, Swanson M, Neil J, Carels R. Majority of female bariatric patients retain an obese identity 18–30 months after surgery. Eat Weight Disord. 2018:1–8.
42. Riva G. Neuroscience and eating disorders: the allocentric lock hypothesis. Med Hypotheses. 2012;78(2):254–7.
43. Fairburn CG, Cooper Z, Shafran R. Cognitive behaviour therapy for eating disorders: a "transdiagnostic" theory and treatment. Behav Res Ther. 2003;41(5):509–28.
44. Masheb RM, Grilo CM. The nature of body image disturbance in patients with binge eating disorder. Int J Eat Disord. 2003;33(3):333–41.
45. Grilo CM, White MA, Masheb RM. Significance of overvaluation of shape and weight in an ethnically diverse sample of obese patients with binge-eating disorder in primary care settings. Behav Res Ther. 2012;50(5):298–303.
46. Lydecker JA, White MA, Grilo CM. Form and formulation: examining the distinctiveness of body image constructs in treatment-seeking patients with binge-eating disorder. J Consult Clin Psychol. 2017;85:1095–103.
47. Wang SB, Jones PJ, Dreier M, Elliott H, Grilo CM. Core psychopathology of treatment-seeking patients with binge-eating disorder: a network analysis investigation. Psychol Med. 2019;49(11):1923–8.
48. Grilo CM, Masheb RM, Crosby RD. Predictors and moderators of response to cognitive behavioral therapy and medication for the treatment of binge eating disorder. J Consult Clin Psychol. 2012;80(5):897.
49. Ivezaj V, Wiedemann AA, Grilo CM. Overvaluation of weight or shape and loss-of-control eating following bariatric surgery. Obesity. 2019;27(8):1239–43.
50. Ballardini D, Schumann R. La riabilitazione psiconutrizionale nei disturbi dell'alimentazione. Carocci Faber; 2011.
51. First MB, Williams JBW, Karg RS, Spitzer RL. Structured clinical interview for DSM-5 disorders, clinician version (SCID-5-CV). Arlington, VA: American Psychiatric Association; 2015.
52. Garner DM. EDI-3, eating disorder inventory-3: Professional manual. Psychological Assessment Resources, Incorporated; 2004.
53. Garner DM, Garfinkel PE. The eating attitudes test: an index of the symptoms of anorexia nervosa. Psychol Med. 1979;9(2):273–9.
54. Stunkard AJ, Messick S. The three-factor eating questionnaire to measure dietary restraint, disinhibition and hunger. J Psychosom Res. 1985;29(1):71–83.
55. Lundell LR, Dent J, Bennett JR, Blum AL, Armstrong D, Galmiche JP, Johnson F, Hongo M, Richter JE, Spechler SJ, Tytgat GN, Wallin L. Endoscopic assessment of esophagitis: clinical and functional correlates and further validation of the Los Angeles classification. Gut. 1999;45(2):172–80.
56. Zentner A. Clinical assessment to determine a patient's suitability for bariatric surgery. B C Med J. 2018;60(3):151–5.
57. Ambwani S, Boeka AG, Brown JD, Byrne TK, Budak AR, Sarwer DB, Fabricatore AN, Morey LC, O'Neil PM. Socially desirable responding by bariatric surgery candidates during psychological assessment. Surg Obes Relat Dis. 2013;9(2):300–5.
58. Sarwer DB, Fabricatore AN. Psychiatric considerations of the massive weight loss patient. Clin Plast Surg. 2008;35(1):1–0.
59. Schag K, Mack I, Giel K, Ölschläger S, Skoda EM, von Feilitzsch M, Zipfel S, Teufel M. The impact of impulsivity on weight loss four years after bariatric surgery. Nutrients. 2016;8(11):721.

60. Ivezaj V, Barnes RD, Cooper Z, Grilo CM. Loss-of-control eating after bariatric/sleeve gastrectomy surgery: similar to binge-eating disorder despite differences in quantities. Gen Hosp Psychiatry. 2018;54:25–30.
61. Pratt JS, Browne A, Browne NT, Bruzoni M, Cohen M, Desai A, Inge T, Linden BC, Mattar SG, Michalsky M. Podkameni D. ASMBS pediatric metabolic and bariatric surgery guidelines, 2018. Surg Obes Relat Dis. 2018;14(7):882–901.
62. Shoar S, Mahmoudzadeh H, Naderan M, Bagheri-Hariri S, Wong C, Parizi AS, Shoar N. Long-term outcome of bariatric surgery in morbidly obese adolescents: a systematic review and meta-analysis of 950 patients with a minimum of 3 years follow-up. Obes Surg. 2017;27(12):3110–7.
63. Mackey ER, Wang J, Harrington C, Nadler EP. Psychiatric diagnoses and weight loss among adolescents receiving sleeve gastrectomy. Pediatrics. 2018;142(1):e20173432.
64. Utzinger LM, Gowey MA, Zeller M, Jenkins TM, Engel SG, Rofey DL, Inge TH, Mitchell JE. Teen Longitudinal Assessment of Bariatric Surgery (Teen-LABS) Consortium. Loss of control eating and eating disorders in adolescents before bariatric surgery. Int J Eat Disord. 2016;49(10):947–52.
65. Goldschmidt AB, Khoury J, Jenkins TM, Bond DS, Thomas JG, Utzinger LM, Zeller MH, Inge TH, Mitchell JE. Adolescent loss-of-control eating and weight loss maintenance after bariatric surgery. Pediatrics. 2018;141(1):e20171659.

Night Eating Syndrome and Nocturnal Sleep-Related Eating Disorder

13

Caterina Lombardo and Silvia Cerolini

13.1 Night Eating Syndrome (NES): Diagnostic Criteria and Clinical Features

The night eating syndrome (NES) is currently classified by the *Diagnostic and Statistical Manual of Mental Disorders 5th Edition* (DSM-5) [1] as an eating disorder, within the category of "Other Specified Feeding or Eating Disorder." According to DSM-5, it is characterized by recurrent episodes of night eating, in terms of eating after awakenings from sleep, or by excessive food consumption after the evening meal. The awareness and the recall of the nocturnal eating episode are present. This pattern of behaviors should not be explained by environmental influences or social norms and should lead to significant impairment and distress. Moreover, the disordered eating pattern must not be explained by other mental disorders, such as binge eating disorder (BED), and is not attributable to another medical disorder or to an effect of medication.

In the 1955, Stunkard and colleagues [2] proposed the first conceptualization of NES, as a disorder including morning anorexia, evening hyperphagia, insomnia, and distress. Since then, diagnostic criteria for NES have evolved over the years. Before the inclusion within the DSM-5, Allison and colleagues [3] summarized the proposed diagnostic criteria concluding that NES is characterized by two core symptoms: (1) evening hyperphagia and/or nocturnal ingestions and (2) the presence of at least three of five descriptor symptoms among the following: morning

---

C. Lombardo (✉) · S. Cerolini
Department of Psychology, Sapienza University of Rome, Rome, Italy
e-mail: caterina.lombardo@uniroma1.it; silvia.cerolini@uniroma1.it

© Springer Nature Switzerland AG 2022
E. Manzato et al. (eds.), *Hidden and Lesser-known Disordered Eating Behaviors in Medical and Psychiatric Conditions*,
https://doi.org/10.1007/978-3-030-81174-7_13

anorexia, post-dinner eating, insomnia, depression, and the belief that one must eat in order to get back to sleep after a nocturnal awakening. Two important features should be acknowledged for NES. The first is that people who have symptoms of evening or nocturnal hyperphagia do clearly remember the eating episodes. The second is that these episodes may be described as the consumption of more than 25% of all calories after the "evening meal" [3]. Considering the "evening meal," instead of a specific time of the day (e.g., 7 PM, as suggested by Stunkard and colleagues [4]), allows to overcome the main difficulty that clinicians who work with this disorder face: The time of the day devoted to the evening meal varies greatly across individuals and cultures. A wide national survey by Striegel-Moore et al. [5] including US 13+-year-old individuals examined the prevalence of three different definitions of night eating: (a) consuming 25% or more of the total daily calories between 7:00 PM and 4:59 AM; (b) consuming 50% or more of the total daily calories between 7:00 PM and 4:59 AM; and (c) consuming anything between 11:00 PM and 4:59 AM, regardless of the amount of calories consumed. Results showed that the estimate of the percentage of individuals exhibiting a possible night eating varied for each definition: the first definition (25%+ kcal after 7 PM) estimated that NES was present in more than one-third of the population; the other two definitions (50%+ kcal after 7 PM and any eating after 11 PM) gave more conservative estimates of fewer than 13% of individuals meeting these criteria. Additionally, a video polysomnographic (VPSG) study from a case series of 20 patients with NES conducted by Loddo et al. [6] found that patients with evening hyperphagia showed significantly longer time delays from awakening to food intake, total eating episode duration, and sleep latency after eating offset, compared to patients with nocturnal ingestion, suggesting the existence of potential NES subtypes.

Due to the lack of a standard definition before the inclusion in the DSM-5, data about prevalence of NES are scarce, but suggest that it may be estimated around 1.5% of the total population [7]. Specifically, a prevalence of 6–16% has been described among obese patients [7], and it seems to rise with increasing body mass index, reaching about 2–20% among bariatric surgery samples [8]. A critical review of the literature by Vander Wal [9] shows that the onset of NES is during early adulthood (ranging from the late teens to late 20s) and its duration is long-lasting, with periods of remission and exacerbation that may coincide with stressful life events. Moreover, NES seems to affect both genders, and its prevalence among persons of various racial groups is almost unknown [9]. A recent narrative review of the literature [10] documents that night eating is also common during pregnancy, with the estimated prevalence in different populations ranging from 15% to 45%. The potential unfavorable nutritional features of night eating may induce aberrant circadian rhythms in pregnant women, resulting in adverse metabolic and pregnancy outcomes.

Empirical findings suggest that female patients with NES show (a) a phase delay in the timing of meals; (b) delayed circadian rhythms for total caloric, fat, and carbohydrate intake; and (c) phase delays in food-regulatory and circadian melatonin rhythms [11]. Moreover, NES has been linked to emotional difficulties such as depression, anxiety, and stress [7, 12, 13].

Several studies provide evidence that NES is clearly a different construct compared to BED [14] and sleep-related eating disorder (SRED) [15], though several symptoms and characteristics overlap.

13.2 Sleep-Related Eating Disorder (SRED) and Differential Diagnosis with NES

For a long time, the distinction between NES and SRED has been unclear since they were considered either the same or distinct disorders. Currently NES is included in the DSM-5 as an eating disorder, while SRED is classified as a NREM-related parasomnia in the third edition of the *International Classification of Sleep Disorders* (ICSD-3) [16], but it is not included within the sleep/wake disorders class of the DSM-5. SRED, first described by Schenck and colleagues in 1991 [17], is characterized by recurrent episodes of dysfunctional eating that occur after an arousal during the main sleep period with partial or complete amnesia for the event. This may result in weight gain from eating high-calorie foods, potentially generating glucosidic or lipidic metabolism destabilization or aggravating pre-existing diabetes mellitus, hypertension, and OSAS [18]. Moreover, it may cause various injuries due to both the non-complete awakening and the consumption of also inedible or toxic items [19]. Usually, individuals who suffer from SRED get out of bed to eat and drink after having normally fallen asleep, describing the episode as an out-of-control behavior, unassociated with any feeling of hunger and thirst, and at the end of which, sleep can be restarted [20]. In the morning, people usually do not remember the episode.

Data on prevalence of SRED in the general population are not available; however, it has been approximately estimated between 0.5 and 4.7%, rising at 16.7% in patients with diurnal eating disorders, affecting both genders and all ages, with a predominant onset in female young adults [20–22]. There is evidence indicating that SRED often occurs in individuals with previous or current episodes of sleep-walking [23]. In addition, it is also important to distinguish the clinical features between drug-induced and primary SRED, which has been documented by Komada et al. [24] as (a) higher mean age of onset (40 years old in drug-induced SRED vs 26 years old in primary SRED), (b) significantly higher rate of patients who had total amnesia during most of their SRED episodes (75.0% vs 31.8%), (c) significantly lower rate of comorbidity of night eating syndrome (0% vs 63.3%), and (d) significantly lower rate of history of sleepwalking (10.0% vs 46.7%).

The main distinction between NES and SRED is definitely the level of consciousness during nighttime eating episode, specifically the presence of awareness in the first condition and the absence or the impairment of full memory of the events in the morning after the final awakening, in the second condition. Despite this main distinction, some individuals with altered level of consciousness during nocturnal eating (with SRED diagnosis) may also have night eating behaviors with full alertness both within a single night and across the longitudinal course of the disorder [21, 25], thus complicating their differentiation. In fact, some patients cannot be easily brought to full consciousness during an episode of eating, as is the case with sleepwalking, and may have no recall of having eaten during the night, whereas other patients have considerable alertness during an episode and have substantial recall in the morning [19]. It has been debated whether NES and SRED should be considered as independent entities or whether they should be considered as a continuum of a single condition. In fact, both SRED and NES share a chronic course, familiar associations, and comorbid neuropsychiatric diseases [18–20]. As suggested by Winkelman [21], SRED and NES may reflect opposite ends of a continuum of impairment of consciousness during nocturnal eating.

Moreover, the differential diagnosis between these two disorders may be challenging due to difficulties related to the referral patterns and biases of the researchers/clinicians: for instance, sleep disorders specialists are facilitated in diagnosing parasomnias and are more concerned with the level of consciousness during nocturnal eating episodes, whereas eating disorders specialists are more focused on eating behavior such as characterized by the timing, type, and number of calories consumed [26]. Winkelman sarcastically distinguished night eating from the two specialists' perspectives: SRED patients are sleepwalkers to whom happens to eat, whereas NES patients are those with binge eating disorder to whom happens to eat at night.

Although the state of consciousness during nocturnal eating can be described as the major distinction, Winkelman et al. [21] suggested that two other potential distinguishing features, described by researchers over the years, are the timing of nocturnal eating and the rate of comorbid sleep disorders present in individuals with nocturnal eating. While individuals with a diagnosis of SRED always report night eating after awakenings that occur during the main sleep period (i.e. during the first sleep cycles), individuals with a diagnosis of NES may report to eat both during nighttime awakenings or after evening meal, before going to bed.

Secondly, the comorbidity between SRED and sleep disorders such as sleepwalking, restless legs syndrome (RLS), periodic limb movements of sleep (PLMS), or obstructive sleep apnea (OSA), but not in NES, can be identified as another main distinguish feature, possibly suggesting different etiologies [21]. Particularly, SRED and sleepwalking share common clinical features such as similar timing of episode (particularly during the first half of the night) and numerous arousals from stage N3 sleep [23]. For these common characteristics, SRED has been considered to occur as a result of a dysfunction in sustaining stable slow-wave sleep, which is similar to sleepwalking [27]. However, empirical evidences are still lacking and heterogeneous, and firm conclusions have not been yet formulated. A recent cross-sectional web-based survey of Japanese young adults aged 19–25 years ($n = 3347$) indicated a prevalence of 4.8% reporting nocturnal eating behavior and a prevalence of 2.2% reporting sleep-related eating disorder-like behavior [28]. Both behaviors were associated with smoking, use of hypnotic medications, and previous and/or current sleepwalking. Nocturnal eating behavior but not sleep-related eating disorder-like behavior was characterized by a sleep-awake phase delay and sleep disturbance. This first epidemiological study offers a novel contribution in exploring the prevalence and the main features of the two behaviors; however, results should be considered preliminary in assessing the pathophysiology of NES and SRED. Confirmation of the reproducibility of these findings and prospective research that includes face-to-face interviews is warranted.

13.3 Comorbidity and Differential Diagnosis Between NES and Other Eating and Weight Disorders

As previously discussed, NES is currently considered a stand-alone construct and diagnosis. However, it has been documented that NES may occur in comorbidity with several medical and psychopathological conditions.

Individuals with NES seem to be more likely to have another eating disorder than members of the general population with prevalence estimates ranging from 5 to 44%. NES is more common among persons with eating disorders than in the general population [9]. A study conducted by Tu et al. [29] comparing multiple subgroups of eating disorder adult patients with anorexia nervosa (AN), bulimia nervosa (BN), BED, and NES and a control group found that NES was identified in 10.3%, 34.9%, and 51.7% of the individuals with AN, BN, and BED, respectively. Clinical patients (specifically NES-only, BN-only, and BN with NES patients) had similar degrees of clinical features (i.e., depression, sleep quality, sleep medication use, and daytime dysfunction) within group comparisons; however, all groups showed significantly more severe degrees than controls. Moreover, a subtype of BN with NES referred the presence of greater eating and weight concerns compared to BN-only group. This evidence may suggest that NES may overlap with BN in several dimensions of psychopathology.

Other studies estimated that approximately 15–20% of patients with NES also have BED [30]. Although some symptoms overlap, compared to individuals with BED, NES participants eat fewer meals during the day and more during the night and report fewer objective bulimic and overeating episodes, disinhibition, hunger, and shape/weight concerns [14], although these concerns may still be significant [31]. According to Vander Wal [9], compared to other eating disorders, such as BED or bulimia nervosa, other clinical features of NES may be considered: the duration of the nocturnal eating episodes (averaging 3.5 min in one study [32]) often accompanied by the goal of returning to sleep, the lower number of calories consumed during the eating episodes, and the absence of compensatory behaviors.

Moreover, as suggested by McCuen-Wurst and colleagues [30], BED and NES overall occur in 5–15% of individuals with obesity, highlighting that both disorders are linked to weight gain and medical comorbidities, such as diabetes and metabolic syndrome.

A population-based twin study conducted by Tholin et al. [33] found that NES was more prevalent in males and females with obesity (respectively, 2.5 times and 2.8 times more prevalent) compared to non-obese men and women. Also other studies documented the association between NES and BMI, weight gain, and obesity, and this eating disorder seems to be more common among weight loss treatment-seeking individuals than in the general community [9, 34–37]. NES prevalence also increases with BMI in psychiatric populations [30, 38]. Some authors proposed that individual differences in emotional regulation, especially the presence of emotional eating, could modulate the relationship between NES and body mass index and other parameters [39]. However, there are some studies producing mixed results and suggesting that NES and BMI/obesity are not necessarily linked, especially at certain ages [e.g., 40–43]. In 2019, a literature review of 11 studies investigating the association between NES and BMI by Bruzas and Allison [44] indicated heterogeneous results: 5 of these studies reported a positive relationship, 5 showed no relationship, and 1 produced mixed findings. The most relevant weakness of the existent literature was that it was almost entirely cross-sectional. Other findings documented that this association may vary along with age: night eating severity seems to be correlated with a higher BMI in middle-age individuals, but not in young adults, suggesting its potential contributive role in the development of obesity [45–47]. Probably, the weight gain may occur after long periods of engaging in night eating [40].

More longitudinal researches are needed to clarify this association [44], especially those connecting obesity and chronodisruption, those analyzing the role of circadian genes involved in the biological drive in NES, and those examining the onset and the symptomology progression related to weight gain and obesity [36].

13.4 Comorbidity of NES with Other Psychopathological Conditions

As anticipated in the previous paragraphs, NES seems to be linked not only to eating- or weight-related syndromes but also with other psychopathological symptoms and disorders such as mood, anxiety, and sleep disorders.

13.4.1 Mood and Anxiety Disorders

Literature reviews support the association between night eating and depression and anxiety [9, 48]. NES has been previously associated with high level of depressive symptoms and physical and emotional abuse and neglect [49]. Less recently, also Gluck et al. [50] reported higher rate of depression and lower self-esteem in overweight participants with NES (diagnosed using Stunkard's proposed criteria in 1996 [4] of (1) skipping breakfast > 4 days/week, interpreted as morning anorexia; (2) consuming more than 50% of total daily calories after 7 PM; and (3) difficulty falling asleep or staying asleep >4 days/week) compared to overweight participants without NES. Later, Lundgren et al. [31] conducted a weight-matched comparison group in which 19 non-obese participants with NES were compared to 22 non-obese healthy controls. They found that NES group reported greater depressed mood, perceived stress, sleep disturbances, decreased quality of life, and more frequent comorbidities, such as anxiety, mood, and substance use disorders. Authors suggested that NES might have negative health implications beyond that associated with obesity. The association of NES and depression was also reported in another study that found that among individuals with NES, 56% had a lifetime history of major depressive disorder [51].

A study by Gül et al. [52] documented a prevalence of NES diagnosis of 13.4% among 216 patients diagnosed with major depressive disorder (MDD) compared to a prevalence of 2.3% in a control group of 216 individuals matched for gender, age, and educational level. These authors also documented that, comparing MDD patients with NES and without NES, the proportion of those with severe depression, suicide attempt narratives, and smoke addiction was higher in the group with NES. Moreover, these patients reported also significantly higher scores of anxiety compared to patients without NES. A study by Kucukgoncu et al. [7] examined the prevalence of NES among 155 depressed outpatients and the difference between NES and non-NES group. NES was identified in 21.3% of the patients. Groups differed for several clinical features, but specifically NES group reported higher scores of depression and anxiety severity.

Another study by Melo et al. [53], conducted on 80 euthymic bipolar patients and 40 controls, reported a prevalence of NES of 8.8% in the patient group, while anyone of the control group reported the presence of NES. Patients with NES showed poorer functioning, higher levels of anxiety, and worse sleep parameters.

The association between NES and anxiety is also supported by a study by Pawlow et al. [13], which indicated that individuals with NES reported both state and trait anxiety levels above the average range for healthy adults and that the highest night eating scores corresponded to the highest trait anxiety scores. Furthermore, a sample of obese patients with NES reported significantly higher symptoms of anxiety than other patients and evening hyperphagia levels and mood and sleep disturbances were all correlated with nocturnal anxiety [54].

De Zwaan et al. [51] documented a 17% prevalence of generalized anxiety disorder and an 18% prevalence of post-traumatic stress disorder in persons with night eating, whereas Lundgren et al. [31] found that 47.7% of participants with NES met criteria for anxiety disorders compared with 9.1% of controls.

We can conclude that a large portion of individuals suffering from night eating also experience clinical levels of depression and anxiety, that, if present, may exacerbate the problem.

13.4.2 Sleep Problems

The results of several studies support the relationship between NES and poor sleep quality in college students [40, 47, 55] and adults [31, 47]. Moreover, students complying with symptoms consistent with any level of NES reported also shorter sleep time than students without any symptoms of NES [40]. A study by Nolan and Gotlieb [56] found that the presence of diagnostic criteria for NES were associated with poor sleep quality, higher depression scores, and food addiction in a community sample of adults. Considering the link between NES and sleep in clinical samples, results of the abovementioned studies including depressed or bipolar patients with NES showed the presence of greater sleep disturbances and worse sleep quality and quantity [7, 53]. Particularly, the study of Melo et al. [53] found that euthymic bipolar patients with NES had higher insomnia severity and poorer sleep quality and more evening preference (eveningness), which has been associated with depressive symptoms in several clinical situations [57]. These authors suggest that therapies improving insomnia and sleep quality may be a helpful addition to treatment of those with NES. However, it is unclear whether nocturnal eating is a response to a lack of sleep or vice versa, and further studies are needed in order to clarify this relationship that could be likely bidirectional.

Deeping this topic, some studies documented that although NES is characterized by a delayed circadian pattern of eating, individuals with NES showed a normal sleep-wake cycle [11, 58]: the timing of the sleep cycles is phase appropriate, with similar bedtimes and morning wake-up times, suggesting that it may be the delayed eating rhythm that secondarily disrupts sleep [48, 58]. Additionally, a study by O'Reardon et al. [59] compared the eating and sleep-wake patterns of 46 overweight/obese NES subjects with 43 matched control subjects. These authors measured sleep parameters for 7 days using the actigraphy (a wrist device worn by the individual) and sleep and food diaries (which measure, respectively, the self-reported quantity of sleep and food intake). They found no significant difference between the two groups on daily food intake, sleep duration, and sleep onset. This suggests that the great difference is in the abnormal timing and pattern of eating: NES subjects reported to eat significantly more after the evening meal and less during the morning. They also showed significantly more nocturnal arousals than did controls and reported to eat during those awakenings. These results suggest that the NES may be characterized by a circadian phase delay in the timing of food intake within a normal sleep-wake cycle.

However, the experience of nighttime sleep disturbances due to multiple awakenings each night has been documented other times, though the numbers and the duration may vary among studies [11, 58, 60], experiencing a high degree of nighttime sleep disturbances compared to controls. A polysomnographic study by Rogers et al. [61] also supported previous findings by O'Reardon and colleagues [59], indicating no significant differences in sleep onset or sleep offset times, but documented the presence of increased sleep disruptions and reduced sleep efficiency.

13.5 Conclusions

Although the study of night eating syndrome (NES) goes back to the 50s of the last century [2], its inclusion within the diagnostic manuals is more recent: it has been included only in the 5th version of the DSM [1] and only within the category of "Other Specified Feeding or Eating Disorder." Knowledge about NES may still be considered partial or preliminary at all levels: diagnostic, epidemiologic, and etiopathologic. At the diagnostic level, DSM-5 includes the presence of recurrent episodes of eating after awakenings from sleep or after the evening meal and the awareness and recall of the nocturnal eating episode in the morning. However, what should be considered nocturnal eating is still unclear. At the beginning, Stunkard and colleagues [4] suggested to consider as nocturnal eating an eating episode that occurs after 7 PM. However, this definition did not take into account individual and cultural differences. For overcoming this problem, some researchers [e.g., 3] suggested that nocturnal eating might be better described as the consumption of more than 25% of all calories of the day after the "evening meal." However, also the "evening meal" needs to be better clarified. For instance, in several cultures, people use to have a dinner at home around 5–7 PM and then spend time outside home eating and drinking with friends or colleagues. Should this be considered as a night eating episode? Or if a person has this habit but his/her cultural norms do not include it, should it be considered a night eating episode?

Data about prevalence of NES are scarce and vary widely. Recent evidence, reviewed in the present chapter, suggests prevalence rates of about 1.5% in the general population and of about 6–16% among patients with obesity, reaching about 2–20% among bariatric surgery samples. It seems that NES prevalence is equally distributed across genders and its prevalence among persons of various racial groups is almost unknown. However, also prevalence estimates are preliminary due to the unclear diagnostic definition.

Findings reviewed in the present chapter evidence that NES is frequently present in comorbidity with sleep, anxiety, and depressive disorders. However, also comorbidity rates may be underestimated due to the unclear diagnostic definition.

Consequences of life stress events need also further investigation. Several findings suggest that they may act as triggers of recurrent episodes. However, more information is needed in order to understand which other triggers could be identified.

Several studies provide evidence that NES is a different syndrome compared to BED and to sleep-related eating disorder, though several symptoms and characteristics overlap. However, also these overlaps, especially with SRED, need further clarification.

For all these reasons, we think that more data are needed for better understanding NES and its determinants and clinical manifestations and for hypothesizing and testing clinical interventions.

References

1. American Psychiatric Association. Diagnostic and statistical manual of mental disorders (DSM-5®). Washington DC: American Psychiatric Pub; 2013.
2. Stunkard AJ, Grace WJ, Wolff HG. The night-eating syndrome: a pattern of food intake among certain obese patients. Am J Med. 1955;19:78–86. https://doi.org/10.1016/0002-9343(55)90276-X.
3. Allison KC, Lundgren JD, O'Reardon JP, Geliebter A, Gluck ME, Vinai P, et al. Proposed diagnostic criteria for night eating syndrome. Int J Eat Disord. 2010;43:241–7. https://doi.org/10.1002/eat.20693.
4. Stunkard A, Berkowitz R, Wadden T, Tanrikut C, Reiss E, Young L. Binge eating disorder and the night-eating syndrome. Int J Obes Relat Metab Disord. 1996;20:1–6.

5. Striegel Moore RH, Franko DL, Thompson D, Affenito S, Kraemer HC. Night eating: prevalence and demographic correlates. Obesity. 2006;14(1):139–47. https://doi.org/10.1038/oby.2006.17.
6. Loddo G, Zanardi M, Caletti MT, et al. Searching food during the night: the role of video-polysomnography in the characterization of the night eating syndrome. Sleep Med. 2019;64:85–91. https://doi.org/10.1016/j.sleep.2019.06.018.
7. Kucukgoncu S, Tek C, Bestepe E, Musket C, Guloksuz S. Clinical features of night eating syndrome among depressed patients. Eur Eat Disord Rev. 2014;22:102–8. https://doi.org/10.1002/erv.2280.
8. de Zwaan M, Marschollek M, Allison KC. The night eating syndrome (NES) in bariatric surgery patients. Eur Eat Disord Rev. 2015;23(6):426–34. https://doi.org/10.1002/erv.2405.
9. Vander Wal JS. Night eating syndrome: a critical review of the literature. Clin Psychol Rev. 2012;32(1):49–59. https://doi.org/10.1016/j.cpr.2011.11.00.
10. Loy SL, Loo RSX, Godfrey KM, et al. Chrononutrition during pregnancy: a review on maternal night-time eating. Nutrients. 2020;12:2783. https://doi.org/10.3390/nu12092783.
11. Goel N, Stunkard AJ, Rogers NL, Van Dongen HP, Allison KC, O'Reardon JP, et al. Circadian rhythm profiles in women with night eating syndrome. J Biol Rhythms. 2009;24(1):85–94. https://doi.org/10.1177/0748730408328914.
12. Kucukgoncu S, Midura M, Tek C. Optimal management of night eating syndrome: challenges and solutions. Neuropsychiatr Dis Treat. 2015;11:751–60. https://doi.org/10.2147/NDT.S70312.
13. Pawlow L, O'Neil P, Malcolm R. Night eating syndrome: effects of brief relaxation training on stress, mood, hunger, and eating patterns. Int J Obes. 2003;27:970–8. https://doi.org/10.1038/sj.ijo.0802320.
14. Allison KC, Grilo CM, Masheb RM, Stunkard AJ. Binge eating disorder and night eating syndrome: a comparative study of disordered eating. J Consult Clin Psychol. 2005;73(6):1107. https://doi.org/10.1037/0022-006X.73.6.1107.
15. Volpe U, Atti AR, Cimino M, Monteleone AM, De Ronchi D, Fernández-Aranda F, Monteleone P. Beyond anorexia and bulimia nervosa: what's "new" in eating disorders. J Psychopathol. 2015;21:415–23.
16. American Academy of Sleep Medicine. International classification of sleep disorders. 3rd ed. Darien, IL: American Academy of Sleep Medicine; 2014.
17. Schenck C, Hurwitz T, Bundlie S, Mahowald M. Sleep-related eating disorders: polysomnographic correlates of a heterogeneous syndrome distinct from daytime eating disorders. Sleep. 1991;14(5):419–31. https://doi.org/10.1093/sleep/14.5.419.
18. Howell MJ, Schenck CH, Crow SJ. A review of night-time eating disorders. Sleep Med Rev. 2009;13(1):23–34. https://doi.org/10.1016/j.smrv.2008.07.005.
19. Auger RR. Sleep-related eating disorders. Psychiatry (Edgmont). 2006;3(11):64–70.
20. Chiaro G, Caletti MT, Provini F. Treatment of sleep-related eating disorder. Curr Treat Options Neurol. 2015;17(8):33. https://doi.org/10.1007/s11940-015-0361-6.
21. Winkelman JW, Johnson EA, Richards LM. Sleep-related eating disorder. Handb Clin Neurol. 2011;98:577–85.
22. Schenck CH, Mahowald MW. Review of nocturnal sleep-related eating disorders. Int J Eat Disord. 1994;15(4):343–56. https://doi.org/10.1002/eat.2260150405.
23. Brion A, Flamand M, Oudiette D, Voillery D, Golmard JL, Arnulf I. Sleep-related eating disorder versus sleepwalking: a controlled study. Sleep Med. 2012;13(8):1094–101. https://doi.org/10.1016/j.sleep.2012.06.012.
24. Komada Y, Takaesu Y, Matsui K, Nakamura M, Nishida S, Kanno M, et al. Comparison of clinical features between primary and drug-induced sleep-related eating disorder. Neuropsychiatr Dis Treat. 2016;12:1275. https://doi.org/10.2147/NDT.S107462.
25. Winkelman JW. Nocturnal binge eating is a familiar disorder (abstract). Sleep Res. 1993;68.
26. Winkelman JW. Sleep-related eating disorder and night eating syndrome: sleep disorders, eating disorders, or both? Sleep. 2006;29:876–7. https://doi.org/10.1093/sleep/29.7.876.

27. Zadra A, Pilon M, Montplaisir J. Polysomnographic diagnosis of sleepwalking: effects of sleep deprivation. Ann Neurol. 2008;63(4):513–9. https://doi.org/10.1002/ana.21339.
28. Matsui K, Komada Y, Nishimura K, et al. Prevalence and associated factors of nocturnal eating behavior and sleep-related eating disorder-like behavior in japanese young adults: results of an internet survey using Munich parasomnia screening. J Clin Med. 2020;9:1243. https://doi.org/10.3390/jcm9041243.
29. Tu C-Y, Meg Tseng M-C, Chang C-H. Night eating syndrome in patients with eating disorders: is night eating syndrome distinct from bulimia nervosa? J Formos Med Assoc. 2019;118:1038–46. https://doi.org/10.1016/j.jfma.2018.10.010.
30. McCuen-Wurst C, Ruggieri M, Allison KC. Disordered eating and obesity: associations between binge eating-disorder, night-eating syndrome, and weight-related co-morbidities. Ann N Y Acad Sci 2018;1411(1):96. doi: https://doi.org/10.1111/nyas.13467.
31. Lundgren JD, Allison KC, O'Reardon JP, Stunkard AJ. A descriptive study of non-obese persons with night eating syndrome and a weight-matched comparison group. Eat Behav. 2008;9(3):343–51. https://doi.org/10.1016/j.eatbeh.2007.12.004.
32. Spaggiari MC, Granella F, Parrino L, Marchesi C, Melli I, Terzano MG. Nocturnal eating syndrome in adults. Sleep. 1994;17(4):339–44. https://doi.org/10.1093/sleep/17.4.339.
33. Tholin S, Lindroos A, Tynelius P, Åkerstedt T, Stunkard AJ, Bulik CM, et al. Prevalence of night eating in obese and nonobese twins. Obesity. 2009;17(5):1050–5. https://doi.org/10.1038/oby.2008.676.
34. Geliebter A. Night-eating syndrome in obesity. Nutrition. 2001;17(6):483–4. https://doi.org/10.1016/S0899-9007(01)00550-0.
35. Meule A, Allison KC, Platte PA. German version of the Night Eating Questionnaire (NEQ): psychometric properties and correlates in a student sample. Eat Behav. 2014a;15(4):523–7. https://doi.org/10.1016/j.eatbeh.2014.07.002.
36. Gallant AR, Lundgren J, Drapeau V. The night-eating syndrome and obesity. Obes Rev. 2012;13(6):528–36. https://doi.org/10.1111/j.1467-789X.2011.00975.x.
37. Aronoff NJ, Geliebter A, Zammit G. Gender and body mass index as related to the night-eating syndrome in obese outpatients. J Acad Nutr Diet. 2001;101(01):102–4. https://doi.org/10.1016/S0002-8223(01)00022-0.
38. Lundgren JD, Rempfer MV, Brown CE, Goetz J, Hamera E. The prevalence of night eating syndrome and binge eating disorder among overweight and obese individuals with serious mental illness. Psychiatry Res. 2010;175(3):233–6. https://doi.org/10.1016/j.psychres.2008.10.027.
39. Meule A, Allison KC, Platte P. Emotional eating moderates the relationship of night eating with binge eating and body mass. Eur Eat Disord Rev. 2014b;22:147–51. https://doi.org/10.1002/erv.2272.
40. Yahia N, Brown C, Potter S, Szymanski H, Smith K, Pringle L, et al. Night eating syndrome and its association with weight status, physical activity, eating habits, smoking status, and sleep patterns among college students. Eat Weight Disord. 2017;22(3):421–33. https://doi.org/10.1007/s40519-017-0403-z.
41. Nolan LJ, Geliebter A. Validation of the Night Eating Diagnostic Questionnaire (NEDQ) and its relationship with depression, sleep quality, "food addiction", and body mass index. Appetite. 2017;111:86–95. https://doi.org/10.1016/j.appet.2016.12.027.
42. Calugi S, Dalle Grave R, Marchesini G. Night eating syndrome in class II–III obesity: metabolic and psychopathological features. Int J Obes (Lond). 2009;33(8):899–904. https://doi.org/10.1038/ijo.2009.105.
43. Andersen GS, Stunkard AJ, Sørensen TI, Petersen L, Heitmann BL. Night eating and weight change in middle-aged men and women. Int J Obes (Lond). 2004;28(10):1338–43. https://doi.org/10.1038/sj.ijo.0802731.
44. Bruzas MB, Allison KC. A review of the relationship between night eating syndrome and body mass index. Curr Obes Rep. 2019;8:145–55. https://doi.org/10.1007/s13679-019-00331-7.
45. Meule A, Allison KC, Brahler E, de Zwaan M. The association between night eating and body mass depends on age. Eat Behav. 2014c;15(4):683–5. https://doi.org/10.1016/j.eatbeh.2014.10.003.

46. Marshall HM, Allison KC, O'Reardon JP, Birketvedt G, Stunkard AJ. Night eating syndrome among nonobese persons. Int J Eat Disord. 2004;35(2):217–22. https://doi.org/10.1002/eat.10241.
47. Nolan LJ, Geliebter A. "Food addiction" is associated with night eating severity. Appetite. 2016;98:89–94. https://doi.org/10.1016/j.appet.2015.12.025.
48. Person S. Perceived stress, psychological functioning and sleep in night eating syndrome. Lakehead University Library. 2014. https://knowledgecommons.lakeheadu.ca/handle/2453/574.
49. Allison KC, Grilo CM, Masheb RM, Stunkard AJ. High self-reported rates of neglect and emotional abuse, by persons with binge eating disorder and night eating syndrome. Behav Res Ther. 2007;45(12):2874–83. https://doi.org/10.1016/j.brat.2007.05.007.
50. Gluck ME, Geliebter A, Satov T. Night eating syndrome is associated with depression, low self-esteem, reduced daytime hunger, and less weight loss in obese outpatients. Obes Res. 2001;9(4):264–7. https://doi.org/10.1038/oby.2001.31.
51. de Zwaan M, Roerig DB, Crosby RD, Karaz S, Mitchell JE. Nighttime eating: a descriptive study. Int J Eat Disord. 2006;39(3):224–32. https://doi.org/10.1002/eat.20246.
52. Gül HK, Aykut DS, Tiryaki A, Arslan FC. Night eating syndrome in patients with major depressive disorder. Klinik Psikofarmakoloji Bulteni. 2018;28(suppl S1):18.
53. Melo MCA, de Oliveira Ribeiro M, de Araújo CFC, de Mesquita LMF, de Bruin PFC, de Bruin VMS. Night eating in bipolar disorder. Sleep Med. 2018;48:49–52. https://doi.org/10.1016/j.sleep.2018.03.031.
54. Sassaroli S, Ruggiero GM, Vinai P, Cardetti S, Carpegna G, Ferrato N, et al. Daily and nightly anxiety among patients affected by night eating syndrome and binge eating disorder. Eat Disord. 2009;17(2):140–5. https://doi.org/10.1080/10640260802714597.
55. Nolan LJ, Geliebter A. Night eating is associated with emotional and external eating in college students. Eat Behav. 2012;13(3):202–6. https://doi.org/10.1016/j.eatbeh.2012.02.002.
56. Nolan LJ, Geliebter A. Factor structure of the Night Eating Diagnostic Questionnaire (NEDQ) and an evaluation of the diagnostic criteria of the night eating syndrome. J Eat Disord. 2019;7:39. https://doi.org/10.1186/s40337-019-0268-9.
57. Hirata FC, Lima MCO, de Bruin VMS, Nóbrega PR, Wenceslau GP, de Bruin PFC. Depression in medical school: the influence of morningness-eveningness. Chronobiol Int. 2007;24(5):939–46. https://doi.org/10.1080/07420520701657730.
58. Stunkard AJ, Allison KC, O'Reardon JP. The night eating syndrome: a progress report. Appetite. 2005;45(2):182–6. https://doi.org/10.1016/j.appet.2005.01.013.
59. O'Reardon JP, Ringel BL, Dinges DF, Allison KC, Rogers NL, Martino NS, et al. Circadian eating and sleeping patterns in the night eating syndrome. Obes Res. 2004;12(11):1789–96. https://doi.org/10.1038/oby.2004.222.
60. Birketvedt GS, Florholmen J, Sundsfjord J, Østerud B, Dinges D, Bilker W, et al. Behavioral and neuroendocrine characteristics of the night-eating syndrome. JAMA. 1999;282(7):657–63. https://doi.org/10.1001/jama.282.7.657.
61. Rogers NL, Dinges DF, Allison KC, Maislin G, Martino N, O'Reardon JP, et al. Assessment of sleep in women with night eating syndrome. Sleep. 2006;29(6):814–9.

When "Healthy" Is Taken Too Far: Orthorexia Nervosa—Current State, Controversies and Future Directions

14

Valeria Galfano, Elena V. Syurina, Martina Valente, and Lorenzo M. Donini

The term orthorexia (from the Greek "ortho" meaning "straight or "correct" and "orexi" meaning appetite) was coined by Steven Bratman, in 1997, to describe a pathological obsession with healthful eating. The first article was published in a peer-reviewed journal in 2004. The authors defined orthorexia nervosa (ON) as a "maniacal obsession" in the pursuit of healthy foods [1]. From this moment, many papers, in particular starting from 2011, have been published, and the ON has assumed a scientific dignity [2].

This chapter aims to summarize the current stand of the scientific knowledge about the disorder and highlight several important avenues for further exploration. Thus, the chapter will broadly consist of two sections. In the first one, we present the current scientific knowledge on ON, including its commonly accepted symptoms, risk factors, proposed diagnostic criteria and assessment tools as well as the latest developments in the field of therapeutic approach to ON. The second part of the chapter aims to highlight the latest controversies and on-going discussions in the field of ON research. Among them are aetiological discussion about ON, potential for presentation of ON as a continuum from healthy orthorexia to orthorexia nervosa and the potential role of culture in the behaviours associated with ON. We will then conclude with some suggested new avenues for scientific exploration of ON.

Valeria Galfano and Elena V. Syurina contributed equally to this work.

V. Galfano · L. M. Donini (✉)
Department of Experimental Medicine, Sapienza University, Rome, Italy
e-mail: lorenzomaria.donini@uniroma1.it

E. V. Syurina · M. Valente
Athena Institute, Faculty of Science, Vrije Universiteit Amsterdam, Amsterdam, The Netherlands
e-mail: e.v.syurina@vu.nl; m.valente@vu.nl

14.1 General Characteristics

"Eating disorders are serious and potentially fatal health problems that constitute a considerable burden of mental health problems" [3]. Societal influences and pressures are continuously changing and cause an evolution of eating patterns and behaviours. The remarkable influence of commercial food advertisements in our media today has contributed to the appearance of "orthorexic" subjects who select their foods based solely on whether or not they are considered to be properly healthful foodstuffs [4]. These individuals will obsessively follow strict diets that selectively avoid certain foods and therefore are insufficient and/or unbalanced. Moreover, this behaviour leads to changes in social and personal relationships, social isolation and finally changes in individual's general psycho-physical condition [5].

Symptoms of ON are related to pathological eating attitude leading to nutritionally unbalanced diet—foods are excluded based on a presumed impurity; these beliefs change from subject to subject and can be extremely variable; therefore, there is no characteristic food pattern of subjects with ON; impairment of physical health due to malnutrition follows the unbalanced diet and obsessive-compulsive symptoms—ritualized preoccupation with buying, preparing and consuming foods; excessive amounts of time are spent reading about, acquiring and/or preparing specific types of foods; guilty feelings and worries after transgressions; intolerance of other's food beliefs; severe distress or impairment of social or vocational functioning [6]. The perceived quality of food for these individuals becomes therefore more important than personal values, interpersonal relations, career plans and social relationships [7]. While other eating disorders such as "anorexia nervosa (AN)" and "bulimia nervosa (BN)" are obsessions about the quantity of food intake, "orthorexia nervosa" is focused on the quality of food intake. Self-esteem in these subjects is linked to the strong willpower that it is necessary to adhere to extreme food selection: they feel morally superior to those who eat "impure" foods [5].

ON is not currently recognized in the *Diagnostic and Statistical Manual of Mental Disorders, Fifth Edition* (DSM-5), but many eating disorder professionals agree on considering it a genuine syndrome in need of more research and awareness [8]. Similarly, in the scientific literature, there is an on-going debate regarding whether or not ON should be classified as being a distinct disorder, as an obsessive-compulsive disorder (OCD), a subtype of an existing eating disorder or a precursor for or a residual of an eating disorder (AN and BN patients may switch from an obsession with the quantity of food to an obsession with its quality, and vice versa) [9, 10]. In fact, a healthy diet may represent a socially acceptable method of weight control for anorexic and bulimic individuals [11].

Studies attempted to explore the relationship between ON and weight loss, in order to distinguish ON from other eating disorders, and therefore gain insights into the classification of ON. Although ON has initially been considered solely driven by health-related reasons, some studies reported an overlap between the driving forces of ON and those of other eating disorders, suggesting that also ON may be triggered by the desire for weight loss. For example, a study conducted in 2015 reported an association between ON and lower appearance evaluation and body area satisfaction: women suffering from ON were more likely to exercise regularly; perpetuate dieting, eating restraint and weight vigilance; and pay attention to appearance [12]. A 2017 study confirmed that ON is significantly correlated with appearance orientation, overweight preoccupation, self-classified weight and lower body area satisfaction [13]. More recently, a 2019 study confirmed these findings, demonstrating that the main motive for ON would be weight control, concluding that ON may be a maladaptive eating strategy driven by appearance-related reasons [14]. These findings suggest that the boundary between ON and other eating disorders may be blurred.

Such behavioural patterns can lead to a broad range of personal and societal consequences. ON may cause nutritional deficiencies due to avoidance of entire food groups. In particular, these patients may experience medical complications such as osteopenia, anaemia, hyponatremia, metabolic acidosis, pancytopenia, testosterone deficiency and bradycardia [15–17].

Psychologically, individuals with ON may feel frustrated when they disregard their food-related prescriptions, disgusted when food purity is apparently compromised and guilty when they commit food transgressions, worried about imperfection and nonoptimal health [11]. Indeed, dietary violations may cause a desire for self-punishment (e.g. stricter diet) or purification (e.g. cleansing fast) [15].

Finally, orthorexic subjects are frequently socially isolated since they are convinced that their health can be maintained only in isolation avoiding the influence of other people towards whom they often take on feelings of superiority [11].

14.2 Risk Factors and Drivers

There is an on-going investigation regarding the reasons why some individuals develop ON, while others do not. The investigation is focusing on the drivers of the ON behaviour and the predisposing factors that make individuals more susceptible to the development of the pathological behavioural patterns. These broadly can be divided into individual and societal groups.

14.2.1 Individual factors

A recent review of the literature identified risk factors for ON, these being perfectionism; obsessive-compulsive thoughts and behaviours; current or past history of other types of psychopathology, following a vegetarian/vegan diet; engaging in disordered eating habits; past dieting experience; Instagram use; and having a health-related background/occupation [18]. The same review also showed the lack of evidence that gender and self-esteem can be seen as factors contributing to increase in ON risk. Mixed findings were reported for the following factors: age, SES, BMI, belonging to a health-related field, exercise engagement, vegetarianism/veganism, body dissatisfaction and alcohol, tobacco, and drug use [18].

Findings linking drive for thinness and weight control to ON remain largely unclear. For example, findings assessing the link between body image, body dissatisfaction, BMI and ON are inconsistent; instead, a few studies confirmed a relationship between drive for thinness and thin-ideal internalization and ON [18]. Notably, a 2019 study reported that ON would be driven by weight control purposes, rather than health-related reasons [14].

One of the most researched predisposing factors is perfectionism. Despite it not being unique to ON and being shown to be implicated in the psychopathology of AN and BN, literature suggests it plays an important role in ON. Perfectionism is defined as a personality trait characterized by the search for excessively high standards, expectations of impeccability and disproportionate criticism of self and others. ON individuals are characterized by perfectionism since they aim to eat a "perfect" diet following strict dietary rules [11, 19].

14.2.2 Societal Drivers

Broader sociocultural trends and forces possibly triggering ON are weight bias and obesity stigma, availability of organic/clean food, high income, access to food research/knowledge, positive reinforcement from others, availability of time for food planning/preparation [18] and internalized fear for chronic conditions and non-communicable diseases [20], all of which seem to be highly related to modern Western culture [21]. This possible link between ON and cultural aspects will be discussed in more details in the second part of the chapter.

Body image, depression, social comparison and disordered eating are negatively affected by social media that are increasingly attended by young adults. The relationship between social media use and ON is controversial. Here, the attention was predominantly concentrated in the possible influence of Instagram on the prominence of ON behaviours. On the one hand, increased Instagram use has been associated with increased ON symptomatology [22]; on the other, positive and supportive conversations about ON were identified on Instagram, which suggest Instagram is also used as a platform to enhance recovery and healthier habits [23]. An online survey conducted among social media users ($N = 680$) following health food accounts found that higher Instagram use was associated with a greater tendency towards orthorexia nervosa, with no other social media channel having this effect. These results highlight the implications that social media, and in particular social media "celebrities", can have on psychological well-being [22].

14.3 Diagnostic Criteria

Although a growing number of articles concerning "orthorexia" have been published, at present, there is no universally shared definition of ON, the diagnostic criteria are under debate, and the psychometric instruments used in the literature revealed some methodological flaws [6].

Two key features should be present among the diagnostic criteria of ON:

(a) Obsessive focus on dietary practices believed to promote optimum well-being through healthy eating (with inflexible dietary rules, recurrent and persistent preoccupations related to food, compulsive behaviours)
(b) Consequent, clinically significant, impairment (e.g. medical or psychological complications, great distress and/or impairment in important areas of functioning) [2]

Specific diagnostic criteria proposed by the authors were used in few studies. Four of them published their proposal, allowing a brief comparison of criteria suggested to diagnose ON [6] (Table 14.1).

Many of the features described above echo symptoms of AN and obsessive-compulsive disorder (OCD), conditions that are themselves highly comorbid and have functionally similar clinical presentations [19].

14.4 Tools for Assessment of ON

The psychometric instruments that have been used in the studies on ON include the Bratman Orthorexia Test (BOT) [15] and the ORTO-15 [24] (that was recently revised and re-validated) [25], but these have revealed some methodological flaws [26, 27].

Additional psychometric tools used are EHQ (Eating Habits Questionnaire) [28], DOS (Dusseldorf Orthorexia Scale) [29], BOS (Barcelona Orthorexia Scale) [30] and TOS (Teruel Orthorexia Scale) [31].

In addition to the lack of a universally shared definition and diagnostic criteria, there are no official tools for evaluating ON tendency. Precisely, seven tools have been constructed, which have been subsequently adapted to other languages: the Orthorexia Self-Test (BOT) [15], the ORTO-15 [1, 24], the Eating Habits Questionnaire (EHQ) [28], the Dusseldorf Orthorexia Scale (DOS) [29], the Barcelona Orthorexia Scale (BOS) [30], the Teruel Orthorexia Scale (TOS) [31] and the Orthorexia Nervosa Inventory (ONI) [32].

The BOT and the ORTO-15 are the first tools constructed to assess ON and the most widely used by scholars. They were translated into different languages; for example, the BOT has been adapted to German [33] and Swedish [34], while the ORTO-15 to Turkish [35, 36], Portuguese [37], Hungarian [38], Polish [39, 40], German [41], English [13, 42], Spanish [43, 44], Arabic [45] and French [46]. Despite their popularity, these tools received criticisms [47, 48].

Table 14.1 Specific diagnostic criteria proposed by the authors

Setnick (2013)

Criterion A: pathological preoccupation with nutrition and diet far beyond that which is necessary for health, and undue influence of diet on self-evaluation, evidenced by characteristics such as:
1. Phobic avoidance of or response to foods perceived to be unhealthy, such as refusal to be in proximity to such food or experiencing panic while watching others eat the food
2. Severe emotional distress or self-harm after eating a food considered unhealthy
3. Persistent failure to meet appropriate nutritional needs leading to nutritional deficit and/or psychological dependence on individual nutrient supplements in place of food intake due to the belief that synthetic nutrients are superior to those found in food or that food is contaminated (except in cases where food is known to be contaminated)
4. Following a restrictive diet prescribed for a medical condition that the individual does not have or to prevent illness not known to be influenced by diet
5. Insisting on the health benefits of the diet in the face of evidence to the contrary
6. Marked interference with social functioning or activities of daily living, such as isolation when eating, avoidance of social functions where food is served or neglect of work, school or family responsibilities due to food-related activities

Criterion B: not the result of a lack of available food or a culturally sanctioned practice

Criterion C: the individual endorses a drive for health or life extension rather than a drive for thinness

Criterion D: the eating disturbance is not attributable to a medical condition or another mental disorder such as anorexia nervosa, bulimia nervosa or obsessive-compulsive disorder

Moroze et al. (2014)

Criterion A: obsessional preoccupation with eating "healthy foods", focusing on concerns regarding the quality and composition of meals (two or more of the following):
1. Consuming a nutritionally unbalanced diet due to preoccupying beliefs about food "purity"
2. Preoccupation and worries about eating impure or unhealthy foods and on the impact of food quality and composition on physical and/or emotional health
3. Rigid avoidance of foods believed by the patient to be "unhealthy", which may include foods containing any fat, preservatives, food additives, animal products or other ingredients considered by the subject to be unhealthy
4. For individuals who are not food professionals, excessive amounts of time (e.g. 3 or more hours per day) spent reading about, acquiring and/or preparing specific types of foods based on their perceived quality and composition
5. Guilty feelings and worries after transgressions in which "unhealthy" or "impure" foods are consumed
6. Intolerance of other's food beliefs
7. Spending excessive amounts of money relative to one's income on foods because of their perceived quality and composition

Criterion B: the obsessional preoccupation becomes impairing by either of the following:
1. Impairment of physical health due to nutritional imbalances, e.g. developing malnutrition due to unbalanced diet
2. Severe distress or impairment of social, academic or vocational functioning due to obsessional thoughts and behaviours focusing on patient's beliefs about "healthy" eating

Criterion C: the disturbance is not merely an exacerbation of the symptoms of another disorder, such as obsessive-compulsive disorder, or of schizophrenia or another psychotic disorder

Criterion D: the behaviour is not better accounted for by the exclusive observation of organized orthodox religious food observance or when concerns with specialized food requirements are in relation to professionally diagnosed food allergies or medical conditions requiring a specific diet

Barthels et al. (2015)

Table 14.1 (continued)

Setnick (2013)
Criterion A: enduring and intensive preoccupation with healthy nutrition, healthy foods and healthy eating **Criterion B**: pronounced anxieties for as well as extensive avoidance of foods considered unhealthy according to subjective beliefs **Criterion C** C1. At least two overvalued ideas concerning the effectiveness and potential health benefits of foods and/or C2. Ritualized preoccupation with buying, preparing and consuming foods, which is not due to culinary reasons but stems from overvalued ideas. Deviation or impossibility to adhere to nutrition rules causes intensive fears, which can be avoided by a rigid adherence to the rules **Criterion D** D1: The fixation on healthy eating causes suffering or impairments of clinical relevance in social, occupational or other important areas of life and/or negatively affects children (e.g. feeding children in an age-inappropriate way) AND/OR D2. Deficiency syndrome due to disordered eating behaviour. Insight into the illness is not necessary; in some cases, the lack of insight might be an indicator for the severity of the disorder **Criterion E**: intended weight loss and underweight may be present, but worries about weight and shape should not dominate the syndrome For diagnosing orthorexia, criteria A, B, C and E must be clearly fulfilled. Criterion D should be fulfilled at least partially. If criterion E is not clearly fulfilled, diagnosing atypical anorexia nervosa is recommended
Dunn and Bratman (2016)
Criterion A: obsessive focus on "healthy" eating, as defined by a dietary theory or set of beliefs whose specific details may vary; marked by exaggerated emotional distress in relationship to food choices perceived as unhealthy; weight loss may ensue as a result of dietary choices, but this is not the primary goal. As evidenced by the following: A1. Compulsive behaviour and/or mental preoccupation regarding affirmative and restrictive dietary practices believed by the individual to promote optimum health A2. Violation of self-imposed dietary rules causing exaggerated fear of disease, sense of personal impurity and/or negative physical sensations, accompanied by anxiety and shame A3. Dietary restrictions escalate over time, up till removing entire food groups, and involve progressively more frequent and/or severe "cleanses" (partial fasts) regarded as purifying or detoxifying. This escalation commonly leads to weight loss, but the desire to lose weight is absent, hidden or subordinated to ideation about healthy eating **Criterion B**: the compulsive behaviour and mental preoccupation become clinically impairing by any of the following: B1. Malnutrition, severe weight loss or other medical complications from restricted diet B2. Intrapersonal distress or impairment of social, academic or vocational functioning secondary to beliefs or behaviours about healthy diet B3. Positive body image, self-worth, identity and/or satisfaction excessively dependent on compliance with self-defined "healthy" eating behaviour

To date, new tools have been proposed, for example, the DOS [29], with its translations into English [49], Chinese [50] and Spanish [51], the newly constructed Orthorexia Nervosa Inventory (ONI) [32] or the ORTO-R [25].

14.5 Prevalence

While attempts to determine the prevalence of ON have been made, the lack of consensus on diagnostic criteria for the condition means there is not yet a reliable estimate available. The prevalence of ON ranges from less than 1 to 88.7%, with studies conducted in different population groups [2]. This range is obviously extremely wide, and no study has yet been conducted which has provided a reliable estimate [3, 35, 52–54]. Partially, this variety is caused by the use of varied assessment tools, which accounts for differences in cut-off scores as some of the instruments are known to be more prone for overestimation of ON behaviour, compared to others (see Sect. 14.4). However, what we also see in the literature is the increasing prominence of highly specific samples used for prevalence estimation. Some studies review the behaviours of general university students, while other studies focus on student in specific departments like nutrition and dietetics or medical students [55–57]. Even when the sample is not limited to university students, often it is fairly specific: for instance, one study focused on gym attendees or yoga practitioners [58, 59]. On the one hand, such sample specification is necessary and often justified by the fact that young adults (i.e. university students) are the group most at risk for development of ON. On the other hand, it also adds to the confusion regarding the actual scale of the issue and conflicting anecdotal evidence about ON. We observe a chicken and egg situation when the lack of official definition leads to confusion about the scale and conflicting evidence about the prevalence leads to discussion about official definitions of ON. Additionally, knowledge on health practitioners' opinions regarding ON is lacking [2, 35, 52–54].

Literature shows no clear correlation between ON and age, gender, education and socio-economic level. However, prevalence of ON seems higher among medical doctors, dietitians, Ashtanga yoga practitioners and exercise science students. It seems that more nutrition education may be related to a greater focus on healthy and correct nutrition and a higher trend for ON [35, 53, 60–62]. A high risk of ON emerged in athletes involved in performing arts [63] and fitness activities [34].

14.6 Current Stand on the Therapeutic Approach

The objective of the therapeutic approach is to make more varied the eating pattern, to improve socialization in particular during meals, to diversify leisure activities to include nonfood themes and to avoid or to treat malnutrition.

However, healthcare professionals agree on the necessity to have a multidisciplinary intervention involving physicians, psychotherapists and dieticians [64, 65].

The therapeutic protocol should combine medications (e.g. serotonin reuptake inhibitors and antipsychotics such as olanzapine), cognitive-behavioural therapy (focused on the symptoms that are prominent), relaxation training (to counteract pre- and postprandial anxiety) and psychoeducation (addressed on what patients eat, buy, prepare and feel about the food they consume while counteracting false food beliefs) with close monitoring in outpatient settings [11, 16, 64–68]. An inpatient approach should be proposed in case of significant malnutrition [16].

No studies concerning psychotherapy for ON have been published until now. ON, AN and OCD are highly comorbid conditions and present functionally similar clinical presentations [19]; therefore, prevention of exposure and response therapy (ERP) is probably an appropriate intervention also for the treatment of ON. According to international guidelines, ERP has become the gold standard psychological intervention for OCD in children and adults. To overcome the anxiety associated with obsessive thoughts, the individual's exposure to stimuli is necessary in the absence of behavioural rituals [69, 70].

ERP also represents a core component of the psychological treatment of AN [71].

Generally, obsessions and compulsions typical of ON, related to healthy eating, can be effectively treated with ERP techniques. Significant family involvement is essential in paediatric and adolescent patients [69]. Parents should have significant control over the domestic food environment and should receive instructions to support the child in following a nutritionally adequate diet. In the early stages of treatment, the patient and therapist work to develop an ERP hierarchy, incorporating exposure scenarios and eliminating compulsions (e.g. search on Google for energy content and nutritional values of food or eating food with unknown ingredients). Patients of all ages, especially those who have eliminated a large number of foods, should create easy/medium/hard food lists and should be encouraged to relatively quickly reintroduce "easy" and then "medium" foods into meals.

A predictable feeding schedule could help reduce pressure on patients by eliminating decision-making about when or if to eat. However, some patients with ON can be overly rigid by joining a structured meal plan. In these cases, deviating from the structure should be treated as an ERP exercise.

A strategy for patients of all ages, especially for paediatric, could be the use of concrete rewards to reinforce participation in ERP.

A key component of treatment is regular weighing, with patients made aware of their weight. To date, there is no evidence in the literature that open weighing has the iatrogenic effect of creating weight concern in patients who deny weight or shape problems [71].

14.7 Controversies and Discussions in the Literature

Despite the fact that ON is receiving an increasing amount of attention in the scientific literature, it continues being in the centre of heated academic debate. In the following section, we would like to highlight a few dimensions of this debate. We will start with the debate about the possible links between ON and other disorders, both eating and non-eating ones. Then we will present the latest argument against the black-and-white definition of the disorder and towards presenting it as a continuum of behaviours. Linked to these two, we will discuss the current stand on the potential role of culture in the development of ON and whether ON can be seen as a separate disorder or more as a cultural manifestation of distress. After a short presentation of the link between ON behaviours and the effects of health systems on these, we will conclude with a small section on our vision on the way forward for ON research.

14.7.1 Aetiological Discussion (ON and Other Disorders)

ON is commonly described in the literature as a new eating disorder or disordered eating pattern due to the fact that the symptoms of the phenomenon are focused on food intake. Individuals with ON behaviours develop obsession with the perceived quality and "healthiness" of the food they consume. Thus, a lot of debate surrounding the prospective introduction of ON as a separate diagnostic entity surrounds the distinctiveness of ON from other eating disorders: AN, BN and AFRID. This is further supported by the studies that have identified that having a history of eating disorders increases the risk of ON behaviour [13, 41, 54]. A recent study used a sample of adults self-reporting symptoms of varied eating disorders to further investigate the differences between ON and other eating disorders. Their findings suggest that ON symptoms were more strongly related to AN than to ARFID while also being a separate distinct entity [72].

However, the debate about the distinctiveness of ON stretches further than just comparing ON to AN, BN and AFRID. ON seems to be associated with BN [2, 60], while different authors found an association with different eating behaviours (restricting attitude [62], dieting [53] vegan and vegetarian diet) [53, 62, 73].

A variety of authors suggest a significant overlap between ON symptoms and obsessive-compulsive disorder (OCD) and obsessive-compulsive personality disorder (OCPD) [74]. This is especially linked to the high prevalence of obsessive thoughts and pre-occupation with certain patterns of food consumption [75]. Currently, there is no evidence definitively either proving or disproving the distinctiveness of ON from OCD and OCPD.

Another prominent disorder that is investigated regarding its possible common underlying aetiology is autism spectrum disorder (ASD). This has been suggested in a study about historical positioning of AN, ON and ASD due to the overlap between behaviours typical of AN and ASD, i.e. rigid attitudes and behaviours [76]. This was further supported, among others, by a study on opinions of the Dutch health professionals regarding the possible classification of ON [3] and the review of the psycho-social risk factors of ON [18]. It is however important to note that the relationship between ON and ASD symptoms is a complicated one as a recent study investigating the link between ON and cognitive inflexibility concluded that despite inflexible thoughts and behaviours specific for healthy eating, the condition does not seem to be associated with inflexibility as an executive function deficit [77].

Despite these discussions, studies that investigated the opinions of the health professionals and people who self-identify with having ON, as well as case studies, report ON being a distinct entity in need for official recognition: i.e. diagnostic criteria [3, 16, 78].

14.7.1.1 Can ON Be Seen as a Continuum?

Part of the diagnostic conversation about ON is linked to the application of the assessment tools, specifically the cut-off point that separates the "normal" from "disordered". It was previously identified that some instruments have a higher sensitivity and thus classify the behaviours more easily as ON compared to others [79, 80]. This was one of the reasons several researchers recently considered the fact the orthorexia may not be a single pathological construct, but rather have two aspects: orthorexia nervosa (linked to disordered behaviours and cognitions) and healthy orthorexia (having a natural interest in food quality and eating healthy). Such division was first introduced by Barrada and Rancero during their research on the development of one of the newer instruments to measure orthorexic tendencies [81]. They discovered that while items geared towards orthorexia nervosa were positively correlated to such phenomena as distress, restrained eating, OCD symptoms and low physical self-esteem, the items designed to measure healthy orthorexia were either unrelated or even negatively correlated to various psychopathological items [81]. The authors concluded that people who score high on the healthy orthorexia scale are in general interested in healthy diets without signs of psychopathology and they link their interest to their "lifestyle" and often are ready to spend considerable resources (time and money) to identify and utilize health alternatives for their meals. In this population, there is no indication of obsessive thoughts or pathological pre-occupations that are observed in the groups scoring high on orthorexia nervosa scales.

Similar findings were found in a recent paper which attempted to disentangle if the two proposed dimensions of orthorexia can be considered new eating styles or basically equivalent to restrained eating behaviour [73]. Following their analysis, they conclude that one should carefully distinguish between orthorexia nervosa and healthy orthorexia. While orthorexia nervosa is related to psychological distress, healthy orthorexia shows a different pattern and is related to well-being and may even serve as protective factor against psychological distress. Their analysis also, among others, showed that orthorexia could be distinguished from restrained eating, emotional eating and external eating. And one of the suggested conclusions was that orthorexia nervosa is offering a new dimension to restrictive eating pattern, which in turn feeds into the discussion about aetiology of orthorexia (see above). Moreover, it was noted that orthorexia nervosa and healthy orthorexia may also have different motivations. In the case of orthorexia nervosa, the main motive noted by the study was weight control, with sensorial appeal and affect regulation also showing significant associations. However, for healthy orthorexia, the main motive was health content, with sensorial appeal and price also showing significant associations [14]. In the recent paper, we reviewed the factors contributing to making choices about healthy eating and reviewed if some of those can potentially be seen as leading to development of orthorexic tendencies. Among the factors contributing to desire to eat healthy were the desire to take care of the body, the desire to have a fit body, the preference for the taste of healthy food, concerns about future chronic conditions and the desire to have a good appearance in adulthood [20]. However, only concerns about future chronic conditions were positively correlated with orthorexia nervosa tendencies. This further underlines the importance of more in-depth investigation about orthorexic behaviour. One solution would be to regard it as a continuum with healthy orthorexia on the one end of the spectrum and orthorexia nervosa on the other end. As with the majority of mental health disorders in general and eating disorders in particular, the transition from behaviours considered normal to those on the pathology spectrum is complex in nature and can take a long time. Thus, we believe it is crucial to further investigate the so-called tipping point: when does a positive intention of being healthy turn to the darker side of obsessive thoughts and behaviours that are harming the everyday life of the individuals?

14.7.2 Cultural Discussion

Another on-going discussion about ON is whether it can be seen as a separate, distinct condition or a more culture-bound disorder or even culturally defined manifestation of distress.

ON has been reported to disproportionally affect "Western" countries and to be directly linked to "Western culture" [19, 82, 83]. "Western culture" refers broadly to values like individualism, capitalism and materialism and is linked to industries like the food and diet industries, as well as the transferring of values and messages through mass media [84, 85]. Currently, it is unclear if ON is a culture-bound disorder and how and whether it should be classified.

Despite the fact that studies about ON have been conducted in many different countries, we can observe a certain trend as a vast majority of the studies have been conducted in the West European countries (i.e. Italy, Germany, Spain, Portugal, the Netherlands and the UK) or North America [86]. Notable exceptions to this rule were studies from Turkey and a small selection of Eastern European countries (i.e. Poland, Hungary) [38, 59, 87] and some studies from non-European countries, i.e. Lebanon [57]. Moreover, some comparative studies have reported significant differences in the prevalence and symptomology of ON between Western and Eastern European countries. For instance, a study comparing Italian, Spanish and Polish samples found difference in prevalence per country with ON behaviours seeming to be more prevalent in Poland [55]. Another interesting study compared the prevalence and symptomology between German and Lebanese samples [88]. This study concludes that culture is playing an important role in the development of eating pathologies and ON in particular. They also identified that prevalence of ON was higher in Lebanese sample, while some distinct patterns of beliefs were linked to higher risk of ON behaviours.

It is however important to note that current cross-cultural studies are commonly using the same measurement instruments that are often only linguistically validated, with no cultural adaptation.

14.8 Directions for Further Investigation: Use of Transdisciplinary Approach

There is a general agreement that more research and more in-depth investigations regarding the phenomenon of ON are needed. Among the areas that get continuous attention are risk factors leading to orthorexic behaviours, strive for a unified definition and diagnostic criteria, validation of the diagnostic instruments and looking into the pathways to help the individuals suffering from ON.

One of the directions we would like to highlight is the possibility of implementation of a new approach to investigation into ON. The fact that there are many sets of diagnostic criteria, none of which has received official recognition as a "golden standard", shed light on an underlying fragmentation of research about ON. The lack of official diagnostic criteria is particularly relevant in that it tells us that an official, shared conceptualization and understanding of ON may be missing. There seems to be a clear need for the scientific community to jointly define what are diagnostic attributes of ON. However, scientists cannot do it alone. The fact of ON being a complex phenomenon, because it is driven by broader societal forces and because it lies at the intersections between health and illness, makes impellent a transdisciplinary approach.

A transdisciplinary approach to research implies the elimination of the distinction between knowledge development and problem resolution. Knowledge co-production from scientific and societal actors is central: different perspectives come together in a learning process, which is required to solve complex issues. Within this approach, participatory techniques are needed to involve not only multiple disciplines but also multiple non-academic stakeholders in the research process [89, 90]. Research on ON may therefore benefit from a transdisciplinary approach, since different academic disciplines (psychology, nutrition, sociology, anthropology, etc.) and different societal actors (patients, food industry, health professionals, etc.) may be involved in understanding ON.

References

1. Donini LM, Marsili D, Graziani MP, Imbriale M, Cannella C. Orthorexia nervosa: a preliminary study with a proposal for diagnosis and an attempt to measure the dimension of the phenomenon. Eat Weight Disord. 2004;9(2):151–7. https://doi.org/10.1007/BF03325060.
2. Dunn TM, Bratman S. On orthorexia nervosa: a review of the literature and proposed diagnostic criteria. Eat Behav. 2016;21:11–7. https://doi.org/10.1016/j.eatbeh.2015.12.006.
3. Ryman FVM, Cesuroglu T, Bood ZM, Syurina EV. Orthorexia nervosa: disorder or not? Opinions of Dutch health professionals. Front Psychol. 2019;10:555. https://doi.org/10.3389/fpsyg.2019.00555.
4. Harris JL, Bargh JA, Brownell KD. Priming effects of television food advertising on eating behavior. Health Psychol. 2009;28(4):404–13. https://doi.org/10.1037/a0014399.
5. Bratman, S. Original essay on orthorexia; 1997. www.orthorexia.comS. Accessed April 2006.
6. Cena H, Barthels F, Cuzzolaro M, Bratman S, Brytek-Matera A, Dunn T, Varga M, Missbach B, Donini LM. Definition and diagnostic criteria for orthorexia nervosa: a narrative review of the literature. Eat Weight Disord. 2018;24 https://doi.org/10.1007/s40519-018-0606-y.
7. ANRED. Less-well-known eating disorders and related problems. http://www.anred.com/defslesser.htmlS. Accessed April 2006.
8. Vandereycken W. Media hype, diagnostic fad or genuine disorder? Professionals' opinions about night eating syndrome, orthorexia, muscle dysmorphia, and emetophobia. Eat Disord. 2011;19(2):145–55. https://doi.org/10.1080/10640266.2011.551634.
9. Dunn TM, Gibbs J, Whitney N, Starosta A. Prevalence of orthorexia nervosa is less than 1%: data from a US sample. Eat Weight Disord. 2017;22(1):185–92. https://doi.org/10.1007/s40519-016-0258-8.
10. Brytek-Matera A. Orthorexia nervosa–an eating disorder, obsessive-compulsive disorder or disturbed eating habit. Arch Psychiatry Psychother. 2012;1:55–60.
11. Mathieu J. What is orthorexia? J Am Diet Assoc. 2005;105(10):1510–2. https://doi.org/10.1016/j.jada.2005.08.021.

12. Brytek-Matera A, Donini LM, Krupa M, Poggiogalle E, Hay P. Erratum to: Orthorexia nervosa and self-attitudinal aspects of body image in female and male university students. J Eat Disord. 2016;4(16) https://doi.org/10.1186/s40337-016-0105-3.
13. Barnes MA, Caltabiano ML. The interrelationship between orthorexia nervosa, perfectionism, body image and attachment style. Eat Weight Disord. 2017;22(1):177–84. https://doi.org/10.1007/s40519-016-0280-x.
14. Depa J, Barrada JR, Roncero M. Are the motives for food choices different in orthorexia nervosa and healthy orthorexia? Nutrients. 2019;11(3):697. https://doi.org/10.3390/nu11030697.
15. Bratman S, Knight D. Health food junkies: orthorexia nervosa–overcoming the obsession with healthful eating. New York, NY: Broadway; 2000.
16. Moroze RM, Dunn TM, Craig Holland J, Yager J, Weintraub P. Microthinking about micronutrients: a case of transition from obsessions about healthy eating to near-fatal "orthorexia nervosa" and proposed diagnostic criteria. Psychosomatics. 2015;56(4):397–403. https://doi.org/10.1016/j.psym.2014.03.003.
17. Park SW, Kim JY, Go GJ, et al. Orthorexia nervosa with hyponatremia, subcutaneous emphysema, pneumomediastinum, pneumothorax, and pancytopenia. Electrolyte Blood Press. 2011;9(1):32–7.
18. McComb SE, Mills JS. Orthorexia nervosa: a review of psychosocial risk factors. Appetite. 2019;140:50–75. https://doi.org/10.1016/j.appet.2019.05.005.
19. Koven NS, Abry AW. The clinical basis of orthorexia nervosa: emerging perspectives. Neuropsychiatr Dis Treat. 2015;11:385–94. https://doi.org/10.2147/NDT.S61665.
20. Valente M, Syurina EV, Muftugil-Yalcin S, Cesuroglu T. "Keep Yourself Alive": from healthy eating to progression to orthorexia nervosa a mixed methods study among young women in the Netherlands. Ecol Food Nutr. 2020:1–20. https://doi.org/10.1080/03670244.2020.1755279.
21. Syurina EV, Bood ZM, Ryman FVM, Muftugil-Yalcin S. Cultural phenomena believed to be associated with orthorexia nervosa—opinion study in dutch health professionals. Front Psychol. 2018;9:1419. https://doi.org/10.3389/fpsyg.2018.01419.
22. Turner PG, Lefevre CE. Instagram use is linked to increased symptoms of orthorexia nervosa. Eat Weight Disord. 2017;22(2):277–84. https://doi.org/10.1007/s40519-017-0364-2.
23. Santarossa S, Lacasse J, Larocque J, Woodruff SJ. #Orthorexia on Instagram: a descriptive study exploring the online conversation and community using the Netlytic software. Eat Weight Disord. 2019;24(2):283–90. https://doi.org/10.1007/s40519-018-0594-y.
24. Donini LM, Marsili D, Graziani MP, Imbriale M, Cannella C. Orthorexia nervosa: validation of a diagnosis questionnaire. Eat Weight Disord. 2005;10:e28–32.
25. Rogoza R, Donini LM. Introducing ORTO-R: a revision of ORTO-15: based on the re-assessment of original data. Eat Weight Disord. 2020; https://doi.org/10.1007/s40519-020-00924-5.
26. Missbach B, Dunn TM, König JS. We need new tools to assess Orthorexia Nervosa. A commentary on "Prevalence of Orthorexia Nervosa among College Students Based on Bratman's Test and Associated Tendencies". Appetite. 2017;108:521–4.
27. Roncero M, Barrada JR, Perpiñá C. Measuring orthorexia nervosa: psychometric limitations of the ORTO-15. Span J Psychol. 2017;20:41.
28. Gleaves DH, Graham EC, Ambwani S. Measuring "orthorexia": development of the Eating Habits Questionnaire. Int J Educ Psychol Assess. 2013;12(2):1–18.
29. Barthels F, Meyer F, Pietrowsky R. Die Düsseldorfer Orthorexie Skala-Konstruktion und Evaluation eines Fragebogens zur Erfassung ortho-rektischen Ernährungsverhaltens. Z Klin Psychol Psychother. 2015;44(2):97–105. https://doi.org/10.1026/1616-3443/a000310.
30. Bauer SM, Fusté A, Andrés A, Saldaña C. The Barcelona Orthorexia Scale (BOS): development process using the Delphi method. Eat Weight Disord. 2018;24:247. https://doi.org/10.1007/s40519-018-0556-4.
31. Roncero M, Barrada JR, Perpiñá C. Measuring orthorexia nervosa: psychometric limitations of the ORTO-15. Span J Psychol. 2017;20:E41. https://doi.org/10.1017/sjp.2017.36.
32. Oberle CD, De Nadai AS, Madrid AL. Orthorexia Nervosa Inventory (ONI): development and validation of a new measure of orthorexic symptomatology. Eat Weight Disord. 2020; https://doi.org/10.1007/s40519-020-00896-6.

33. Kinzl JF, Hauer K, Traweger C, Kiefer I. Orthorexia nervosa: eine häufige essstörung bei diätassistentinnen. Ern Umschau. 2005;52(11):436–9.
34. Eriksson L, Baigi A, Marklund B, Lindgren EC. Social physique anxiety and sociocultural attitudes toward appearance impact on orthorexia test in fitness participants. Scand J Med Sci Sports. 2008;18(3):389–94. https://doi.org/10.1111/J.1600-0838.2007.00723.x.
35. Bosi ATB, Çamur D, Güler Ç. Prevalence of orthorexia nervosa in resident medical doctors in the faculty of medicine (Ankara, Turkey). Appetite. 2007;49(3):661–6. https://doi.org/10.1016/j.appet.2007.04.007.
36. Arusoğlu G, Kabakçi E, Köksal G, Merdol TK. Ortoreksiya nervoza ve Orto-11'in türkçeye uyarlama çalişmasi [Orthorexia nervosa and adaptation of ORTO-11 into Turkish]. Turk Psikiyatri Derg. 2008;19(3):283–91.
37. Alvarenga MS, Martins MC, Sato KS, Vargas SV, Philippi ST, Scagliusi FB. Orthorexia nervosa behavior in a sample of Brazilian dietitians assessed by the Portuguese version of ORTO-15. Eat Weight Disord. 2012;17(1):e29–35. https://doi.org/10.1007/BF03325325.
38. Varga M, Thege BK, Dukay-Szabó S, Túry F, van Furth EF. When eating healthy is not healthy: orthorexia nervosa and its measurement with the ORTO-15 in Hungary. BMC Psychiatry. 2014;14(59) https://doi.org/10.1186/1471-244X-14-59.
39. Brytek-Matera A, Krupa M, Poggiogalle E, Donini LM. Adaptation of the ORTHO-15 test to Polish women and men [published correction appears in Eat Weight Disord. 2014 Jun;19(2):271]. Eat Weight Disord. 2014;19(1):69–76. https://doi.org/10.1007/s40519-014-0100-0.

Fine Modulo

40. Stochel M, Janas-Kozik M, Zejda JE, Hyrnik J, Jelonek I, Siwiec A. Validation of ORTO-15 questionnaire in the group of urban youth aged 15–21. Psychiatr Pol. 2015;49(1):119–34. https://doi.org/10.12740/PP/25962.
41. Missbach B, Hinterbuchinger B, Dreiseitl V, Zellhofer S, Kurz C, König J. When eating right, is measured wrong! A validation and critical examination of the ORTO-15 questionnaire in German. PLoS One. 2015;10(8):e0135772. https://doi.org/10.1371/journal.pone.0135772.
42. Moller S, Apputhurai P, Knowles SR. Confirmatory factor analyses of the ORTO 15-, 11- and 9-item scales and recommendations for suggested cut-off scores [published correction appears in Eat Weight Disord. 2019;24(5):981]. Eat Weight Disord. 2019;24(1):21–8. https://doi.org/10.1007/s40519-018-0515-0.
43. Parra-Fernandez ML, Rodríguez-Cano T, Perez-Haro MJ, Onieva-Zafra MD, Fernandez-Martinez E, Notario-Pacheco B. Structural validation of ORTO-11-ES for the diagnosis of orthorexia nervosa, Spanish version. Eat Weight Disord. 2018;23(6):745–52. https://doi.org/10.1007/s40519-018-0573-3.
44. Parra-Fernandez ML, Rodríguez-Cano T, Onieva-Zafra MD, Perez-Haro MJ, Casero-Alonso V, Camargo JCM, Notario-Pacheco B. Adaptation and validation of the Spanish version of the ORTO-15 questionnaire for the diagnosis of orthorexia nervosa. PLoS One. 2018;13(1):e0190722. https://doi.org/10.1371/journal.pone.0190722.
45. Haddad C, Hallit R, Akel M. Validation of the Arabic version of the ORTO-15 questionnaire in a sample of the Lebanese population. Eat Weight Disord. 2019; https://doi.org/10.1007/s40519-019-00710-y.
46. Babeau C, Le Chevanton T, Julien-Sweerts S, Brochenin A, Donini LM, Fouques D. Structural validation of the ORTO-12-FR questionnaire among a French sample as a first attempt to assess orthorexia nervosa in France. Eat Weight Disord. 2019; https://doi.org/10.1007/s40519-019-00835-0.
47. Meule A, Holzapfel C, Brandl B, et al. Measuring orthorexia nervosa: a comparison of four self-report questionnaires. Appetite. 2020:146, 104512. https://doi.org/10.1016/j.appet.2019.104512.

48. Moller S, Apputhurai P, Knowles SR. Confirmatory factor analyses of the ORTO 15-, 11- and 9-item scales and recommendations for suggested cut-off scores [published correction appears in Eat Weight Disord. 2019 Oct;24(5):981]. Eat Weight Disord. 2019;24(1):21–8. https://doi.org/10.1007/s40519-018-0515-0.
49. Chard CA, Hilzendegen C, Barthels F, Stroebele-Benschop N. Psychometric evaluation of the English version of the Düsseldorf orthorexie scale (DOS) and the prevalence of orthorexia nervosa among a US student sample. Eat Weight Disord. 2018;24(2):275–81. https://doi.org/10.1007/s40519-018-0570-6.
50. He J, Ma H, Barthels F, Fan X. Psychometric properties of the Chinese version of the Düsseldorf Orthorexia Scale: prevalence and demographic correlates of orthorexia nervosa among Chinese university students. Eat Weight Disord. 2019;24(3):453–63. https://doi.org/10.1007/s40519-019-00656-1.
51. Parra-Fernández ML, Onieva-Zafra MD, Fernández-Muñoz JJ, Fernández-Martínez E. Adaptation and validation of the Spanish version of the DOS questionnaire for the detection of orthorexic nervosa behavior. PLoS One. 2019;14(5):e0216583. https://doi.org/10.1371/journal.pone.0216583.
52. Fidan T, Ertekin V, Sikay S, Kirpinar I. Prevalence of orthorexia among medical students in Erzurum, Turkey. Compr Psychiatry. 2010;51:49–54. https://doi.org/10.1016/j.comppsych.2009.03.001.
53. Valera JH, Ruiz PA, Valdespino BR, Visioli F. Prevalence of orthorexia nervosa among ashtanga yoga practitioners: a pilot study. Eat Weight Disord. 2014;19:469–72. https://doi.org/10.1007/s40519-014-0131-6.
54. Segura-Garcia C, Ramacciotti C, Rania M, Aloi M, Caroleo M, Bruni A. The prevalence of orthorexia nervosa among eating disorder patients after treatment. Eat Weight Disord. 2015;20:161–6. https://doi.org/10.1007/s40519-014-0171-y.
55. Gramaglia C, Gambaro E, Delicato C, et al. Pathways to and results of psychiatric consultation for patients referred from the emergency department. Are there differences between migrant and native patients? Transcult Psychiatry. 2019;56(1):167–86. https://doi.org/10.1177/1363461518798844.
56. Agopyan A, Kenger EB, Kermen S. The relationship between orthorexia nervosa and body composition in female students of the nutrition and dietetics department. Eat Weight Disord. 2019;24:257–66. https://doi.org/10.1007/s40519-018-0565-3.
57. Farchakh Y, Hallit S, Soufia M. Association between orthorexia nervosa, eating attitudes and anxiety among medical students in Lebanese universities: results of a cross-sectional study. Eat Weight Disord. 2019;24:683–91. https://doi.org/10.1007/s40519-019-00724-6.
58. Erkin Ö, Göl I. Determination of health status perception and orthorexia nervosa tendencies of Turkish yoga practitioners: a cross-sectional descriptive study. Progr Nutr. 2019;21(1):105–12.
59. Bóna E, Szél Z, Kiss D. An unhealthy health behavior: analysis of orthorexic tendencies among Hungarian gym attendees. Eat Weight Disord. 2019;24:13–20.
60. Asil E, Sürücüoğlu MS. Orthorexia nervosa in Turkish dietitians. Ecol Food Nutr. 2015;54(4):303–13.
61. Malmborg J, Bremander A, Olsson MC, Bergman S. Health status, physical activity, and orthorexia nervosa: a comparison between exercise science students and business students. Appetite. 2017;109:137–43.
62. Bo S, Zoccali R, Ponzo V, Soldati L, De Carli L, Benso A, Fea E, Rainoldi A, Durazzo M, Fassino S. University courses, eating problems and muscle dysmorphia: are there any associations? J Transl Med. 2014;12:221. https://doi.org/10.1186/s12967-014-0221-2.
63. Aksoydan E, Camci N. Prevalence of orthorexia nervosa among Turkish performance artists. Eat Weight Disord. 2009;14:33–7.
64. Bartrina JA. Ortorexia o la obsesión por la dieta saludable [Orthorexia or when a healthy diet becomes an obsession]. Arch Latinoam Nutr. 2007;57(4):313–5. Spanish.
65. Borgida A. In sickness and in health: orthorexia nervosa, the study of obsessive healthy eating [dissertation]. USA: ProQuest Information and Learning; 2012, pp/ 6376–6376. http://gradworks.umi.com/34/67/3467161.html. Accessed 15 Dec 2014.

66. Simpson HB, Wetterneck CT, Cahill SP, et al. Treatment of obsessive-compulsive disorder complicated by comorbid eating disorders. Cogn Behav Ther. 2013;42(1):64–76.
67. Schröder A, Heider J, Zaby A, et al. Cognitive behavioral therapy versus progressive muscle relaxation training for multiple somatoform symptoms: results of a randomized controlled trial. Cogn Ther Res. 2013;37(2):296–306.
68. Barsky AJ, Ahern DK, Bauer MR, et al. A randomized trial of treatments for high-utilizing somatizing patients. J Gen Intern Med. 2013;28(11):1396–404.
69. Freeman J, Sapyta J, Garcia A, Compton S, Khanna M, Flessner C, et al. Family-based treatment of early childhood obsessive-compulsive disorder: The pediatric obsessive-compulsive disorder treatment study for young children (POTS Jr)da randomized clinical trial. JAMA Psychiat. 2014;71(6):689–98.
70. Torp NC, Dahl K, Skarphedinsson G, Thomsen PH, Valderhaug R, Weidle B, Wentzel-Larsen T. Effectiveness of cognitive behavior treatment for pediatric obsessive-compulsive disorder: acute outcomes from the Nordic Long-term OCD Treatment Study (NordLOTS). Behav Res Ther. 2015;64:15–23.
71. Fairburn CG. Cognitive behavior therapy and eating disorders. New York: Guilford Press; 2008.
72. Zickgraf HF, Ellis JM, Essayli JH. Disentangling orthorexia nervosa from healthy eating and other eating disorder symptoms: relationships with clinical impairment, comorbidity, and self-reported food choices. Appetite. 2019;134:134–40. https://doi.org/10.1016/j.appet.2018.12.006.
73. Barthels F, Barrada JR, Roncero M. Orthorexia nervosa and healthy orthorexia as new eating styles. PLoS One. 2019;14(7):e0219609. https://doi.org/10.1371/journal.pone.0219609.
74. Scarff JR. Orthorexia nervosa: an obsession with healthy eating. Federal Practitioner. 2017;34(6):36–9.
75. Koven NS, Senbonmatsu N. A neuropsychological evaluation of orthorexia nervosa. Open J Psychiatry. 2013;3:214–22. https://doi.org/10.4236/ojpsych.2013.32019.
76. Dell'Osso L, Abelli M, Carpita B, et al. Historical evolution of the concept of anorexia nervosa and relationships with orthorexia nervosa, autism, and obsessive-compulsive spectrum. Neuropsychiatr Dis Treat. 2016;12:1651–60. https://doi.org/10.2147/NDT.S108912.
77. Hayatbini N, Oberle CD. Are orthorexia nervosa symptoms associated with cognitive Inflexibility? Psychiatry Res. 2019;271:464–8. https://doi.org/10.1016/j.psychres.2018.12.017.
78. Reynolds R, McMahon S. Views of health professionals on the clinical recognition of orthorexia nervosa: a pilot study. Eat Weight Disord. 2019; https://doi.org/10.1007/s40519-019-00701-z.
79. Reynolds R. Is the prevalence of orthorexia nervosa in an Australian university population 6.5%? Eat Weight Disord. 2018;23(4):453–8.
80. Gramaglia C, Brytek-Matera A, Rogoza R, Zeppegno P. Orthorexia and anorexia nervosa: two distinct phenomena? A cross-cultural comparison of orthorexic behaviours in clinical and non-clinical samples. BMC Psychiatry. 2017;17(1):75. https://doi.org/10.1186/s12888-017-1241-2.
81. Barrada R, Roncero M. Bidimensional structure of the orthorexia: development and initial validation of a new instrument. Anales De Psicología/Annals of Psychology. 2018;34(2):283–91.
82. Varga M, Dukay-Szabó S, Túry F, van Furth EF. Evidence and gaps in the literature on orthorexia nervosa [published correction appears in Eat Weight Disord. 2013;18(2):113. van Furth Eric, F [corrected to van Furth, Eric F]]. Eat Weight Disord. 2013;18(2):103–11. https://doi.org/10.1007/s40519-013-0026-y.
83. Oberle CD, Samaghabadi RO, Hughes EM. Orthorexia nervosa: assessment and correlates with gender, BMI, and personality. Appetite. 2017;108:303–10. https://doi.org/10.1016/j.appet.2016.10.021.
84. Eckersley R. Is modern Western culture a health hazard. Int J Epidemiol. 2006;35:252–8. https://doi.org/10.1093/ije/dyi235.
85. Hesse-Biber S, Leavy P, Quinn CE, Zoino J. The mass marketing of disordered eating and eating disorders: the social psychology of women, thinness and culture. Paper Presented at the Women's Studies International Forum, New York, NY; 2006, pp. 208–224. https://doi.org/10.1016/j.wsif.2006.03.007.

86. Domingues RB, Carmo C. Orthorexia nervosa in yoga practitioners: relationship with personality, attitudes about appearance, and yoga engagement. Eat Weight Disord. 2020; https://doi.org/10.1007/s40519-020-00911-w.
87. Tóth-Király I, Gajdos P, Román N, Vass N, Rigó A. The associations between orthorexia nervosa and the sociocultural attitudes: the mediating role of basic psychological needs and health anxiety. Eat Weight Disord. 2019; https://doi.org/10.1007/s40519-019-00826-1.
88. Strahler J, Haddad C, Salameh P, Sacre H, Obeid S, Hallit S. Cross-cultural differences in orthorexic eating behaviors: associations with personality traits. Nutrition. 2020;110811:77. https://doi.org/10.1016/j.nut.2020.110811.
89. Swaans K, Broerse J, Meincke M, Mudhara M, Bunders J. Promoting food security and well-being among poor and HIV/AIDS affected households: lessons from an interactive and integrated approach. Eval Program Plann. 2009;32(1):31–42. https://doi.org/10.1016/j.evalprogplan.2008.09.002.
90. Stock P, Burton RJF. Defining terms for integrated (multi-inter-trans-disciplinary) sustainability research. Sustainability. 2011;3(8):1090–113.

Pica

15

Alexandra Höger and Andrea Sabrina Hartmann

15.1 Symptomatic Presentation of Pica Disorder

Individuals diagnosed with pica disorder all share the same core symptom: the consumption of substances that are considered as non-food. Substances consumed are very idiosyncratic and may range from clay, raw starch, ice, body fluids (e.g., feces, vomit) to hair (for an overview, see [1]). Pica can be fatal, as was highlighted by Cruz and colleagues [2], who collected data on inpatient mortality over a 15-year period in a Portuguese community hospital and found a mortality rate of 9.1% ($n = 3$ out of $n = 31$) in pica, compared to, e.g., 0.9% ($n = 25$ out of $n = 1.750$) in anorexia nervosa (AN). Risks associated with pica depend on the substance ingested [1] and may include an iron and/or zinc deficiency [3], parasitic infections [4], (gastro)intestinal obstruction, and constipation [5].

Historically, pica behavior has been documented since the sixteenth century [6]. Its first appearance in a diagnostic manual was within the *Diagnostic and Statistical Manual of Mental Disorders* (DSM)-III [7], under the category of "Infancy, Childhood or Adolescence Disorders." In the DSM-IV [8], it remained in the similar category of "Disorders Usually First Diagnosed in Infancy, Childhood or Adolescence," up until the introduction of the DSM-5 in 2013, whereupon pica disorder was classified in "Feeding and Eating Disorders" alongside more commonly known disorders such as AN or bulimia nervosa [9]. This switch in classification highlights that the onset of the disorder may occur not only in childhood or adolescence but also over the entire lifespan [5, 9].

A. Höger (✉) · A. S. Hartmann
Department of Human Sciences, Institute of Psychology, Clinical Psychology and Psychotherapy, Osnabrück University, Osnabrück, Germany
e-mail: ahoeger@uos.de; andrea.hartmann@uos.de; andrea.hartmann@uni-osnabrueck.de

© Springer Nature Switzerland AG 2022
E. Manzato et al. (eds.), *Hidden and Lesser-known Disordered Eating Behaviors in Medical and Psychiatric Conditions*,
https://doi.org/10.1007/978-3-030-81174-7_15

According to the DSM-5, a diagnosis of pica disorder can only be given if the affected individual is older than 2 years in terms of developmental age and if the pica behavior is shown over the duration of at least 1 month [9]. The former criterion aims to exclude children in whom the oral exploration of non-food substances is considered as age-appropriate due to their lower developmental status. Furthermore, to warrant a diagnosis, the pica behavior should be neither socially nor culturally accepted [9]. In regions like sub-Saharan Africa, South America, and the Caribbean, the consumption of earth-like substances (e.g., clay, soil) is believed to heal different kinds of medical issues (e.g., nausea, infections; [10, 11]) and would therefore not justify a diagnosis of pica disorder. Lastly, a pica diagnosis in the context of another medical condition or mental disorder should only be given if the pica severity warrants additional clinical focus [9]. Not listed in the DSM-5 criteria, but repeatedly reported, is a craving for the ingested substance comparable to substance use disorders [12]. People with pica disorder sometimes spend a lot of their time and monetary resources obtaining the craved substance [13]. On top of this, affected individuals are often confronted with (self-)stigmatization [14], possibly leading to the development of secondary comorbidities (e.g., [15]).

15.2 Prevalence Rates

Reported worldwide prevalence rates for the general population range from 0.02 to 76.5% [12] and up to 27.8% for pregnant women [16], although studies in Western countries have found lower prevalence rates of pica behavior during pregnancy, ranging from 0.2% in Denmark [17] to 8.2% in the USA [18]. In children, single pica behavior incidents often present selectively (20.30%, [1]; 12.30%, [19]; 10%, [20]), but much less in a recurrent form (4.98%, [19]), and even less so above a clinical cut-off score (3.90%, [20]; 3.5 [21]). Specifically, 0.3–25% of children with intellectual disabilities (ID) are reported to have shown pica behavior depending on the setting [21, 22], 14–36% of children with autism spectrum disorders (ASD) [21, 23], as well as 28% of children with both ASD and ID [21].

When interpreting these studies, it should be noted that the criteria and diagnostic tools used to identify pica behavior or disorder vary strongly [24]. Furthermore, generalizing the prevalence rates is only possible to a limited degree, since most studies are community-based and not representative (e.g., [19, 25]).

15.3 Etiology

To date, no integrative etiological model of pica disorder exists. Rather, some etiological theories have been postulated, e.g., by Young [12], who attributes the development of pica behavior to three main reasons: (1) hunger, which might explain the elevated prevalence rates in African communities; (2) compensation for nutritional deficiencies; and (3) protection against other harmful matters. None of these theories have been confirmed empirically. First, pica behavior is shown not only in

African communities but also in societies with unlimited access to food (see Sect. 15.2), and it is not (only) triggered by hunger but rather by aspects such as the taste of the substance, indulgence, curiosity, the release of internal tension, or simply boredom [26]. Second, even though people with pica have an increased risk of anemia as well as lower hemoglobin, hematocrit, and plasma zinc levels, especially when consuming earth-like substances [3], these findings are correlational and do not allow for causal interpretations. And lastly, notwithstanding that some of the commonly ingested pica items have absorbing, detoxifying characteristics (e.g., clay, raw starch), substances consumed are also items that could directly cause injuries or lead to toxic reactions [13].

Despite being identified as often comorbid with anorexia nervosa (AN) in young adults in treatment centers [14], no correlations between pica eating and eating disorder psychopathology in general could be found in youth [19]. Thus, one might argue that hallmark features of the other eating disorders, e.g., body image disturbance and weight control, are not driving factors in the development and maintenance of pica eating [26]. Similarly, pica behavior has been reported to exist alongside learning disabilities [27], schizophrenia [28], obsessive-compulsive disorder [29], and depression [30], although it remains unclear whether there are shared etiological factors at work.

15.4 Diagnostic Assessment and Treatment

Previous studies did not reach consensus on the definitions of pica behavior or the diagnostic criteria for pica disorder. Only a small number of validated diagnostic and screening instruments for pica behavior or pica disorder exist. These can generally be divided into clinical interviews, which aim to confer a diagnosis, and questionnaires, which are either used as screening instruments or to examine the pathological behavior dimensionally, e.g., through self-constructed questionnaires (e.g., [25, 26]). To date, there are no standardized questionnaire-based instruments for adults [31], and only a few recent studies have tried to assess pica by using checklists in accordance with the DSM-5 criteria (e.g., [14]). Furthermore, the existing diagnostic interviews and questionnaires were constructed separately for children and adults [31], thus impeding the comparability of the measures across the age span. For instance, both the Screening Tool of Feeding Problems [32] and the Eating Disorders in Youth-Questionnaire [33] include pica behavior, but only focus on children. One step toward a standardized diagnostic instrument based on DSM-5 criteria was recently undertaken through the development of the semi-structured Pica, Avoidant Restrictive Food Intake Disorder (ARFID) and Rumination Disorder Interview (PARDI; [31]), which is applicable for both children and adults. Although reliability and internal validity of the PARDI have only been tested for ARFID and not yet for pica, it has shown promising results, which warrant further research attention. The PARDI, the Eating Disorder Assessment for DSM-5 (EDA-5; [34]), and the Diagnostic Interview Schedule for Children (DISC-IV; [35]) are the only approaches to an interview-based diagnosis of pica disorder. The most established diagnostic instrument for mental disorders, namely, the Structured Clinical Interview for DSM-5 (SCID-5; [36]), does not include a diagnostic segment on pica. Another diagnostic tool that can be used to achieve a better understanding of the functional properties and severity of pica is a behavioral analysis. According to the majority of the functional analyses carried out in reported (case) studies, pica behavior appears to be highly automatically reinforcing (e.g., [13, 37–40]). While the underlying mechanisms are not yet fully understood, self-stimulation or self-reassurance has been mentioned (e.g., [19]).

In terms of treatment, Sturmey and Williams [13] formulated five goals based on their review of the literature: (1) reducing the rate of pica, (2) increasing alternative behavior, (3) achieving a generalization and maintenance of the effects, (4) reducing behavior management strategies, and (5) preserving the safety of the patient. In order to achieve these goals, effective interventions are necessary. So far, only two randomized controlled trials assessing the treatment effects of micronutrient or iron supplementation on pica behavior in children have been published. Iron supplementation did not show significant effects in terms of treating pica behavior when compared to the administration of saline solution [41]; neither did the placebo-controlled administration of iron or micronutrient supplementation show significant predictive value for a reduction in geophagy [42]. Based on a systematic literature review of treatment studies, consisting predominantly of case studies, Moline and colleagues recommended a combination of reinforcement-based treatment techniques [37]. Notably, most of the studies included in the review targeted youth, meaning that these recommendations need to be taken with caution when referring to adult patients. In more detail, non-contingent reinforcement (NCR), differential reinforcement (DR), and environmental enrichment (EE) showed promising effects [37]. In NCR, a desired stimulus is added on a time-based schedule to provide an alternative to the automatic reinforcement of the pica substance. When used in combination with response blocking (RB), NCR has been found to lead to an initial 80% reduction in pica behavior in youth compared to baseline [43] and to result in an immediate reduction of pica behavior to near-zero levels [44]. By contrast, other studies did not yield such promising results (e.g., [45]). When using DR, only desired behaviors (e.g., not showing pica behavior, engaging in alternate behaviors) are reinforced, while the unwanted behaviors are extinguished. Even though one study found that DR led to initial decreases in pica ([46]), and another study reported short-term effects of DR combined with response blocking (RB) [47], long-term effects still need to be assessed [37]. EE works through the permanent availability of alternative reinforcing stimuli and seems to be more effective as part of a combination of treatments [48, 49] than as a solitary treatment approach [37].

Punishment-based techniques are often mentioned in older case studies (e.g., [50]), while it is nowadays mostly agreed that they should only be used if the pica behaviors endanger the patient and other strategies did not work. Methods like time-out, the use of contingent aversive stimuli, and physical restraint have proven to be effective in initially reducing pica behavior (e.g., [51–53]), but with limited maintenance of the effects [37].

15.5 Outlook

In sum, knowledge about pica disorder, and its etiological and maintaining factors, is limited, and studies on prevalence rates and treatment outcomes are restricted to certain target populations. Given the potentially fatal outcome of the disorder, there is a pressing need to better understand both its development and its treatment. Future research should therefore include patient groups that are diagnosed by standardized structured interviews based on DSM-5 criteria and should examine different combinations of the promising treatment techniques in order to gain a deeper understanding of their applicability across age groups, ethnicities, and comorbidities. Additionally, longitudinal studies are needed in order to better understand both the development and course of the disorder. And finally, randomized controlled trials to evaluate treatment options are called for.

References

1. Leung AKC, Hon KL. Pica: a common condition that is commonly missed—an update review. Curr Pediatr Rev. 2019;15(3):164–9. https://doi.org/10.2174/1573396315666190313163530.
2. Cruz AM, Goncalves-Pinho M, Santos JV, Coutinho F, Brandao I, Freitas A. Eating disorders-related hospitalizations in Portugal: a nationwide study from 2000 to 2014. Int J Eat Disord. 2018;51(10):1201–6. https://doi.org/10.1002/eat.22955.
3. Miao D, Young SL, Golden CD. A meta-analysis of pica and micronutrient status. Am J Hum Biol. 2015;27(1):84–93. https://doi.org/10.1002/ajhb.22598.
4. Rose EA, Porcerelli JH, Neale AV. Pica: common but commonly missed. J Am Board Fam Pract. 2000;13(5):353–8. https://doi.org/10.3122/15572625-13-5-353.
5. Hartmann AS, Becker AE, Hampton C, Bryant-Waugh R. Pica and rumination disorder in DSM-5. Psychiatric Ann. 2012;42(11):426–30. https://doi.org/10.3928/00485713-20121105-09.
6. Parry-Jones WL, Parry-Jones B. Implications of historical evidence for the classification of eating disorders. Br J Psychiatry. 1994;165:287–92.
7. American Psychiatric Association. Diagnostic and statistical manual of mental disorders (DSM-3). Washington, DC: American Psychiatric Association; 1975.
8. American Psychiatric Association. Diagnostic and statistical manual of mental disorders (DSM-4). Washington, DC: American Psychiatric Association; 1994.
9. American Psychiatric Association. Diagnostic and statistical manual of mental disorders (DSM-5). Washington, DC: American Psychiatric Association; 2013.
10. Kosuke Kawai K, Saathoff E, Antelman G, Msamanga G, Fawzi WW. Geophagy (soil-eating) in relation to anemia and helminth infection among HIV–infected pregnant women in Tanzania. Am J Trop Med Hyg. 2009;80(1):36–43.
11. Young SL. Pica in pregnancy: new ideas about an old condition. Annu Rev Nutr. 2010;30:403–22.
12. Young SL. Craving earth. Understanding pica. The use to eat clay, starch, ice and chalk. New York: Columbia University Press; 2011.
13. Sturmey P, Williams DE. Pica in individuals with developmental disabilities. Autism and child psychopathology series. Basel: Springer International Publishing; 2016.
14. Delaney CB, Eddy KT, Hartmann AS, Becker AE, Murray HB, Thomas JJ. Pica and rumination behavior among individuals seeking treatment for eating disorders or obesity. Int J Eat Disord. 2015;48(2):238–48. https://doi.org/10.1002/eat.22279.

15. Boyd JE, Adler EP, Otilingam PG, Peters T. Internalized stigma of mental illness (ISMI) scale: a multinational review. Compr Psychiatry. 2014;55(1):221–31. https://doi.org/10.1016/j.comppsych.2013.06.005.
16. Fawcett EJ, Fawcett JM, Mazmanian D. A meta-analysis of the worldwide prevalence of pica during pregnancy and the postpartum period. Int J Gynaecol Obstet. 2016;133(3):277–83. https://doi.org/10.1016/j.ijgo.2015.10.012.
17. Mikkelsen TB, Andersen AM, Olsen SF. Pica in pregnancy in a privileged population: myth or reality. Acta Obstet Gynecol Scand. 2006;85(10):1265–6. https://doi.org/10.1080/00016340600676425.
18. Rainville AJ. Pica practices of pregnant women are associated with lower maternal hemoglobin level at delivery. J Am Diet Assoc. 1998;98(3):293–6. https://doi.org/10.1016/S0002-8223(98)00069-8.
19. Hartmann AS, Poulain T, Vogel M, Hiemisch A, Kiess W, Hilbert A. Prevalence of pica and rumination behaviors in German children aged 7-14 and their associations with feeding, eating, and general psychopathology: a population-based study. Eur Child Adolesc Psychiatry. 2018;27(11):1499–508. https://doi.org/10.1007/s00787-018-1153-9.
20. Murray HB, Thomas JJ, Hinz A, Munsch S, Hilbert A. Prevalence in primary school youth of pica and rumination behavior: the understudied feeding disorders. Int J Eat Disord. 2018;51(8):994–8. https://doi.org/10.1002/eat.22898.
21. Fields V, Soke G, Reynolds A, Tian L, Wiggins L, Maenner M, et al. Pica, autism and other disabilities. Pediatrics. 2021; https://doi.org/10.1542/peds.2020-0462. Online ahead of print.
22. Ali Z. Pica in people with intellectual disability: a literature review of aetiology, epidemiology and complications. J Intellect Dev Disabil. 2001;26(3):205–15. https://doi.org/10.1080/13668250020054486.
23. LoVullo SV, Matson JL. Comorbid psychopathology in adults with autism spectrum disorders and intellectual disabilities. Res Dev Disabil. 2009;30(6):1288–96. https://doi.org/10.1016/j.ridd.2009.05.004.
24. Cooper SA, Smiley E, Morrison J, Williamson A, Allan L. Mental ill-health in adults with intellectual disabilities: prevalence and associated factors. Br J Psychiatry. 2007;190:27–35. https://doi.org/10.1192/bjp.bp.106.022483.
25. Ardeshirian KA, Howarth DA. Esperance pica study. Aust Fam Physician. 2017;46(4):243.
26. Hartmann AS. Pica behaviors in a German community-based online adolescent and adult sample: an examination of substances, triggers, and associated pathology. Eat Weight Disord. 2019; https://doi.org/10.1007/s40519-019-00693-w.
27. McNaughten B, Bourke T, Thompson A. Fifteen-minute consultation: the child with pica. Arch Dis Child Educ Pract Ed. 2017;102(5):226–9.
28. Tracy JI, de Leon J, Qureshi G, McCann EM, McGrory A, Josiassen RC. Repetitive behaviors in schizophrenia: a single disturbance or discrete symptoms? Schizophr Res. 1996;20(1-2):221–9.
29. Bharti A, Mishra AK, Sinha V, Anwar Z, Kumar V, Mitra S. Paper eating: an unusual obsessive-compulsive disorder dimension. Ind Psychiatry J. 2015;24(2):189.
30. Jawed SH, Krishnan VH, Prasher VP, Corbett JA. Worsening of pica as a symptom of depressive illness in a person with severe mental handicap. Br J Psychiatry. 1993;162(6):835–7.
31. Bryant-Waugh R, Micali N, Cooke L, Lawson EA, Eddy KT, Thomas JJ. Development of the pica, ARFID, and rumination disorder interview, a multi-informant, semi-structured interview of feeding disorders across the lifespan: a pilot study for ages 10-22. Int J Eat Disord. 2019;52(4):378–87. https://doi.org/10.1002/eat.22958.
32. Matson JL, Kuhn DE. Identifying feeding problems in mentally retarded persons: development and reliability of the screening tool of feeding problems (STEP). Res Dev Disabil. 2001;22(2):165–72.
33. Hilbert A, van Dyck Z. Eating disorders in youth questionnaire. Leipzig: University of Leipzig; 2016. Retrieved from: http://www.qucosa.de/recherche/frontdoor/?tx_slubopus4frontend%5bid%5d=urn:nbn:de:bsz:15-qucosa-197246.

34. Sysko R, Glasofer DR, Hildebrandt T, Klimek P, Mitchell JE, Berg KC, et al. The Eating Disorder Assessment for DSM-5 (EDA-5): development and validation of a structured interview for feeding and eating disorders. Int J Eat Disord. 2015;48(5):452–63.
35. Shaffer D, Fisher P, Lucas CP, Dulcan MK, Schwab-Stone ME. NIMH diagnostic interview schedule for children version IV (NIMH DISC-IV): description, differences from previous versions, and reliability of some common diagnoses. J Am Acad Child Adolesc Psychiatry. 2000;39(1):28–38.
36. First MB. Structured clinical interview for the DSM (SCID). Encyclopedia Clin Psychol. 2014:1–6.
37. Moline R, Hou S, Chevrier J, Thomassin KA. Systematic review of the effectiveness of behavioral treatments for pica in youths. Clin Psychol Psychother. 2020; https://doi.org/10.1002/cpp.2491. Online ahead of print.
38. McAdam DB, Breibord J, Levine M, Williams DE. Pica. handbook of evidence-based practice in clinical psychology. New York: Wiley; 2012.
39. Piazza CC, Roane HS, Keeney KM, Boney BR, Abt KA. Varying response effort in the treatment of pica maintained by automatic reinforcement. J Appl Behav Anal. 2002;35(3):233–46.
40. Wasano LC, Borrero JC, Kohn CS. Brief report: a comparison of indirect versus experimental strategies for the assessment of pica. J Autism Dev Disord. 2009;39(11):1582.
41. Gutelius MF, Millican FK, Layman EM, Cohen GJ, Dublin CC. Nutritional studies of children with pica: I. Controlled study evaluating nutritional status, II. Treatment of pica with iron given intramuscularly. Pediatrics. 1962;29(6):1012–23.
42. Nchito M, Wenzel Geissler P, Mubila L, Friis H, Olsen A. Effects of iron and multimicronutrient supplementation on geophagy: a two-by-two factorial study among Zambian schoolchildren in Lusaka. Trans R Soc Trop Med Hyg. 2004;98(4):218–27. https://doi.org/10.1016/s0035-9203(03)00045-2.
43. Call NA, Simmons CA, Mevers JEL, Alvarez JP. Clinical outcomes of behavioral treatments for pica in children with developmental disabilities. J Autism Dev Disord. 2015;45(7):2105–14.
44. Saini V, Greer BD, Fisher WW, Lichtblau KR, DeSouza AA, Mitteer DR. Individual and combined effects of noncontingent reinforcement and response blocking on automatically reinforced problem behavior. J Appl Behav Anal. 2016;49(3):693–8.
45. Piazza CC, Fisher WW, Hanley GP, LeBlanc LA, Worsdell AS, Lindauer SE, et al. Treatment of pica through multiple analyses of its reinforcing functions. J Appl Behav Anal. 1998;31(2):165–89.
46. Napolitano D, Blakkman L, Kohl L, Vallese H, McAdam D. The use of functional communication training to reduce pica. J Speech Lang Pathol Appl Behav Anal. 2007;2(1):25.
47. Slocum SK, Mehrkam LR, Peters KP, Vollmer TR. Using differential reinforcement of a discard response to treat pica. Behav Interven. 2017;32(3):234–41.
48. Horner RD. The effects of an environmental "enrichment" program on the behavior of institutionalized profoundly retarded children. J Appl Behav Anal. 1980;13(3):473–91.
49. Falcomata TS, Roane HS, Pabico RR. Unintentional stimulus control during the treatment of pica displayed by a young man with autism. Res Autism Spectr Disord. 2007;1(4):350–9.
50. Foxx R, Martin E. Treatment of scavenging behavior (coprophagy and pica) by overcorrection. Behav Res Ther. 1975;13(2-3):153–62.
51. Carter SL, Wheeler JJ, Mayton MR. Pica: a review of recent assessment and treatment procedures. Educ Training Dev Disabilities. 2004:346–58.
52. Ferreri SJ, Tamm L, Wier KG. Using food aversion to decrease severe pica by a child with autism. Behav Modif. 2006;30(4):456–71.
53. Singh NN, Bakker LW. Suppression of pica by overcorrection and physical restraint: a comparative analysis. J Autism Dev Disord. 1984;14(3):331–41.

Purging Disorder

16

Norbert Quadflieg

16.1 Introduction

The term purging disorder (PurD) was used only in the fifth edition of the *Diagnostic and Statistical Manual of Mental Disorders* (DSM-5; [1]). Actually, PurD as a clinical phenomenon is not new and was already described in earlier editions of the DSM (DSM-III-R, DSM-IV; [2, 3]) as an eating disorder not otherwise specified. DSM-IV defined PurD as "the regular use of inappropriate compensatory behavior (e.g. self-induced vomiting) by an individual of normal body weight after consumption of a small amount of food (e.g. two cookies)." The current DSM-5 named PurD and placed it under the heading of "Other specified feeding or eating disorders." Following the generally broad diagnostic approach of the DSM-5, the definition of PurD reads "recurrent purging behavior to influence weight or shape (e.g., self-induced vomiting, misuse of laxatives, diuretics, or other medications) in the absence of binge eating." This definition added two important extensions to the earlier definition: (1) PurD is no longer restricted to individuals with normal weight but covers all weight groups. (2) The amount of food consumed before purging is no longer restricted to being small but includes any amount of food below the threshold of a regular eating binge which by definition may be rather large. Essentially, PurD according to DSM-5 covers any inappropriate compensatory purging behavior without additional requirements concerning amount of food or body weight. As both anorexia nervosa (AN) and bulimia nervosa (BN) include purging behavior as a

N. Quadflieg (✉)
Department of Psychiatry and Psychotherapy, University of Munich (LMU), Munich, Germany
e-mail: Norbert.Quadflieg@med.uni-muenchen.de

© Springer Nature Switzerland AG 2022
E. Manzato et al. (eds.), *Hidden and Lesser-known Disordered Eating Behaviors in Medical and Psychiatric Conditions*,
https://doi.org/10.1007/978-3-030-81174-7_16

possible symptom, at this time, it is not clear if PurD is more typical for a restrictive-anorexic or for a bulimic eating disorder (ED).

Within this frame, Keel and Striegel-Moore [4] proposed a more stringent set of criteria putting PurD more clearly into the context of ED:

> "A Recurrent purging in order to influence weight or shape, such as self-induced vomiting, misuse of laxatives, diuretics, or enemas.
>
> B Purging occurs, on average, at least once a week for 3 months.
>
> C Self-evaluation is unduly influenced by body shape or weight or there is an intense fear of gaining weight or becoming fat.
>
> D The purging is not associated with objectively large binge episodes.
>
> E The purging does not occur exclusively during the course of anorexia nervosa or bulimia nervosa."

Studies on PurD applied varying definitions concerning the frequency and type of purging behavior, and empirical evidence on PurD is limited. This summary, therefore, will report existing evidence accepting the study-specific definitions of PurD without discussing the definitions in detail.

16.2 Prevalence

Several community studies addressed the prevalence of PurD. One study reported a point prevalence of 0.4% in girls aged 9–12; 1.9% in female adolescents aged 13–15; 2.5% each in age groups 16–18, 19–22, and 23–27; and 1.3% in females older than 27 years [5]. Another study [6] found a prevalence of 2.7% at age 14 in a mixed sample of male and female adolescents. A third study [7] reported 1-month prevalence separately for 11–19-year-old girls (4.8%) and boys (1.6%). Interestingly, this study also reported a 1-month prevalence of 4.5% in participants giving their sex as "other" (i.e., neither girl nor boy).

Community studies reported lifetime prevalence for young adult females as 6.2% [5], 3.8% until age 22 [8], and 5.3% at ages 28–39 [9].

Some data exist on lifetime prevalence in clinical samples. In a registry of adult females receiving specialized ED treatment, 8.2% were treated for PurD [10]. In adolescent outpatients aged 7–18 years, 4.5% were treated for PurD [11]. Tasca et al. [12] reported a prevalence of 6.7% (purging once a week) and 5.6% (purging twice a week) of PurD in a female tertiary care sample. For calendar years 1985–2004, a chart review of mostly females treated for an ED found a lifetime prevalence of 2.8% [13].

Most studies limit research to females, and little is known on the number of males affected by PurD. One study included 5.3% males in a sample of inpatients, a percentage higher than in AN, binge/purge type (1.9%) and BN, purging type (2.4%) in the same sample [14]. In another sample, 9.7% of adolescent outpatients were male [11].

Concluding, PurD is rare in young girls and shows a peak prevalence of 2–4% in adolescents and a decreasing prevalence in older adults. Between 6 and 8% of ED patients are treated for PurD.

16.3 Clinical Correlates

16.3.1 Compensatory Behaviors

In a large sample of treated females with PurD [10], vomiting was the most frequent purging behavior (82%), followed by laxative (18%) and diuretics (7%) use. Female twins with PurD from a population study reported vomiting (71%), laxative use (26%), diuretics use (36%), strict dieting (55%), fasting (50%), and vigorous exercise (55%) as compensatory measures [8].

16.3.2 Loss of Control Eating

Although by definition no large objective binges should occur in PurD, loss of control eating (subjective binges) is not uncommon. Of 79 adolescent outpatients with PurD, 23 (29%) reported loss of control eating. Those with and without loss of control eating did not differ in restraint, shape/weight/eating concerns and depression [15]. The level of subjective binge eating in PurD is higher than in BN [16].

16.3.3 Body Weight

Generally, the body mass index in PurD is in the normal range and comparable to the body mass index of BN [9, 10, 14, 17].

16.3.4 Weight/Shape/Eating Concerns

Individuals with PurD show elevated weight, shape, and eating concerns compared to controls without an ED [16, 18–20]. Generally, the level of these concerns seems to be similar in PurD and BN [15, 16, 18]. However, Smith and Crowther [20] reported lower concerns in PurD than in BN with high effect sizes.

16.3.5 Restraint

Restraint or cognitive control of eating is elevated in PurD compared to controls without an ED [18, 19] and on a similar level as BN [18].

16.3.6 Medical Complications

Purging behavior has a high potential to cause adverse medical conditions. Affection areas are the musculoskeletal, gastrointestinal, and cardiovascular system, skin, kidneys, and esophagus and teeth [21].

16.4 Comorbidity

Only very few studies report on comorbidity in PurD. Mood disorders are the most frequently found comorbid diagnoses at the time of treatment for PurD (69% [14], 36% [10]). Prevalence of anxiety disorders was 25% [14] and 19% [10]. Koch et al. [14] also reported 4% somatoform disorders and 11% personality disorders, mostly of the borderline type. Substance use disorder was reported by 11% in Ekeroth et al.'s [10] sample. In the female twin sample of Munn-Chernoff et al. [8], lifetime prevalence was 37% for major depressive disorder, 38% for alcohol use disorder, 4% for cannabis use disorder, and 32% for nicotine dependence. In a small sample of PurD ($N = 37$), 15% were found to have a personality disorder, a rate not higher than in BN [8].

16.5 Treatment

Treatment for PurD is not different from treatment for other EDs. Riesco et al. [22] reported a high drop-out rate from outpatient group cognitive-behavioral therapy for PurD. No RCT for the treatment of PurD exists. One RCT of cognitive-behavioral therapy included eight individuals with PurD in a mixed sample, but did not report results separately [23].

16.6 Outcome

Diagnostic outcome 1 year after treatment for PurD in a sample of 39 females was 15% PurD, 3% AN binge/purge type, 3% AN restricting type, 5% BN, and 31% subthreshold ED. No binge eating disorder (BED) was reported at follow-up. Remission rate was 44% [10].

In a larger sample ($N = 147$) of males and females treated for PurD, 5-year diagnostic outcome was 25% PurD, 5% AN binge/purge type, 1% AN restricting type, 5% BN purging type, 1% BED, and 22% subthreshold ED. No BN non-purging type was reported at follow-up. Remission rate was 42% [14].

A community study reported the 10-year diagnostic outcome in 56 adult females with PurD at the baseline assessment. At follow-up, 18% of the participants were diagnosed with PurD, 7% with BN, and 38% with other specified feeding or eating disorders (DSM-5). An additional 38% had no ED diagnosis. Interestingly, no significant changes from baseline to follow-up were reported for depression and state and trait anxiety [24].

In these studies, there was a considerable percentage of patients who retained the PurD diagnosis after 1–10 years. Cross-over to AN was rare, but some patients developed a full diagnosis of BN. Remission was not very high (less than half of the samples) in these studies. In adolescents, PurD showed little stability. Of 37 adolescents diagnosed with a PurD at age 14, 8% retained this diagnosis at age 17, and none retained this diagnosis at age 20. About one fifth of the sample crossed over to AN or BN, and no ED was found in 62% at age 17 and in 65% at age 20 [6].

Koch et al. [14] reported higher depression and somatization scores as well as a higher age at treatment to predict higher ED pathology scores. Stice et al. [25] addressed risk factors in adolescence for developing a PurD and found no specific predictors for PurD. According to the results of this study, risk factors for PurD seem to be the same as for other EDs. Analyzing weight suppression as single risk factor, however, showed that the increase of weight suppression by one standard deviation increased the risk of onset of PurD 1.5-fold, with an odds ratio of 1.46 (95% confidence interval 1.23–1.74). A similarly increased risk was found for the onset of AN and BN, but not for the onset of BED [26].

No deaths were reported over 10 years in PurD in a community sample [24]. There is only one study reporting standardized mortality in PurD. Out of 219 inpatients, 11 (5%) had died about 9 years later [27]. The standardized mortality ratio (SMR) was 3.90 (2.05–7.21), indicating a nearly fourfold risk for death in individuals with PurD compared to the general population of the same sex and age. This SMR is lower than in AN (5.35; 4.34–6.52) and higher than in BN (1.49; 1.10–1.97) [28].

16.7 Conclusion

PurD is a severe ED with a high potential of deadly outcome. It seems that purging behavior in its own is a point needing special attention in therapy, independent of the more impressing presence of eating binges.

References

1. American Psychiatric Association. Diagnostic and statistical manual of mental disorders. 5th ed. Arlington, VA.: American Psychiatric Association; 2013.
2. American Psychiatric Association. Diagnostic and statistical manual of mental disorders. 3rd ed. Washington DC: American Psychiatric Association; 1987, Revised.
3. American Psychiatric Association. Diagnostic and statistical manual of mental disorders. 4th ed. Washington DC: American Psychiatric Association; 1994, DSM-IV.
4. Keel PK, Striegel-Moore RH. The validity and clinical utility of purging disorder. Int J Eat Disord. 2009;42:706–19. https://doi.org/10.1002/eat.20718.
5. Glazer KB, Sonneville KR, Micali N, Swanson SA, Crosby R, Horton NJ, Eddy KT, Field AE. The course of eating disorders involving bingeing and purging among adolescent girls: prevalence, stability, and transitions. J Adolesc Health. 2019;64:165–71. https://doi.org/10.1016/j.jadohealth.2018.09.023.
6. Allen KL, Byrne SM, Oddy WH, Crosby RD. Early onset binge eating and purging eating disorders: course and outcome in a population-based study of adolescents. J Abnorm Child Psychol. 2013;41:1083–96. https://doi.org/10.1007/s10802-013-9747-7.
7. Mitchison D, Mond J, Bussey K, Griffiths S, Trompeter N, Lonergan A, Pike KM, Murray SB, Hay P. DSM-5 full syndrome, other specified, and unspecified eating disorders in Australian adolescents: prevalence and clinical significance. Psychol Med. Epub ahead of print. https://doi.org/10.1017/S0033291719000898.

8. Munn-Chernoff MA, Keel PK, Klump KL, Grant JD, Bucholz KK, Madden PA, et al. Prevalence of and familial influences on purging disorder in a community sample of female twins. Int J Eat Disord. 2015;48:601–6. https://doi.org/10.1002/eat.22378.
9. Wade TD, Bergin JL, Tiggemann M, Bulik CM, Prevalence FCG. Long-term course of lifetime eating disorders in an adult australian twin cohort. Aust New Zeal J Psychiatry. 2006;40:121–8. https://doi.org/10.1080/j.1440-1614.2006.01758.x.
10. Ekeroth K, Clinton D, Norring C, Birgegård A. Clinical characteristics and distinctiveness of DSM-5 eating disorder diagnoses: findings from a large naturalistic clinical database. J Eat Disord. 2013;1 https://doi.org/10.1186/2050-2974-1-31.
11. Vo M, Accurso EC, Goldschmidt AB, Le Grange D. The impact of DSM-5 on eating disorder diagnoses. Int J Eat Disord. 2017;50:578–81. https://doi.org/10.1002/eat.22628.
12. Tasca GA, Maxwell H, Bone M, Trinneer A, Balfour L, Bissada H. Purging disorder: psychopathology and treatment outcomes. Int J Eat Disord. 2012;45:36–42. https://doi.org/10.1002/eat.20893.
13. Nakai Y, Nin K, Noma S, Teramukai S, Fujikawa K, Wonderlich SA. Changing profile of eating disorders between 1963 and 2004 in a Japanese sample. Int J Eat Disord. 2018;51:953–8. https://doi.org/10.1002/eat.22935.
14. Koch S, Quadflieg N, Fichter M. Purging disorder: a comparison to established eating disorders with purging behaviour. Eur Eat Disord Rev. 2013;21:265–75. https://doi.org/10.1002/erv.2231.
15. Goldschmidt AB, Accurso EC, O'Brien S, Fitzpatrick KK, Lock JD, Le Grange D. The importance of loss of control while eating in adolescents with purging disorder. Int J Eat Disord. 2016;49:801–4. https://doi.org/10.1002/eat.22525.
16. Brown TA, Haedt-Matt AA, Keel PK. Personality pathology in purging disorder and bulimia nervosa. Int J Eat Disord. 2011;44:735–40. https://doi.org/10.1002/eat.20904.
17. Wade TD. A retrospective comparison of purging type disorders: eating disorder not otherwise specified and bulimia nervosa. Int J Eat Disord. 2007;40:1–6. https://doi.org/10.1002/eat.20314.
18. Keel PK, Haedt A, Edler C. Purging disorder: an ominous variant of bulimia nervosa? Int J Eat Disord. 2005;38:191–9. https://doi.org/10.1002/eat.20179.
19. Keel PK, Holm-Denoma JM, Crosby RD. Clinical significance and distinctiveness of purging disorder and binge eating disorder. Int J Eat Disord. 2011;44:311–6. https://doi.org/10.1002/eat.20821.
20. Smith KE, Crowther JH. An exploratory investigation of purging disorder. Eat Behav. 2013;14:26–34. https://doi.org/10.1016/j.eatbeh.2012.10.006.
21. Forney KJ, Buchman-Schmitt JM, Keel PK, Frank GK. The medical complications associated with purging. Int J Eat Disord. 2016;49:249–59. https://doi.org/10.1002/eat.22504.
22. Riesco N, Agüera Z, Granero R, Jiménez-Murcia S, Menchón JM, Fernández-Aranda F. Other specified feeding or eating disorders (OSFED): Clinical heterogeneity and cognitive-behavioral therapy outcome. Eur Psychiatry. 2018;54:109–16. https://doi.org/10.1016/j.eurpsy.2018.08.0010924-9338.
23. Macdonald DE, McFarlane TL, Dionne MM, David L, Olmsted MP. Rapid response to intensive treatment for bulimia nervosa and purging disorder: a randomized controlled trial of a CBT intervention to facilitate early behavior change. J Consult Clin Psychol. 2017;85:896–908. https://doi.org/10.1037/ccp0000221.
24. Forney KJ, Crosby RD, Brown TA, Klein KM, Keel PK. A naturalistic, long-term follow-up of purging disorder. Psychol Med. 2020:1–8. https://doi.org/10.1017/S0033291719003982.
25. Stice E, Gau JM, Rohde P, Shaw H. Risk factors that predict future onset of each DSM–5 eating disorder: predictive specificity in high-risk adolescent females. J Abnorm Psychol. 2017;126:38–51. https://doi.org/10.1037/abn0000219.

26. Stice E, Rohde P, Shaw H, Desjardins C. Weight suppression increases odds for future onset of anorexia nervosa, bulimia nervosa, and purging disorder, but not binge eating disorder. Am J Clin Nutr. 2020;112:941–7. https://doi.org/10.1093/ajcn/nqaa146.
27. Koch S, Quadflieg N, Fichter M. Purging disorder: a pathway to death? A review of 11 cases. Eat Weight Disord. 2013;19:21–9. https://doi.org/10.1007/s40519-013-0082-3.
28. Fichter MM, Quadflieg N. Mortality in eating disorders—results of a large prospective clinical longitudinal study. Int J Eat Disord. 2016;49:391–401. https://doi.org/10.1002/eat.22501.

Rumination Disorder 17

C. Laird Birmingham

17.1 Definition

Rumination disorder is the syndrome in which a patient repeatedly regurgitates the food they have swallowed up into their mouth, followed by chewing and swallowing it and then regurgitating it, over and over again [1–8]. The regurgitation is "partial vomiting" in that the vomitus doesn't leave the mouth.

This behavior is a reflex, only as conscious as a smile or a facial tic [9]. It is not accompanied by retching or distress. The patient who suffers from rumination disorder almost never reports it because they perceive it as disgusting. It is performed in a way that does not attract attention, but it is accompanied by an apparent calmness. The patient may be recurrently regurgitating and swallowing in front of you—without you noticing!

17.2 Case

A 21-year-old female, with a past history of anorexia nervosa, is admitted to a residential treatment center for bulimia nervosa. She had a medical, nursing, psychological, and psychiatric assessment on admission and has had a number of times in the past. Since admission she has had constant meal support with observation. After 2 weeks of treatment, she was asked specifically whether she "brought food back up into her mouth to be chewed and then swallowed as a habit to calm herself." She confirmed the habit but said she had not mentioned it because people would not understand and she felt disgusted with herself for doing it. Various treatments

---

C. L. Birmingham (✉)
Department of Psychiatry, University of British Columbia, Vancouver, BC, Canada
e-mail: Carl.birmingham@ubc.ca; http://www.drbirmingham.com

including psycho-education, chewing gum after meals, domperidone, warming, knitting, and cognitive behavioral therapy were tried with some success. The calming sensation that the rumination disorder caused was difficult for the patient to give up.

17.3 Prevalence

Uncertain, but likely 2–3% of eating disorder patients [10–13]

17.4 Associations

Less likely: restrictive anorexia nervosa

More likely: chronic bulimia nervosa or anorexia nervosa with bingeing purging and eating disorder patients who have mental disabilities

Making the Diagnosis [14–19]
1. You must ask! You must ask every patient you assess whether they regurgitate and then chew and swallow. To do this you must find a way of wording your question so it sounds routine and innocuous. For example:
   (a) You might say, "Many patients with eating disorders develop a habit—they may vomit food into their mouth and then chew and swallow it again." The patient may ask, "Why would they do that?" You respond, "It may cause a feeling of calmness." They might reply, "That happens to me sometimes, but not that often." Or they may respond, "I don't think the food comes all the way up into my mouth."
   (b) If the patient's description is consistent with rumination syndrome, the next step is psycho-education—telling them the pros and cons of this subconscious habit. The particularly devastating effect of this habit on teeth is usually enough to cause them to want to undertake treatment. During interventions the patient will report exactly what is happening, how often, how long, the benefits, and their concerns.
2. When is there a high index of suspicion?
   (a) In the "high-risk associations" listed above.
   (b) Calmness: Consider the diagnosis if the patient appears to be unusually calm after meals. Rumination disorder is not accompanied by retching or distress. It is performed in a way that does not attract attention but is accompanied by an apparent calmness.
   (c) Rapid erosion of teeth. The repeated regurgitation and prolonged presence of gastric contents in the stomach rapidly erode teeth.
   (d) Husky voice. The frequent regurgitation often causes chronic inflammation of the vocal cords that causes the voice to have a husky quality.
3. Don't assume the diagnosis has been excluded!

(a) A patient with rumination disorder may have been assessed by many healthcare professionals in the past. That does not lessen your obligation to consider the diagnosis when you see the patient. The "case report" above is typical of how often the diagnosis is missed.

17.5 Treatment [20]

1. Psychoeducation
   (a) Regurgitation stimulates the parasympathetic (relaxing) part of the brain. This can also be stimulated by knitting, warming, vagus nerve stimulation, and behaviors or habits that the patient can develop with their therapist.
   (b) Rumination disorder causes the coating of the teeth to rapidly decrease. Many patients will need to have dentures or dental reconstruction by their early 30s.
   (c) The esophagus will become weaker and weaker resulting in regurgitation and reflux throughout the day and night. This will cause the patient to experience anxiety rather than calmness.
   (d) Aspiration of the regurgitated material into their lungs becomes more likely over time, especially with inebriation or sedation caused by recreational or doctor-prescribed pills.
   (e) Chronic inflammation of the esophagus is associated with an increased risk of cancer of the esophagus.
   (f) Their vocal cords will become inflamed causing their voice to become hoarse.
2. Gum chewing
   (a) Gum chewing causes air to be swallowed down the esophagus. This can interfere with the food being regurgitated. However, too much air in the stomach can cause burping that may cause regurgitation. If gum chewing helps, continue it. If the gas becomes too great, simethicone tablets (usually a few at a time) can be taken to break up the gastric air bubbles, and the gum chewing can continue.
3. Prokinetic agent
   (a) Medications like domperidone and metoclopramide cause the lower esophageal sphincter to tighten and the stomach to empty, which decreases the likelihood of regurgitation. These medications take effect within 15–30 min, so they should be taken that long before a meal. They last for 6–8 h, so they can be taken three times a day before meals. Their effectiveness in rumination disorder is variable. Both are major tranquilizers with all of the attendant side effects of that class of medications. However, domperidone crosses the blood–brain barrier very little compared to metoclopramide, so domperidone is preferred.
   (b) Alternative methods of producing calmness: The use of warming with a warming pad on medium applied to the skin for 1 h at mealtime [21]; knitting [22]; yoga; and vagus nerve stimulation can be tried.
   (c) Cognitive behavioral therapy [23]

4. Treatments to avoid
    (a) Gastric surgical procedures such as fundo-plication have complications that outweigh any potential benefit.

17.6 Prognosis

In those with mental disabilities where the benefit of rumination disorder is learned, the prognosis for stopping the regurgitation is poor. Often, behavioral techniques that depend on aversive associations rather than rewards are tried—but I do not recommend them.

In eating disorder patients of normal mental ability, the prognosis is highly related to the presence of a reward of equal or greater value that is equally accessibility as compared to the benefits and complications of the rumination disorder. This is similar to treating substance use. Often, focusing on the negative consequences of the rumination disorder in the context of their text, hope for relationships and perhaps pregnancy is the key to successful treatment.

References

1. Birmingham CL, Firoz T. Rumination in eating disorders: literature review. Eat Weight Disord. 2006;11(3):e85–9.
2. Delaney CB, Eddy KT, Hartmann AS, Becker AE, Murray HB, Thomas JJ. Pica and rumination behavior among individuals seeking treatment for eating disorders or obesity. Int J Eat Disord. 2015;48(2):238–48.
3. Dahlgren CL, Wisting L, Ro O. Feeding and eating disorders in the DSM-5 era: a systematic review of prevalence rates in non-clinical male and female samples. J Eat Disord. 2017;5
4. Call C, Walsh BT, Attia E. From DSM-IV to DSM-5: changes to eating disorder diagnoses. Curr Opin Psychiatry. 2013;26(6):532–6.
5. Bryant-Waugh R, et al. Psychiatr Clin North Am. 2019;42(1):157.
6. Kelly NR, Shank LM, Bakalar JL, Tanofsky-Kraff M. Pediatric feeding and eating disorders: current state of diagnosis and treatment. Curr Psychiatry Rep. 2014;16(5)
7. Goleb PC. Rumination disorder resulting in severe malnutrition. J Invest Med. 2017;65(2):416.
8. Hartmann AS, Becker AE, Hampton C, Bryant-Waugh R. Pica and rumination disorder in DSM-5. Psychiatric Ann. 2012;42(11):426–30.
9. Lukas KE, Hamor G, Bloomsmith MA, Horton CL, Maple TL. Removing milk from captive gorilla diets: the impact on regurgitation and reingestion (R/R) and other behaviors. Zoo Biol. 1999;18(6):515–28.
10. Hartmann AS, Poulain T, Vogel M, Hiemisch A, Kiess W, Hilbert A. Prevalence of pica and rumination behaviors in German children aged 7-14 and their associations with feeding, eating, and general psychopathology: a population-based study. Eur Child Adolesc Psychiatry. 2018;27(11):1499–508.
11. Cruz AM, Goncalves-Pinho M, Santos JV, Coutinho F, Brandao I, Freitas A. Eating disorders-related hospitalizations in portugal: a nationwide study from 2000 to 2014. Int J Eat Disord. 2018;51(10):1201–6.
12. Murray HB, Thomas JJ, Hinz A, Munsch S, Hilbert A. Prevalence in primary school youth of pica and rumination behavior: the understudied feeding disorders. Int J Eat Disord. 2018;51(8):994–8.

13. Reis S. Rumination in 2 developmentally normal-children - case-report and review of the literature. J Fam Practice. 1994;38(5):521–3.
14. Kacar M, Hocaoglu C. What is pica and rumination disorder? diagnosis and treatment approaches. Klinik Psikiyatri Dergisi-Turkish J Clin Psychiatry. 2019;22(3):347–54.
15. Kliem S, Schmidt R, Vogel M, Hiemisch A, Kiess W, Hilbert A. An 8-item short form of the Eating Disorder Examination-Questionnaire adapted for children (ChEDE-Q8). Int J Eat Disord. 2017;50(6):679–86.
16. Kondo DG, Sokol MS. Eating disorders in primary care—a guide to identification and treatment. Postgrad Med. 2006;119(2):59–65.
17. Mairs R, Nicholls D. Assessment and treatment of eating disorders in children and adolescents. Arch Dis Child. 2016;101(12):1168–U134.
18. Mayes SD, Humphrey FJ, Handford HA, Mitchell JF. Rumination disorder—differential-diagnosis. J Am Acad Child Adolesc Psychiatry. 1988;27(3):300–2.
19. Thangavelu K, O'Brien P. Case report: recognizing first onset of rumination disorder in adults. Gen Hosp Psychiatry. 2006;28(5):446–7.
20. Fredericks DW, Carr JE, Williams WL. Overview of the treatment of rumination disorder for adults in a residential setting. J Behav Ther Exp Psychiatry. 1998;29(1):31–40.
21. Birmingham CL, Gutierrez E, Jonat L, Beaumont P. Randomized in controlled trial of warming anorexia nervosa. Int J Eat Disord. 2004;35(2):234–8.
22. Clave-Brule M, Mazloum A, Park RJ, Harbottle EJ, Birmingham CL. Managing anxiety in eating disorders with knitting. Eat Weight Disord. 2009;14(1):e1–5.
23. Thomas JJ, Murray HB. Cognitive-behavioral treatment of adult rumination behavior in the setting of disordered eating: a single case experimental design. Int J Eat Disord. 2016;49(10):967–72.

Achalasia and Disordered Eating Behaviours

18

Aurélie Letranchant

18.1 Introduction

Achalasia is a motor disorder of the oesophagus characterized by the absence of oesophageal peristalsis with hypertonia of the inferior oesophageal sphincter (IOS) and the absence of IOS relaxation following deglutition.

Firstly, this chapter will develop the epidemiology, the pathogenesis, the clinical characteristics, the additional examinations and the therapeutic strategies of achalasia. Secondly, we will consider the intricacies between achalasia and eating disorders (ED). Indeed, it is well-known that several feeding or eating disturbances can be primarily explained by or associated with medical conditions.

18.2 Achalasia

18.2.1 Epidemiology

Achalasia has an annual incidence of approximately 1/100,000 worldwide [1, 2]. It is a rare condition in children and adolescents, with an incidence of 0.11/100,000 [3]. Because of its chronicity, the estimated prevalence of achalasia is approximately 9/100,000 to 10/100,000 [1, 2]. Most studies have shown an equal gender distribution, with a diagnosis made on average between 30 and 60 years old [4]. No racial predilection has been highlighted [5]. The mean delay between onset of symptoms and diagnosis has been described to an average of 4–5 years [6].

A. Letranchant (✉)
Adolescent and Young Adult Psychiatry Unit, Institut Mutualiste Montsouris, Paris, France
e-mail: Aurelie.Letranchant@imm.fr

18.2.2 Pathogenesis

Achalasia is a motor disorder induced by a loss of nonadrenergic, noncholinergic, inhibitory ganglion cells in the myenteric plexus, causing unopposed cholinergic activity [7]. The loss of normal muscular functioning is progressive and irreversible.

Genetic, neurodegenerative, infectious and autoimmune mechanisms have been reported as triggers for the inflammatory destruction of inhibitory neurons in the myenteric plexus. Yet, the exact mechanism underlying neuronal loss remains unknown [8].

Genetic factors with an autosomal recessive mode of inheritance can be implicated. Achalasia has been depicted to be associated with Allgrove syndrome or triple A syndrome (achalasia, alacrymia and adrenal insufficiency) [9], Down's syndrome [10] and congenital central hypoventilation syndrome [11].

Several studies have implied a potential association between viral infections and achalasia [12, 13]. Indeed, Chagas disease, caused by Trypanosoma cruzi, very closely resembles the pathophysiology of primary achalasia [14].

Furthermore, achalasia patients are more likely to have concomitant autoimmune diseases [15], and the prevalence of serum neural antibodies is higher, giving more credit to an autoimmune aetiology [16]. Some studies have suggested possible roles of interleukin polymorphisms (IL-10 and IL-23) [17, 18].

Multiple case-control studies have reported a significant association with HLA class II antigens in idiopathic achalasia [19, 20]. A recent genetic association study imputed classical HLA haplotype and amino acid polymorphisms, suggesting immune-mediated processes in achalasia [21].

18.2.3 Clinical Characteristics

At the beginning of the disease, dysphagia can be very subtle and be misinterpreted as dyspepsia, poor gastric emptying or stress. As achalasia develops, difficulty to swallow typically appears with both solid foods and liquids. Other frequent symptoms identified are chest pain, regurgitation of indigested foods, coughing or asthma, odynophagia and epigastric pain [22]. Patients with achalasia can change their eating habits to facilitate the progression of the food bolus, by eating slower or adopting specific movements such as arching their back or raising their arms [23]. Impairments associated with achalasia are elevated risk of secondary oesophageal squamous cell carcinoma [24], respiratory problems due to airway compression or aspiration of undigested food [25] and a massively dilated and tortuous oesophagus [4].

18.2.4 Additional Examinations

Differential diagnosis first focuses on distinguishing a structural mechanical obstruction and a motility disorder.

18.2.4.1 Oesophagogastroduodenoscopy

Oesophagogastroduodenoscopy with mucosal biopsy should be carried out on most patients with either solid or liquid food dysphagia or both. One goal is to rule out gastroesophageal reflux disease, eosinophilic esophagitis, structural lesions (strictures or rings) and oesophageal cancer or "pseudoachalasia" [2]. Endoscopic findings in achalasia may range from a seemingly normal examination to resistance to intubation of the gastro-oesophageal junction [2] or a tortuous dilated oesophagus with retained food and secretions [23].

18.2.4.2 Barium Oesophagram

Signs of achalasia can be dilation of the oesophagus, a narrow esophagogastric junction with a "bird beak" appearance, aperistalsis and poor emptying of barium. The oesophagram also helps assess late- or end-stage achalasia changes (tortuosity, angulation, megaoesophagus) that impact the treatment course [23].

18.2.4.3 Manometry

Barium oesophagram and oesophagogastroduodenoscopy are complementary tests to manometry in the diagnosis and care of achalasia. However, neither of these two tests is subtle enough on its one to guarantee the diagnosis of achalasia [23].

As matter of fact, oesophageal manometry has become the standard for diagnosing and classifying achalasia, by monitoring oesophageal pressures and contractions along the length of a flexible catheter [26]. The manometric finding of aperistalsis and incomplete LES relaxation without evidence of a mechanical obstruction underlines the diagnosis of achalasia [23].

Three different subtypes of achalasia (types I, II and III) are singled out with high-resolution manometry and have both prognostic and potential therapeutic implications [27]. Type I includes impaired inferior oesophageal sphincter (IOS) relaxation, absent peristalsis and normal oesophageal pressure. Type II is defined by impaired IOS relaxation, absent peristalsis and increased pan-oesophageal pressure. Type III shows impaired IOS relaxation, absent peristalsis and distal oesophageal spastic contractions.

18.2.5 Therapeutic Strategies

Achalasia is a chronic condition with no curative therapies. Current treatment courses are focused on reducing the hypertonicity of the IOS by pharmacologic, endoscopic or surgical methods. The treatment aims at relieving patients' symptoms, easing oesophageal evacuation and preserving remaining oesophageal structure and function [2].

18.2.5.1 Medical Treatment

Oral calcium channel blockers or nitrates induce a swift decrease in IOS pressure with moderate benefit for dysphagia [2]. 5-Phosphodiesterase inhibitors, like sildenafil, have also been used to cut down oesophagogastric junction pressure and lower distal oesophageal contractions [28].

18.2.5.2 Botulinum Toxin
Injecting botulinum toxin into the muscle of the IOS can block the release of acetylcholine from nerve endings, thereby restoring the balance between excitatory and inhibitory neurotransmitters [2].

18.2.5.3 Pneumatic Dilation
A pneumatic dilator is a noncompliant cylindrical balloon, positioned fluoroscopically across the IOS and inflated with air using a handheld manometer. Even though surgical myotomy has a better response rate than a single pneumatic dilation, a series of dilations appears to be a sensible alternative to surgery [2].

18.2.5.4 Myotomy
The standard surgical approach for achalasia is laparoscopic Heller myotomy, which divides the circular muscle fibres of the IOS [2]. It has been established that an associated antireflux repair significantly decreases gastroesophageal reflux disease [29].

18.2.5.5 Per-Oral Endoscopic Myotomy
A recent treatment for achalasia is per-oral endoscopic myotomy (POEM) [30]. The procedure implies making a small mucosal incision in the mid-oesophagus and building a submucosal tunnel all the way to the gastric cardia. Selective myotomy of the circular muscle is accomplished with electrocautery [2].

18.2.5.6 Therapeutic Decisions
The treatment of achalasia is not curative, and up to one fifth of patients show symptoms that can require further treatments within 5 years [31, 32]. Laparoscopic Heller myotomy, pneumatic dilation and POEM are effective therapeutic processes [23]. The choice between these three treatment courses should depend on the achalasia type, local expertise and patient preference. Initial success rates of the POEM procedure are similar to those of laparoscopic Heller myotomy [30, 33]. POEM could be the favoured treatment for patients with type III achalasia [34]. Unfit surgical candidates should start by receiving a botulinum toxin injection in the IOS and should be aware that repeated therapy is often necessary. Other therapies with nitrates or calcium channel blockers may be proposed if there is no clinical response to the botulinum toxin. Oesophagectomy may be needed for patients with a dilated oesophagus (>8 cm) and a low responsiveness to an initial myotomy [23].

18.3 Achalasia and Eating Disorders

The diagnosis of achalasia is often achieved several years after onset, when the symptoms worsen with spontaneous or provoked vomiting and the resulting ionic imbalance, food restrictions and weight loss [35, 36].

Several physical, behavioural and psychosocial features of achalasia are similar to an eating disorder (ED) [36]. Food restriction and avoidance may represent a conditioned negative response to pain related to abnormal oesophageal emptying.

Patients with achalasia may have ritualistic ways to eat by eating slowly, chewing thoroughly or mashing or pureeing food [37]. Marked psychosocial disability, such as academic or athletic disability, is also mentioned, due to poor concentration and low energy levels [35].

Moreover, gastrointestinal symptoms such as delayed gastric emptying, postprandial distress, early satiety, constipation, oral or pharyngeal dysphagia and gastric reflux are often reported by individuals with ED [38–40], as are dysphagia, regurgitation and heartburn [41].

Various distinctive features of achalasia different from ED might assist the differential diagnosis. Achalasia may come to mind if the patient states that the regurgitated food tastes non-acidic or includes "bubbly saliva" between meals, as it is coherent with regurgitation of undigested food [42]. Achalasia may also come to mind if swallowing difficulties occur in public, which differs with the secret purging behaviour in bulimia nervosa [43]. Hunger and desire to gain weight are often reported in achalasia, unlike in patients with ED, for example, anorexia nervosa [36]. Clinicians should also be highly vigilant to unusual, stereotyped behaviours like raising the arms, arching the neck and shoulders or standing or sitting up straight during meals [44]. Individuals suffering from achalasia may also loosen belts and scarves or remove necklaces or neckties during meals, due to pain or discomfort.

Finally, a pre-existing ED could be complicated by secondary oesophageal achalasia [45]. In patients with bulimia nervosa, symptoms of eating disorder may predispose to achalasia through decreasing gastric motility and triggering myenteric plexus damage because of repeated vomiting [46]. Previous studies have suggested that these two disorders may trigger each other and create a vicious circle [46].

Therefore, excluding any organic disorder should be a priority when diagnosing an ED.

18.4 Conclusion

Achalasia is a rare chronic condition with a progressive and irreversible loss of normal muscular functioning. The diagnosis is often reached several years after onset, when the symptoms worsen. The earliest appropriate diagnosis and treatment are thus needed. We encourage an increased awareness on achalasia as an important diagnosis to consider, especially in the field of eating disorders (ED). Indeed, achalasia and ED share numerous clinical features, and the diagnosis can be mistaken. Furthermore, achalasia can occur in a pre-existing history of ED. It is important to ensure a multidisciplinary approach (including internists and psychiatrists) to the diagnosis and treatment of complex cases with interwoven somatic and psychiatric features [47].

Acknowledgements This work did not receive any specific grant from funding agencies in the public, commercial, or not-for-profit sectors.

Conflicts of Interest There is no conflict of interest.

References

1. Birgisson S, Richter JE. Achalasia in Iceland, 1952-2002: an epidemiologic study. Dig Dis Sci. 2007;52:1855–60. https://doi.org/10.1007/s10620-006-9286-y.
2. Pandolfino JE, Gawron AJ. Achalasia: a systematic review. JAMA. 2015;313:1841–52. https://doi.org/10.1001/jama.2015.2996.
3. Franklin AL, Petrosyan M, Kane TD. Childhood achalasia: a comprehensive review of disease, diagnosis and therapeutic management. World J Gastrointest Endosc. 2014;6:105–11. https://doi.org/10.4253/wjge.v6.i4.105.
4. Vaezi MF, Pandolfino JE, Vela MF. ACG clinical guideline: diagnosis and management of achalasia. Am J Gastroenterol. 2013;108:1238–49; quiz 1250. https://doi.org/10.1038/ajg.2013.196.
5. Sadowski DC, Ackah F, Jiang B, Svenson LW. Achalasia: incidence, prevalence and survival. A population-based study. Neurogastroenterol Motil. 2010;22:e256–61. https://doi.org/10.1111/j.1365-2982.2010.01511.x.
6. Eckardt VF, Köhne U, Junginger T, Westermeier T. Risk factors for diagnostic delay in achalasia. Dig Dis Sci. 1997;42:580–5. https://doi.org/10.1023/a:1018855327960.
7. O'Neill OM, Johnston BT, Coleman HG. Achalasia: a review of clinical diagnosis, epidemiology, treatment and outcomes. World J Gastroenterol. 2013;19:5806–12. https://doi.org/10.3748/wjg.v19.i35.5806.
8. Chuah SK, Hsu PI, Wu KL, Wu DC, Tai WC, Changchien CS. 2011 update on esophageal achalasia. World J Gastroenterol. 2012;18:1573–8. https://doi.org/10.3748/wjg.v18.i14.1573.
9. Alhussaini B, Gottrand F, Goutet JM, Scaillon M, Michaud L, Spyckerelle C, et al. Clinical and manometric characteristics of Allgrove syndrome. J Pediatr Gastroenterol Nutr. 2011;53:271–4. https://doi.org/10.1097/MPG.0b013e31821456ba.
10. Zárate N, Mearin F, Gil-Vernet JM, Camarasa F, Malagelada JR. Achalasia and Down's syndrome: coincidental association or something else? Am J Gastroenterol. 1999;94:1674–7. https://doi.org/10.1111/j.1572-0241.1999.01161.x.
11. Faure C, Viarme F, Cargill G, Navarro J, Gaultier C, Trang H. Abnormal esophageal motility in children with congenital central hypoventilation syndrome. Gastroenterology. 2002;122:1258–63. https://doi.org/10.1053/gast.2002.33062.
12. Jones DB, Mayberry JF, Rhodes J, Munro J. Preliminary report of an association between measles virus and achalasia. J Clin Pathol. 1983;36:655–7. https://doi.org/10.1136/jcp.36.6.655.
13. Robertson CS, Martin BA, Atkinson M. Varicella-zoster virus DNA in the oesophageal myenteric plexus in achalasia. Gut. 1993;34:299–302. https://doi.org/10.1136/gut.34.3.299.
14. de Oliveira RB, Rezende Filho J, Dantas RO, Iazigi N. The spectrum of esophageal motor disorders in Chagas' disease. Am J Gastroenterol. 1995;90:1119–24.
15. Booy JD, Takata J, Tomlinson G, Urbach DR. The prevalence of autoimmune disease in patients with esophageal achalasia. Dis Esophagus. 2012;25:209–13. https://doi.org/10.1111/j.1442-2050.2011.01249.x.
16. Kraichely RE, Farrugia G, Pittock SJ, Castell DO, Lennon VA. Neural autoantibody profile of primary achalasia. Dig Dis Sci. 2010;55:307–11. https://doi.org/10.1007/s10620-009-0838-9.
17. De León AR, de la Serna JP, Santiago JL, Sevilla C, Fernández-Arquero M, de la Concha EG, et al. Association between idiopathic achalasia and IL23R gene. Neurogastroenterol Motil. 2010;22:734–738.e218. https://doi.org/10.1111/j.1365-2982.2010.01497.x.
18. Nuñez C, García-González MA, Santiago JL, Benito MS, Mearín F, de la Concha EG, et al. Association of IL10 promoter polymorphisms with idiopathic achalasia. Hum Immunol. 2011;72:749–52. https://doi.org/10.1016/j.humimm.2011.05.017.
19. Verne GN, Hahn AB, Pineau BC, Hoffman BJ, Wojciechowski BW, Wu WC. Association of HLA-DR and -DQ alleles with idiopathic achalasia. Gastroenterology. 1999;117:26–31. https://doi.org/10.1016/s0016-5085(99)70546-9.
20. Wong RK, Maydonovitch CL, Metz SJ, Baker JR. Significant DQw1 association in achalasia. Dig Dis Sci. 1989;34:349–52. https://doi.org/10.1007/bf01536254.

21. Gockel I, Becker J, Wouters MM, Niebisch S, Gockel HR, Hess T, et al. Common variants in the HLA-DQ region confer susceptibility to idiopathic achalasia. Nat Genet. 2014;46:901–4. https://doi.org/10.1038/ng.3029.
22. Tsuboi K, Hoshino M, Srinivasan A, Yano F, Hinder RA, Demeester TR, et al. Insights gained from symptom evaluation of esophageal motility disorders: a review of 4,215 patients. Digestion. 2012;85:236–42. https://doi.org/10.1159/000336072.
23. Ates F, Vaezi MF. The pathogenesis and management of achalasia: current status and future directions. Gut Liver. 2015;9:449–63. https://doi.org/10.5009/gnl14446.
24. Zendehdel K, Nyrén O, Edberg A, Ye W. Risk of esophageal adenocarcinoma in achalasia patients, a retrospective cohort study in Sweden. Am J Gastroenterol. 2011;106:57–61. https://doi.org/10.1038/ajg.2010.449.
25. Miyamoto S, Konda Y, Matsui M, Sawada K, Ikeda K, Watanabe N, et al. Acute airway obstruction in a patient with achalasia. Intern Med Tokyo Jpn. 2011;50:2333–6. https://doi.org/10.2169/internalmedicine.50.5603.
26. Pandolfino JE, Kahrilas PJ. American Gastroenterological Association. American Gastroenterological Association medical position statement: clinical use of esophageal manometry. Gastroenterology. 2005;128:207–8. https://doi.org/10.1053/j.gastro.2004.11.007.
27. Pandolfino JE, Kwiatek MA, Nealis T, Bulsiewicz W, Post J, Kahrilas PJ. Achalasia: a new clinically relevant classification by high-resolution manometry. Gastroenterology. 2008;135:1526–33. https://doi.org/10.1053/j.gastro.2008.07.022.
28. Bortolotti M, Mari C, Lopilato C, Porrazzo G, Miglioli M. Effects of sildenafil on esophageal motility of patients with idiopathic achalasia. Gastroenterology. 2000;118:253–7. https://doi.org/10.1016/s0016-5085(00)70206-x.
29. Richards WO, Torquati A, Holzman MD, Khaitan L, Byrne D, Lutfi R, et al. Heller myotomy versus Heller myotomy with Dor fundoplication for achalasia: a prospective randomized double-blind clinical trial. Ann Surg. 2004;240:405–12; discussion 412-415. https://doi.org/10.1097/01.sla.0000136940.32255.51.
30. Inoue H, Minami H, Kobayashi Y, Sato Y, Kaga M, Suzuki M, et al. Peroral endoscopic myotomy (POEM) for esophageal achalasia. Endoscopy. 2010;42:265–71. https://doi.org/10.1055/s-0029-1244080.
31. Bonatti H, Hinder RA, Klocker J, Neuhauser B, Klaus A, Achem SR, et al. Long-term results of laparoscopic Heller myotomy with partial fundoplication for the treatment of achalasia. Am J Surg. 2005;190:874–8. https://doi.org/10.1016/j.amjsurg.2005.08.012.
32. Zaninotto G, Costantini M, Rizzetto C, Zanatta L, Guirroli E, Portale G, et al. Four hundred laparoscopic myotomies for esophageal achalasia: a single centre experience. Ann Surg. 2008;248:986–93. https://doi.org/10.1097/SLA.0b013e3181907bdd.
33. von Renteln D, Inoue H, Minami H, Werner YB, Pace A, Kersten JF, et al. Peroral endoscopic myotomy for the treatment of achalasia: a prospective single center study. Am J Gastroenterol. 2012;107:411–7. https://doi.org/10.1038/ajg.2011.388.
34. Khashab MA, Vela MF, Thosani N, Agrawal D, Buxbaum JL, Abbas Fehmi SM, et al. ASGE guideline on the management of achalasia. Gastrointest Endosc. 2019; https://doi.org/10.1016/j.gie.2019.04.231.
35. Däbritz J, Domagk D, Monninger M, Foell D. Achalasia mistaken as eating disorders: report of two children and review of the literature. Eur J Gastroenterol Hepatol. 2010;22:775–8. https://doi.org/10.1097/MEG.0b013e3283325d71.
36. Reas DL, Zipfel S, Rø Ø. Is it an eating disorder or achalasia or both? A literature review and diagnostic challenges. Eur Eat Disord Rev. 2014;22:321–30. https://doi.org/10.1002/erv.2307.
37. Richterich A, Brunner R, Resch F. Achalasia mimicking prepubertal anorexia nervosa. Int J Eat Disord. 2003;33:356–9. https://doi.org/10.1002/eat.10144.
38. Bern EM, O'Brien RF. Is it an eating disorder, gastrointestinal disorder, or both? Curr Opin Pediatr. 2013;25:463–70. https://doi.org/10.1097/MOP.0b013e328362d1ad.
39. Mehler PS. Medical complications of bulimia nervosa and their treatments. Int J Eat Disord. 2011;44:95–104. https://doi.org/10.1002/eat.20825.

40. Zipfel S, Sammet I, Rapps N, Herzog W, Herpertz S, Martens U. Gastrointestinal disturbances in eating disorders: clinical and neurobiological aspects. Auton Neurosci. 2006;129:99–106. https://doi.org/10.1016/j.autneu.2006.07.023.
41. Benini L, Todesco T, Frulloni L, Dalle Grave R, Campagnola P, Agugiaro F, et al. Esophageal motility and symptoms in restricting and binge-eating/purging anorexia. Dig Liver Dis. 2010;42:767–72. https://doi.org/10.1016/j.dld.2010.03.018.
42. Cook IJ. Diagnostic evaluation of dysphagia. Nat Clin Pract Gastroenterol Hepatol. 2008;5:393–403. https://doi.org/10.1038/ncpgasthep1153.
43. Gravier V, Naja W, Blaise M, Cremniter D. Achalasia and megaesophagus misdiagnosed as anorexia nervosa. Eur Psychiatry. 1998;13:315–6. https://doi.org/10.1016/S0924-9338(98)80050-3.
44. Blam ME, Delfyett W, Levine MS, Metz DC, Katzka DA. Achalasia: a disease of varied and subtle symptoms that do not correlate with radiographic findings. Am J Gastroenterol. 2002;97:1916–23. https://doi.org/10.1111/j.1572-0241.2002.05900.x.
45. Kutuk MO, Guler G, Tufan AE, Toros F, Kaytanli U. Achalasia as a complication of bulimia nervosa: a case report. S Afr J Psychiatr. 2017;23:996. https://doi.org/10.4102/sajpsychiatry.v23.996.
46. Teufel M, Lamprecht G, Zipfel S, Schrauth M, Rapps N, Martens U, et al. Vomiting and feeling fat—coincidence of achalasia and bulimia nervosa. Int J Eat Disord. 2009;42:90–2. https://doi.org/10.1002/eat.20582.
47. De Hert M, Correll CU, Bobes J, Cetkovich-Bakmas M, Cohen D, Asai I, et al. Physical illness in patients with severe mental disorders. I. Prevalence, impact of medications and disparities in health care. World Psychiatry. 2011;10:52–77. https://doi.org/10.1002/j.2051-5545.2011.tb00014.x.

Cancer and Disordered Eating Behavior: The Issue of Anorexia

19

Alessio Molfino, Maria Ida Amabile, Giovanni Imbimbo, Antonella Giorgi, and Maurizio Muscaritoli

19.1 Introduction

Appetite is the physiological desire to eat. Altered eating behavior, determining the reduction or loss of the desire to eat, is defined as *anorexia*. Although commonly classified as a symptom, anorexia should be rather considered a complex, multifactorial syndrome with negative clinical effects during the course of several acute and chronic clinical conditions [1].

Interestingly, while experimental and clinical studies have documented that anorexia determines a protective effect, conferring survival advantage following acute stress and/or trauma [2], the prolonged loss of appetite represents a negative prognostic factor when it develops in patients affected by chronic diseases, in particular cancer [3]. Anorexia in cancer patients may lead to body weight loss and may reduce quality of life and survival and increase complications [4]. Besides the underlying mechanisms determining the loss of appetite, several factors contribute to reduced food intake, in part due to the physical location of the primary cancer, especially in case of involvement of the digestive tract, and due to factors affecting nutrient absorption which can be determined by mouth ulcers, altered bowel habit, vomiting, and pain, and in part due to the impact of systemic antineoplastic therapy (i.e., chemotherapy), radiotherapy, or malabsorption [3, 5, 6].

Moreover, appetite alterations during cancer are often associated with increased inflammatory response. Elevation in inflammatory markers may be determined by the presence of cancer itself or by the effects for chemo- and radiotherapies [7].

A. Molfino · M. I. Amabile · G. Imbimbo · A. Giorgi · M. Muscaritoli (✉)
Department of Translational and Precision Medicine, Sapienza University of Rome, Rome, Italy
e-mail: alessio.molfino@uniroma1.it; mariaida.amabile@uniroma1.it; imbimbo.1638090@studenti.uniroma1.it; antonella.giorgi@uniroma1.it; maurizio.muscaritoli@uniroma1.it

© Springer Nature Switzerland AG 2022
E. Manzato et al. (eds.), *Hidden and Lesser-known Disordered Eating Behaviors in Medical and Psychiatric Conditions*,
https://doi.org/10.1007/978-3-030-81174-7_19

The pathophysiology of cancer anorexia is complex and involves different domains influencing eating behavior [7] and recognizing mechanisms altering appetite control within the central nervous system [5, 6]. Low appetite may be induced by molecules produced by the tumor, such as pro-inflammatory cytokines, small peptides and metabolites, and others that are able to alter food intake, including increased serum levels of the amino acid tryptophan (the precursor of the neurotransmitter serotonin); hormones such as ghrelin and leptin have been investigated in several experimental and clinical conditions showing direct and indirect effects on appetite levels during cancer [8].

Specific nutrient deficiency (i.e., low zinc circulating levels) may be associated with reduced appetite. In addition, chemotherapy can alter taste perception determining nausea, vomiting, mucositis, and abdominal pain, symptoms that can lead to the loss of appetite [6].

More recently, a role has been identified for the growth/differentiation factor (GDF 15), a cytokine implicated in cancer-associated weight loss, which acts to reduce food intake through activation of its high-affinity binding brain receptor (GFRAL-RET) and has become a target of interest for anti-obesity therapies. Robust data, obtained in multiple patient cohorts, have linked elevated serum levels of GDF-15 to the presence of anorexia and cachexia during the course of several chronic diseases, including cancer, through a direct action of the GDF-15 on brain feeding centers [9]. Elevated circulating GDF-15 levels were associated with energy balance disturbances, cancer development and progression, and chemotherapy-induced anorexia [10]. Moreover, it has been hypothesized that GDF-15 may cause emesis itself and consequently trigger anorectic effects [10].

It is evident that the pathogenesis of cancer anorexia is multifactorial and reflects the complexity of the mechanisms controlling energy homeostasis under physiological conditions [11]. Within the central nervous system, tumors create a variety of alterations in neurotransmitters, neuropeptides, and prostaglandins that modulate eating behavior [6] and alterations in serotonin and corticotrophin releasing factor [12, 13]. Moreover, during cancer, disturbances of the hypothalamic pathways controlling energy homeostasis may occur, which lead to profound metabolic changes in peripheral tissues.

In particular, evidence exists that the hypothalamic melanocortin system does not respond appropriately to peripheral inputs, and its activity is directed to promote catabolic stimuli (i.e., reduced energy intake and increased energy expenditure) [14]. Hypothalamic proinflammatory cytokines and serotonin play a key role in triggering hypothalamic resistance. These catabolic effects represent the central response to peripheral challenges that are likely sensed by the brain through the vagus nerve. Also, disease-induced changes in fatty acid oxidation within hypothalamic neurons may contribute to the dysfunction of the hypothalamic melanocortin system [14]. Ultimately, sympathetic outflow mediates the metabolic changes in peripheral tissues [14].

Persistence of cancer anorexia for months or longer implies that the adaptive feeding response fails. In particular, tumor-released molecules, i.e., proinflammatory cytokines, contribute to anorexia [15]. Several cytokines (interleukin (IL)-1α,

IL-1β, IL-6, IL-8, and tumor necrosis factor-α) have a known effect on appetite by modulating central nervous system neurotransmitter cascades [15, 16], and it has been hypothesized that low appetite may be the final result in the derangements among neurohormonal signals (central and peripheral) controlling appetite [16, 17].

19.2 Anorexia Assessment

Although cancer anorexia is well defined as a clinical entity, identifying patients at risk to develop this condition remains a challenge for most physicians due to several reasons, including the different way each patient describes the anorexia symptoms (quantitatively and qualitatively) during medical consultation [18] and because of the absence of widely accepted validated appetite assessment tools. In addition, even when anorexia is diagnosed, most of physicians, particularly those not expert in clinical nutrition, consider this as condition with low priority in clinical practice [18].

One of the challenges of anorexia assessment is to identify the potential pathogenic factors (i.e., inflammation, depression, etc.) and then provide a correct and multimodal interventional approach [16, 19, 20].

Considering the clinical relevance of anorexia, several diagnostic tools have been proposed.

As previously described, relating the presence of anorexia with patients' eating behaviors plays a key role, even if their specific domains may not completely overlap considering that anorexia reflects the loss of the desire to eat, and actual food intake may not be affected when, for example, anorexic patients are forced to eat [21].

Notwithstanding, reduced food intake is frequently used as a potential marker (indicator) of the presence of anorexia and its severity [22]. In this view, the presence of anorexia may be more effectively characterized by identifying specific symptoms, including early satiety, nausea, and taste alterations, and by assessing its severity [22, 23]. Moreover, in daily clinical practice, a visual analog scale (VAS) is often utilized, which is a reliable tool but may be not clinically meaningful if small modifications in appetite need to be diagnosed [24].

The use of questionnaires to assess the presence of appetite loss is nowadays increasing, thus highlighting their reliability and utility. Moreover, considering that questionnaires provide only a qualitative evaluation of appetite, it is also recommended to quantify the degree of anorexia by using a VAS [8, 25, 26].

The Functional Assessment of Anorexia/Cachexia Therapy (FAACT) questionnaire provides a qualitative and quantitative assessment of anorexia and may be considered as a valid instrument for assessing anorexia in different clinical settings including cancer [27].

A clinical study [25] involving inpatients affected by different type of diseases utilized four appetite tools to diagnose anorexia. The authors observed that its prevalence significantly varied according to the diagnostic tool used, supporting the concept that, in clinical practice, disorders of appetite reflect different underlying mechanisms whose impact on clinical outcome measures may differ [25]. A clinical study, conducted on cancer patients to determine the prevalence of different appetite disorders and their influence on dietary intake and nutritional status, documented that around 62% presented changes in appetite; in particular, patients with a combination of anorexia and early satiety presented the worse overall health perception and fatigue, indicating that appetite disorders have a significant impact on nutritional status and quality of life, especially when anorexia and early satiety were combined [5].

A recent prospective, observational study investigated prevalence of malnutrition in cancer patients at their first medical oncology visit [28]. Appetite loss was evaluated with a two-step questionnaire, to determine the presence of appetite loss first using a modified version of the FAACT questionnaire and then using a VAS adapted for appetite. Based on FAACT scores, poor appetite was present in 41% of patients, with mean scores varying by tumor type and stage of disease. According to FAACT score, pancreatic and gastroesophageal cancer patients resulted anorectic already since the non-metastatic phase of the disease; by contrast, all metastatic patients resulted anorectic based on the FAACT questionnaire. By VAS scoring, 44.5% of patients perceived appetite impairment. All patients in metastatic stage were anorectic based on the VAS [28].

Appetite disorders are highly prevalent among cancer patients at risk of malnutrition and have a definitive impact on nutritional status and quality of life. The coexistence of anorexia and early satiety represents the poorest condition, with serious psychological implications. Most of patients believe "not eating is dying," which is a symbol of progressive weakness and death.

In summary, it is apparent that the concomitant assessment of different anorexia aspects with reliable and dedicated tools is of crucial importance to early detect anorexia and to evaluate the efficacy of its therapeutic strategies.

19.3 Anorexia and Impact on Clinical Outcomes

During the last few years, increased emphasis has been placed on the mechanisms underlying body weight loss in cancer that can be induced by either cancer metabolism and inflammation or the several side effects of the anticancer treatments [29]. This led to consider clinical parameters, such as body mass index, body weight change and food intake, and their modification overtime, in predicting patient's overall survival [29].

In this respect, it is important to elucidate how anorexia associates itself with weight loss and other consequences to influence survival.

Abraham et al. conducted a study on naïve patients with esophageal/gastroesophageal junction or gastric cancer who were assessed using the FAACT Anorexia/Cachexia Subscale (FAACT A/CS) [30]. Patients with a FAACT A/CS score ≤37 over to 48 were considered to be anorexic, and the prevalence of anorexia resulted 69% among the cohort. The median overall survival of patients with a score >37 was longer than in those with score ≤37, while there was no statistical difference in overall survival between those patients who lost ≥5% weight in the 6 months prior to cancer diagnosis and those that had not. In this light, the FAACT A/CS resulted a better predictor of overall survival, in particular in metastatic patients, with respect to body mass index alone or to weight loss [30]. This suggests that anorexia, as assessed by the FAACT A/CS score, is a predictor of survival independently of body weight loss.

Effective nutritional intervention can be achieved by the assessment not only of weight loss history but also of eating behavior and changes in appetite and the consequent impairment in nutritional intake. We believe that nutritional aspects should be carefully considered when managing cancer patients, in particular during anti-cancer treatments. Also, reduced food intake and nutritional issues negatively impact on patients' quality of life in every stage of cancer journey [4]. On the basis of these evidences, reduction in food intake should be early recognized and managed, and oral energy intake should be assessed at least qualitatively and, if possible, quantitatively [20, 21, 31]. Implementing awareness about prevalence and clinical impact of cancer anorexia among healthcare professionals is therefore deemed crucial [19].

Malnutrition is prevalent in cancer and contributes to poor prognosis through progressive depletion of the body's energy and protein reserves determining body weight loss. In particular, percent of weight loss and BMI predict survival independently of conventional prognostic factors [29]. Martin et al. proposed that the severity of weight loss should be evaluated based on the rate of WL and the level of depletion of body reserves [29] identifying a tool, the BMI-adjusted WL grading system, which was useful in efforts to predict survival because its independence of cancer site and stage and performance status.

Interestingly, a recent multicenter study, conducted in lung cancer patients and investigating several aspects for detection of early stages of cachexia, showed that the skeletal muscle mass was the most important component to detect pre-cachexia in more than 65% of patients with no clinically important weight loss (<2%) and the only criterion for detecting pre-cachexia in more than 40% of patients without either anorexia or weight loss [32]. The authors noted that, while the assessment of anorexia was carried out at a specific point in time, muscle mass and weight loss resulted from a process developing over time [32]. In this light, anorexia, as the only symptom to define pre-cachexia patients, should be further investigated.

According to the European Society for Clinical Nutrition and Metabolism (ESPEN) recommendations on actions to be implemented against cancer-related malnutrition [33], three key points have to be highlighted in nutritional care: (i) to screen all cancer patients for nutritional risk early in the course of their management, with specific attention to BMI and body weight change in the previous months; (ii) to include in the clinical practice the assessment of anorexia, body composition, and physical function; and (iii) to use multimodal nutritional support in a "stepwise manner" with individualized plans, including care aimed at improving nutritional intake and physical activity [33].

19.4 What's Next in Terms of Therapeutic Options?

Nutritional status affects tolerability of anticancer treatments and leads to alter therapeutic choices [34]. Therefore, an accurate assessment of nutritional status is of paramount importance in treating cancer patients, and anorexia should be considered as part of this assessment. The ESPEN recommendations on nutrition in cancer patients [33] highlight the importance of moving the treatment's focus from end-stage wasting to support patient's nutritional and functional state throughout the entire anti-cancer treatment, starting immediately at its beginning. This should ensure sufficient energy intake and maintain physical activity to avoid loss of muscle mass, along with reducing systemic inflammation.

Several factors may contribute to the development of anorexia, and each factor should be addressed individually [34]. A "one-size-fits-all" approach appears difficult to be successful [35].

Recently, two randomized phase 3 trials [36], ROMANA 1 and ROMANA 2, using a novel ghrelin-receptor agonist in advanced non-small-cell lung cancer patients with anorexia and cachexia showed improvement in appetite scores (likely leading to increased food intake) in the treatment group as well as an increase in body weight and lean mass compared with the placebo group.

Other several potential targets for cancer anorexia treatment have been identified through preclinical and clinical studies [37, 38]. A novel anti-inflammatory drug, the peptide-nucleic acid OHR118, has been proposed in the management of cancer-related anorexia. A phase 2 trial examined the effects of daily administration of OHR118 for 28 days to patients with advanced solid cancers ($n = 11$) [39], documenting an improvement in anorexia and gastrointestinal symptoms, although this was a single-arm interventional study without a placebo group as control and with a small sample size.

Omega-3 fatty acids, such as eicosapentaenoic acid (EPA) and docosahexaenoic acid (DHA), are able to attenuate and resolve inflammatory response [40] and present effects in reducing fatigue and appetite loss and improving global quality of life [41]. An interesting phase 2 study has been conducted in a population of advanced cancer patients with cancer-related anorexia/cachexia to assess the efficacy and safety of an integrated treatment based on oral EPA and DHA oral supplementation + a diet with high polyphenol content, antioxidants, and drugs (medroxyprogesterone acetate and selective cyclooxygenase-2 inhibitor celecoxib) [42]. The treatment given induced a significant increase in appetite and body weight, and also in lean body mass, although more than half of the enrolled patients was in the range of normal body weight at baseline (even if most of them suffered a significant loss of body weight compared with pre-illness) [42].

Megestrol acetate has showed a benefit compared with placebo, particularly with regard to appetite improvement and body weight gain in cancer patients, but lack of benefit when compared to other drugs [43]. Megestrol acetate combined with formoterol fumarate, a beta2-receptor agonist with high degree of selectivity for skeletal muscle beta2-receptors, was orally administered for 8 consecutive weeks in a phase I/II not-controlled trial in a cohort of cachectic advanced cancer patients [44].

The two drugs combined were safe and well tolerated. The results of the trial showed an increase in mean quadriceps volume and an improvement in appetite. However, the patients who reached the evaluation at 8 weeks were only 7 out of the 13 enrolled. Also, it was not possible to determine whether the documented gain in muscle mass and the improvement in appetite symptoms were due to the combination with megestrol acetate or to the formoterol alone [44].

Cannabinoids represent a class of drugs which includes different chemical molecules [45]. Studies showed that cannabinoids have the potential to improve appetite, calorie and protein intake, and body weight in cancer patients [45], in particular increasing pre-meal appetite and food "tasted better" [46].

Given the complex pathophysiology of cancer anorexia, the combination of drugs treatment with metabolic and nutritional interventions may optimize the cancer therapeutic approach [34]. In this way, earlier screening for anorexia with subsequent nutrition intervention (with or without therapeutic agents that target appetite), if appropriate, may enhance the quality of life of patients with advanced cancers. In addition, this may also provide an opportunity to improve response to anticancer treatments. In clinical practice, it is important to have easily applicable measurements/assessments of anorexia, to measure it objectively and identify patients suitable for early nutritional interventions in cancer journey.

Moreover, eating-related distress in cancer patients determines social and emotional consequences due to their inability to maintain stable food intake and in family relationships [47]. Only an integrated approach pursued by clinicians and all the healthcare team may lead to alleviate eating-related distress and improve quality of life and the altered perceptions of nutritional aspect for cancer patients and their families [18, 31, 47].

Considering the successes obtained in multimodal care research, an integrated model of supportive and nutritional care to alleviate eating-related distress based on the management of nutrition impact symptoms, psychosocial and nutritional support, and advice/education regarding cancer cachexia has been proposed [47]. The aim is to improve quality of life and promote the advanced care planning among patients and family members and the involvement and cooperation between healthcare physicians, nurses, dietitians, and other healthcare professionals [47].

In this light, all the stakeholders involved in cancer patients' management should actively cooperate to ameliorate global health status, bearing in mind that the patient is at the center of our care.

References

1. Laviano A, Koverech A, Seelaender M. Assessing pathophysiology of cancer anorexia. Curr Opin Clin Nutr Metab Care. 2017;20:340–5.
2. Laviano A, Di Lazzaro L, Correia MITD. To feed or not to feed in ICU: evidence based medicine versus physiology-based medicine. Nutrition. 2017;38:6–7.
3. Molfino A, Laviano A, Rossi Fanelli F. Contribution of anorexia to tissue wasting in cachexia. Curr Opin Support Palliat Care. 2010;4:249–53.

4. Molfino A, Amabile MI, Muscaritoli M. Nutrition support for treating cancer-associated weight loss: an update. Curr Opin Support Palliat Care. 2018;12:434–8.
5. Barajas Galindo DE, Vidal-Casariego A, Calleja-Fernández A, Hernández-Moreno A, Pintor de la Maza B, Pedraza-Lorenzo M, et al. Appetite disorders in cancer patients: impact on nutritional status and quality of life. Appetite. 2017;114:23–7.
6. Cooper C, Burden ST, Cheng H, Molassiotis A. Understanding and managing cancer-related weight loss and anorexia: insights from a systematic review of qualitative research. J Cachexia Sarcopenia Muscle. 2015;6:99–111.
7. Molfino A, Amabile MI, Laviano A. Anorexia in cancer: appetite, physiology, and beyond. In: Preedy VR, editor. Handbook of nutrition and diet in palliative care. 2nd ed. Boca Raton, FL: CRC Press; 2019.
8. Molfino A, Iannace A, Colaiacomo MC, Farcomeni A, Emiliani A, Gualdi G, et al. Cancer anorexia: hypothalamic activity and its association with inflammation and appetite-regulating peptides in lung cancer. J Cachexia Sarcopenia Muscle. 2017;8:40–7.
9. Tsai VW, Brown DA, Breit SN. Targeting the divergent TGFβ superfamily cytokine MIC-1/GDF15 for therapy of anorexia/cachexia syndromes. Curr Opin Support Palliat Care. 2018;12:404–9. https://doi.org/10.1097/SPC.0000000000000384.
10. Borner T, Shaulson ED, Ghidewon MY, Barnett AB, Horn CC, Doyle RP, Grill HJ, Hayes MR, De Jonghe BC. GDF15 induces anorexia through nausea and emesis. Cell Metab. 2020;31:351–362.e5. https://doi.org/10.1016/j.cmet.2019.12.004.
11. Baracos VE, Martin L, Korc M, Guttridge DC, Fearon KCH. Cancer-associated cachexia. Nat Rev Dis Primers. 2018;4:17105. https://doi.org/10.1038/nrdp.2017.105.
12. Fearon K, Strasser F, Anker SD, Bosaeus I, Bruera E, Fainsinger RL, et al. Definition and classification of cancer cachexia: an international consensus. Lancet Oncol. 2011;12:489–95.
13. Wallengren O, Lundholm K, Bosaeus I. Diagnostic criteria of cancer cachexia: relation to quality of life, exercise capacity and survival in unselected palliative care patients. Support Care Cancer. 2013;21:1569–77.
14. Laviano A, Inui A, Marks DL, Meguid MM, Pichard C, Rossi Fanelli F, Seelaender M. Neural control of the anorexia-cachexia syndrome. Am J Physiol Endocrinol Metab. 2008;295:E1000–8. https://doi.org/10.1152/ajpendo.90252.2008.
15. Ezeoke CC, Morley JE. Pathophysiology of anorexia in the cancer cachexia syndrome. J Cachexia Sarcopenia Muscle. 2015;6:287–302.
16. Peixoto da Silva S, Santos JMO, Costa E, Silva MP, Gil da Costa RM, Medeiros R. Cancer cachexia and its pathophysiology: links with sarcopenia, anorexia and asthenia. J Cachexia Sarcopenia Muscle. 2020; https://doi.org/10.1002/jcsm.12528.
17. Davis MP, Dreicer R, Walsh D, Lagman R, LeGrand SB. Appetite and cancer associated anorexia: a review. J Clin Oncol. 2004;22:1510–7.
18. Muscaritoli M, Molfino A, Scala F, Christoforidi K, Manneh-Vangramberen I, De Lorenzo F. Nutritional and metabolic derangements in Mediterranean cancer patients and survivors: the ECPC 2016 survey. J Cachexia Sarcopenia Muscle. 2019;10:517–25. https://doi.org/10.1002/jcsm.12420.
19. Muscaritoli M, Molfino A, Lucia S, Rossi Fanelli F. Cachexia: a preventable comorbidity of cancer. A T.A.R.G.E.T. approach. Crit Rev Oncol Hematol. 2015;94:251–9. https://doi.org/10.1016/j.critrevonc.2014.10.014.
20. Muscaritoli M, Molfino A, Gioia G, Laviano A, Rossi Fanelli F. The "parallel pathway": a novel nutritional and metabolic approach to cancer patients. Intern Emerg Med. 2011;6:105–12. https://doi.org/10.1007/s11739-010-0426-1.
21. Molfino A, Muscaritoli M, Rossi Fanelli F. Anorexia assessment in patients with cancer: a crucial issue to improve the outcome. J Clin Oncol. 2015;33:1513.
22. Laviano A, Meguid MM, Inui A, Muscaritoli M, Rossi-Fanelli F. Therapy insight: cancer anorexia cachexia syndrome—when all you can eat is yourself. Nat Clin Pract Oncol. 2005;2:158–65.
23. Rossi Fanelli F, Cangiano C, Ceci F, Cellerino R, Franchi F, Menichetti ET, et al. Plasma tryptophan and anorexia in human cancer. Eur J Cancer Clin Oncol. 1986;22:89–95.

24. Stubbs RJ, Hughes DA, Johnstone AM, Rowley E, Reid C, Elia M, et al. The use of visual analogue scales to assess motivation to eat in human subjects: a review of their reliability and validity with an evaluation of new hand-held computerized systems for temporal tracking of appetite ratings. Br J Nutr. 2000;84:405–15.
25. Arezzo di Trifiletti A, Misino P, Giannantoni P, Giannantoni B, Cascino A, Fazi L, et al. Comparison of the performance of four different tools in diagnosing disease-associated anorexia and their relationship with nutritional, functional and clinical outcome measures in hospitalized patients. Clin Nutr. 2013;32:527–32.
26. Molfino A, Kaysen GA, Chertow GM, Doyle J, Delgado C, Dwyer T, Laviano A, Rossi Fanelli F, Johansen KL. Validating appetite assessment tools among patients receiving hemodialysis. J Ren Nutr. 2016;26:103–10. https://doi.org/10.1053/j.jrn.2015.09.002.
27. Muscaritoli M, Anker SD, Argilés J, Aversa Z, Bauer JM, Biolo G, et al. Consensus definition of sarcopenia, cachexia and pre-cachexia: Joint document elaborated by Special Interest Groups (SIG) "cachexia-anorexia in chronic wasting diseases" and "nutrition in geriatrics". Clin Nutr. 2010;29:154–9.
28. Muscaritoli M, Lucia S, Farcomeni A, Lorusso V, Saracino V, Barone C, et al. Prevalence of malnutrition in patients at first medical oncology visit: the PreMiO study. Oncotarget. 2017;8:79884–96. https://doi.org/10.18632/oncotarget.20168.
29. Martin L, Senesse P, Gioulbasanis I, Antoun S, Bozzetti F, Deans C, et al. Diagnostic criteria for the classification of cancer-associated weight loss. J Clin Oncol. 2015;33:90–9.
30. Abraham M, Kordatou Z, Barriuso J, Lamarca A, Weaver JMJ, Cipriano C, et al. Early recognition of anorexia through patient generated assessment predicts survival in patients with oesophagogastric cancer. PLoS One. 2019;e0224540:14.
31. Muscaritoli M, Rossi Fanelli F, Molfino A. Perspectives of healthcare professionals on cancer cachexia: results from three global surveys. Ann Oncol. 2016;27:2230–6.
32. Antoun S, Morel H, Souquet PJ, Surmont V, Planchard D, Bonnetain F, et al. Staging of nutrition disorders in non-small-cell lung cancer patients: utility of skeletal muscle mass assessment. J Cachexia Sarcopenia Muscle. 2019;10:782–93. https://doi.org/10.1002/jcsm.12418.
33. Arends J, Baracos V, Bertz H, Bozzetti F, Calder PC, Deutz NEP, et al. ESPEN expert group recommendations for action against cancer-related malnutrition. Clin Nutr. 2017;36:1187–96.
34. Molfino A, Amabile MI, Giorgi A, Monti M, D'Andrea V, Muscaritoli M. Investigational drugs for the treatment of cancer cachexia: a focus on phase I and phase II clinical trials. Expert Opin Investig Drugs. 2019;28:733–40. https://doi.org/10.1080/13543784.2019.1646727.
35. Abraham M, Kordatou Z, Barriuso J, Lamarca A, Weaver JMJ, Cipriano C, Papaxoinis G, Backen A, Mansoor W. Early recognition of anorexia through patient-generated assessment predicts survival in patients with oesophagogastric cancer. PLoS One. 2019;14(11):e0224540. https://doi.org/10.1371/journal.pone.0224540.
36. Temel JS, Abernethy AP, Currow DC, Friend J, Duus EM, Yan Y, et al. Anamorelin in patients with nonsmall-cell lung cancer and cachexia (ROMANA 1 and ROMANA 2): results from two randomised, double-blind, phase 3 trials. Lancet Oncol. 2016;17:519–31.
37. Fearon KC, Glass DJ, Guttridge DC. Cancer cachexia: mediators, signaling, and metabolic pathways. Cell Metab. 2012;16:153–66.
38. Garcia JM. What is next after anamorelin? Curr Opin Support Palliat Care. 2017;11:266–71.
39. Chasen M, Hirschman SZ, Bhargava R. Phase II study of the novel peptide-nucleic acid OHR118 in the management of cancer-related anorexia/cachexia. J Am Med Dir Assoc. 2011;12:62–7.
40. Molfino A, Amabile MI, Monti M, Muscaritoli M. Omega-3 polyunsaturated fatty acids in critical illness: anti-inflammatory, proresolving, or both? Oxid Med Cell Longev. 2017;2017:5987082.
41. Sánchez-Lara K, Turcott JG, Juárez-Hernández E, Nuñez-Valencia C, Villanueva G, Guevara P, et al. Effects of an oral nutritional supplement containing eicosapentaenoic acid on nutritional and clinical outcomes in patients with advanced non-small cell lung cancer: randomised trial. Clin Nutr. 2014;33:1017–23.

42. Mantovani G, Macciò A, Madeddu C, Gramignano G, Lusso MR, Serpe R, et al. A phase II study with antioxidants, both in the diet and supplemented, pharmaconutritional support, progestagen, and anti-cyclooxygenase-2 showing efficacy and safety in patients with cancer-related anorexia/cachexia and oxidative stress. Cancer Epidemiol Biomarkers Prev. 2006;15:1030–4.
43. Ruiz Garcia V, Lopez-Briz E, Carbonell Sanchis R, Gonzalvez Perales JL, Bort-Marti S. Megestrol acetate for treatment of anorexia-cachexia syndrome. Cochrane Database Syst Rev. 2013;3:CD004310. https://doi.org/10.1002/14651858.CD004310.pub3.
44. Greig CA, Johns N, Gray C, MacDonald A, Stephens NA, Skipworth RJ, et al. Phase I/II trial of formoterol fumarate combined with megestrol acetate in cachectic patients with advanced malignancy. Support Care Cancer. 2014;22:1269–75.
45. Wang J, Wang Y, Tong M, Pan H, Li D. New prospect for cancer cachexia: medical cannabinoid. J Cancer. 2019;10:716–20.
46. Brisbois TD, de Kock IH, Watanabe SM, Mirhosseini M, Lamoureux DC, Chasen M, et al. Delta-9-tetrahydrocannabinol may palliate altered chemosensory perception in cancer patients: results of a randomized, double-blind, placebo-controlled pilot trial. Ann Oncol. 2011;22:2086–93.
47. Amano K, Baracos VE, Hopkinson JB. Integration of palliative, supportive, and nutritional care to alleviate eating-related distress among advanced cancer patients with cachexia and their family members. Crit Rev Oncol Hematol. 2019;143:117–23. https://doi.org/10.1016/j.critrevonc.2019.08.006.

Celiac Disease and Eating and Weight Disorders

Patrizia Calella and Giuliana Valerio

Celiac disease (CD) is a chronic, immune-mediated, and systemic disorder triggered by exposure to dietary gluten in genetically predisposed individuals [1]. Epidemiological research reveals a worldwide prevalence of CD ranging between 1% and 2% in the general population; women are more affected than men [2]. The CD prevalence has increased in the last years [3], albeit most affected individuals remain undiagnosed because they are asymptomatic or have atypical manifestations [4]. In the past it was believed that CD developed only in childhood, but subsequently it was proven to occur at any age. At the onset, patients may present the classic intestinal manifestations (diarrhea, malabsorption, abdominal distention, weight loss) caused by the small intestinal villous atrophy. Alternatively, they may present non-classic symptoms, such as headache, osteoporosis, bloating, chronic fatigue, and psychiatric disturbances, and finally they may be asymptomatic [5]. Undiagnosed and untreated CD might result in considerable adverse effects, such as chronic nutritional deficiencies, progressive bone loss, increased risk of non-traumatic fractures of hip and vertebrae, and intestinal lymphoma. Therefore, diagnosis of CD requires a high degree of suspicion, followed by accurate screening procedure and duodenal biopsy in selected cases [6]. Once CD is diagnosed, a strict gluten-free diet (GFD) is necessary lifelong, inducing significant changes in the lifestyle of the affected individuals. All the aspects of day life may be influenced, at school, at work, in the sport participation, and in the spare time, causing social and emotional distress [7]. Individuals with CD need to be greatly aware about the changes required in their food habits and social life, especially in the initial stages of diet adjustment. Adherence to GFD requires high attention regarding food, a careful reading of food labels, and avoiding unsafe cross-contact with

P. Calella (✉) · G. Valerio
Department of Movement Sciences and Wellbeing, University of Naples "Parthenope", Naples, Italy
e-mail: patrizia.calella@collaboratore.uniparthenope.it; giuliana.valerio@uniparthenope.it

gluten-containing foods and tableware, cutlery, and cookware. These constrictions are hardly accepted, especially by adolescents, who desire feeling just like their peers [8], and hinder participation to social eating and special occasions. For these reasons, individuals with CD commonly display the "fear to appear ill," because they constantly need to be aware about the ingredients of the food they eat. This feeling may induce stress, anxiety, depression, and embarrassment [9].

Individuals with chronic illness that demands attention to dietary intake are at high risk for engaging in unhealthy weight control behaviors. The worry about dietary intake can be excessive, leading to the development of an eating disorder (ED). Evidences show that the focus on food and food habits, and probably the level of adherence to GFD, may be associated with an increased risk of psychosocial problems and ED patterns in individuals with CD [10, 11]. Most articles showing a positive association between CD and ED focused on case reports [10, 13–16]. Female gender, older age, and being overweight were identified as the main risk factors. Several studies performed either in adolescents or in adults with CD found elevated symptoms of EDs compared with healthy controls [17–21]. Tokatly Latzer et al. [21] investigated symptoms and concerns due to EDs in a cohort of 136 adolescents with CD through a web-mediated survey including the Eating Attitudes Test (EAT-26); they found that 19% females and 7% males scored >20, which is suggestive of an ED. Using the same questionnaire, Satherly et al. [19] reported that the percentage of pathological scores was significantly higher in CD women compared to healthy controls (15.7% versus 3.8%); furthermore, bulimic behavior, explored by the Binge Eating Staircases, was found in 19.4% of CD individuals compared to 2.3% of healthy controls. Another study by Passananti et al. [20] reported that the percentage of pathological scores was significantly higher in newly diagnosed CD patients compared to healthy controls (16% versus 4%); on the contrary, bulimic behavior was found only in men with CD (6%). Similarly Arigo et al. [17] found that 22% out of 177 women with CD met the threshold for ED symptoms of clinical significance. Lastly, Merild et al. [18] on a register-based cohort of women with CD found that the hazard ratio for later development of anorexia nervosa was 1.46 (95% CI 1.08–1.98).

Recent research indicates that either poor or extreme adherence to the GFD may be associated with ED patterns in CD [22, 23]. After the treatment with GFD, a general trend toward an increased body mass index has been reported [24]. This was probably due to the significantly higher amount of lipids and sugar and lower content of fiber than the equivalent gluten-containing food [25]. In subjects with CD, the higher body mass index may be associated with the belief that the diet is responsible of weight gain, which might increase body dissatisfaction and lead to dysfunctional illness beliefs and poor dietary management [19]. In these cases, compensatory behaviors or consuming gluten-rich food is used to obtain purging effect [23, 26]. On the contrary, the presence of several symptoms at the time of diagnosis has been associated with better dietary adherence in order to get relief. These individuals are supposed to be overanxious of suffering CD symptoms again and tend to limit food choices or eat only when they can have a complete control over food preparation [19, 27]. Maladaptive eating behaviors characterized by rigidity, avoidance, controlling behavior, and preoccupation were reported by approximately 53% adolescents with CD [28]. These characteristics have notable resemblances to personality traits of those supposed to be at risk of EDs.

With few exceptions [12] several studies reported that CD was also significantly higher in patient with EDs, indicating a possible bidirectional association [18, 29, 30].

Wotton et al. [30] showed that there was a three-fold elevation of risk of subsequent CD in patients admitted to hospital with anorexia nervosa and a two-fold elevation in individuals with bulimia nervosa. Furthermore, the nationwide study by Marild et al. [18] found a doubled risk for anorexia nervosa after CD diagnosis (odds ratio 2.18, 95% CI 1.45–3.29) compared with controls. A shared genetic susceptibility with common molecular pathways may be hypothesized [30, 31]. Indeed, a recent study found two genes involved in anorexia (AKAP6, NTNG1) differently expressed in the small intestinal tissue of individuals with CD compared with control patients [31].

The concomitance between the two disorders might be also explained by the fact that diagnosis of CD peaks in the first two decades, when EDs are more frequent. In fact, more than 90% of individuals with EDs present this condition before the age of 25 years. Furthermore, symptoms associated to CD, such as abdominal discomfort, dizziness, vomiting, or weight loss, may hamper the diagnosis of EDs [32]. Ultimately, recent interest in the gut–brain axis has led to the discovery of changes in the composition of the gut microbiome in both anorexia nervosa and CD [33, 34]. Future studies are needed to explore the risk of autoimmune diseases and the immunological mechanisms in individuals with various EDs and their family members.

In addition, depression may mediate the link between CD and EDs. Lifetime comorbidity between depression and EDs is high, ranging between 50% in bulimia nervosa and 40% in anorexia nervosa [35]. The risk of significant depressive symptoms in individuals with CD has been assessed [17] and may increase the susceptibility for developing ED behavior [36]. This psychological status is associated with changes in appetite and weight [37].

The treatment of EDs and CD requires different competences and a multidisciplinary approach. Clinicians should be aware of the co-occurrence of these conditions and consider that the two conditions reciprocally worsen the clinical course. Given the health risk of undiagnosed and untreated CD, it is important to consider serological screening for CD in any adolescent and young adult suspected for an ED. Both CD and ED can present non-specific gastrointestinal discomfort leading to undiagnosed or misdiagnosed that may be overwhelming, especially during a particularly susceptible period of growth. These conditions can be misdiagnosed interchangeably, but they can also coexist, making management challenging. Practitioners should educate patients about the importance of attending every follow-up control as well as specialized dietitians should encourage GFD adherence with a positive behavioral approach in order to promote a better quality of life. Early intervention may prevent further complications. Furthermore, it is important that practitioners periodically evaluate anthropometric parameters, since the pathology may modulate such values even in a GFD impacting the state of health. Regular monitoring of both the anthropometric parameters and the psychological status, including the assessment of the body image, should be implemented in adolescents with CD in order to prevent ED from developing. Special attention should be drawn to female adolescents who are at higher risk of depressive symptoms, overweight, and less compliant with the GFD, as these factors are associated with ED status.

The discovery of possible immunological, genetic, and environmental factors common to CD and EDs will increase our competency to approach and manage these conditions. When both diseases coexist, a multidisciplinary approach is often needed to address the additional complexities posed.

References

1. Ludvigsson JF, Leffler DA, Bai JC, Biagi F, Fasano A, Green PHR, Hadjivassiliou M, Kaukinen K, Kelly CP, Leonard JN, et al. The Oslo definitions for coeliac disease and related terms. Gut. 2013;62(1):43–52. https://doi.org/10.1136/gutjnl-2011-301346.
2. Singh P, Arora A, Strand TA, Leffler DA, Catassi C, Green PH, Kelly CP, Ahuja V, Makharia GK. Global prevalence of celiac disease: systematic review and meta-analysis. Clin Gastroenterol Hepatol. 2018;
3. Ludvigsson JF, Rubio-Tapia A, Van Dyke CT, Melton LJ, Zinsmeister AR, Lahr BD, Murray JA. Increasing incidence of celiac disease in a north American population. Am J Gastroenterol. 2013;
4. Fasano A. Celiac disease—how to handle a clinical chameleon. N Engl J Med. 2003;
5. Lebwohl B, Sanders DS, Green PHR. Seminar coeliac disease. Lancet. 2018;
6. Husby, S.; Koletzko, S.; Korponay-Szabó, I.; Kurppa, K.; Mearin, M.L.; Ribes-Koninckx, C.; Shamir, R.; Troncone, R.; Auricchio, R.; Castillejo, G.; et al. European Society Paediatric Gastroenterology, Hepatology and nutrition guidelines for diagnosing coeliac disease 2020. J. Pediatr. Gastroenterol. Nutr. 2019.
7. Van Hees NJM, Van d, Does W, Giltay EJ. Coeliac disease, diet adherence and depressive symptoms. J Psychosom Res. 2013;
8. Rosén A, Ivarsson A, Nordyke K, Karlsson E, Carlsson A, Danielsson L, Högberg L, Emmelin M. Balancing health benefits and social sacrifices: a qualitative study of how screening-detected celiac disease impacts adolescents' quality of life. BMC Pediatr. 2011;
9. Häuser W, Janke KH, Klump B, Gregor M, Hinz A. Anxiety and depression in adult patients with celiac disease on a gluten-free diet. World J Gastroenterol. 2010;
10. Karwautz A, Wagner G, Berger G, Sinnreich U, Grylli V, Huber WD. Eating pathology in adolescents with celiac disease. Psychosomatics. 2008;
11. Wagner G, Zeiler M, Berger G, Huber WD, Favaro A, Santonastaso P, Karwautz A. Eating Disorders in Adolescents with Celiac Disease: Influence of Personality Characteristics and Coping. Eur Eat Disord Rev. 2015;
12. Basso MS, Zanna V, Panetta F, Caramadre AM, Ferretti F, Ottino S. Diamanti, A. Is the screening for celiac disease useful in anorexia nervosa? Eur J Pediatr. 2013;
13. Leffler DA, Dennis M, Edwards George JB, Kelly CP. The interaction between eating disorders and celiac disease: an exploration of 10 cases. Eur J Gastroenterol Hepatol. 2007;
14. Martínez-Olmos MA, Peinō R, Prieto-Tenreiro A, Lage M, Nieto L, Lord T, Molina-Pérez E, Domínguez-Muñoz JE, Casanueva FF. Intestinal absorption and pancreatic function are preserved in anorexia nervosa patients in both a severely malnourished state and after recovery. Eur Eat Disord Rev. 2013;
15. Ricca V, Mannucci E, Calabrò A, Di Bernardo M, Cabras PL, Rotella CM. Anorexia nervosa and celiac disease: two case reports. Int J Eat Disord. 2000;

16. Yucel B, Ozbey N, Demir K, Polat A, Yager J. Eating disorders and celiac disease: a case report. Int J Eat Disord. 2006;
17. Arigo D, Anskis AM, Smyth JM. Psychiatric comorbidities in women with celiac disease. Chronic Illn. 2012;
18. Marild K, Stordal K, Bulik CM, Rewers M, Ekbom A, Liu E, Ludvigsson JF. Celiac disease and anorexia nervosa: a nationwide study. Pediatrics. 2017;
19. Satherley RM, Howard R, Higgs S. The prevalence and predictors of disordered eating in women with coeliac disease. Appetite. 2016;
20. Passananti V, Siniscalchi M, Zingone F, Bucci C, Tortora R, Iovino P, Ciacci C. Prevalence of eating disorders in adults with celiac disease. Gastroenterol Res Pract. 2013;
21. Tokatly Latzer I, Lerner-Geva L, Stein D, Weiss B, Pinhas-Hamiel O. Disordered eating behaviors in adolescents with celiac disease. Eat Weight Disord. 2018;
22. Hommer RE, Swedo SE. Anorexia and autoimmunity: challenging the etiologic constructs of disordered eating. Pediatrics. 2017;
23. Golden NH, Park KT. Celiac disease and anorexia nervosa: an association well worth considering. Pediatrics. 2017;
24. Barone M, Della Valle N, Rosania R, Facciorusso A, Trotta A, Cantatore FP, Falco S, Pignatiello S, Viggiani MT, Amoruso A, et al. A comparison of the nutritional status between adult celiac patients on a long-term, strictly gluten-free diet and healthy subjects. Eur J Clin Nutr. 2016;70:23–7.
25. Miranda J, Lasa A, Bustamante MA, Churruca I, Simon E. Nutritional differences between a gluten-free diet and a diet containing equivalent products with gluten. Plant Foods Hum Nutr. 2014;69:182–7.
26. Zerwas S, Larsen JT, Petersen L, Thornton LM, Quaranta M, Koch SV, Pisetsky D, Mortensen PB, Bulik CM. Eating disorders, autoimmune, and autoinflammatory disease. Pediatrics. 2017;
27. Sverker A, Hensing G, Hallert C. "Controlled by food"—lived experiences of coeliac disease. J Hum Nutr Diet. 2005;
28. Cadenhead JW, Wolf RL, Lebwohl B, Lee AR, Zybert P, Reilly NR, Schebendach J, Satherley R, Green PHR. Diminished quality of life among adolescents with coeliac disease using maladaptive eating behaviours to manage a gluten-free diet: a cross-sectional, mixed-methods study. J Hum Nutr Diet. 2019;
29. Nacinovich R, Tremolizzo L, Corbetta F, Conti E, Neri F, Bomba M. Anorexia nervosa of the restrictive type and celiac disease in adolescence. Neuropsychiatr Dis Treat. 2017;
30. Wotton CJ, James A, Goldacre MJ. Coexistence of eating disorders and autoimmune diseases: record linkage cohort study, UK. Int J Eat Disord. 2016;
31. Mostowy J, Montén C, Gudjonsdottir AH, Arnell H, Browaldh L, Nilsson S, Agardh D, Naluai ÅT. Shared genetic factors involved in celiac disease, type 2 diabetes and anorexia nervosa suggest common molecular pathways for chronic diseases. PLoS One. 2016;
32. Avila JT, Park KT, Golden NH. Eating disorders in adolescents with chronic gastrointestinal and endocrine diseases. Lancet Child Adolesc Heal. 2019;
33. Bascuñán KA, Araya M, Roncoroni L, Doneda L, Elli L. Dietary gluten as a conditioning factor of the gut microbiota in celiac disease. Adv Nutr. 2019;1–15.
34. Borgo F, Riva A, Benetti A, Casiraghi MC, Bertelli S, Garbossa S, Anselmetti S, Scarone S, Pontiroli AE, Morace G, et al. Microbiota in anorexia nervosa: the triangle between bacterial species, metabolites and psychological tests. PLoS One. 2017;
35. Rodgers RF, Paxton SJ. The impact of indicated prevention and early intervention on co-morbid eating disorder and depressive symptoms: a systematic review. J Eat Disord. 2014;
36. Manaf NA, Saravanan C, Zuhrah B. The prevalence and inter-relationship of negative body image perception, depression and susceptibility to eating disorders among female medical undergraduate students. J Clin Diagn Res. 2016;
37. Hamel AE, Zaitsoff SL, Taylor A, Menna R, le Grange D. Body-related social comparison and disordered eating among adolescent females with an eating disorder, depressive disorder, and healthy controls. Nutrients. 2012;

Craniopharyngioma and Eating Disorders

21

Marta Bondanelli, Emilia Manzato, Irene Gagliardi, and Maria Rosaria Ambrosio

21.1 Epidemiology and Pathology

Craniopharyngiomas (CPs) are rare brain tumours arising from embryonic remnants of the craniopharyngeal duct epithelium (known as Rathke's pouch), with incidence of 0.5–2.5 cases per million per year in the general population. CPs have a bimodal age distribution, with a peak in children aged 5–15 years and a second peak in adults between 50 and 74 years of age, accounting for 5–11% of intracranial tumours in childhood and adolescence [1]. The tumour includes two histological subtypes, adamantinomatous craniopharyngioma (ACP) and papillary craniopharyngioma (PCP). ACP with cyst formation is the most common, presenting with the typical bimodal age distribution, and it appears to be driven by activating mutations in CTNNB1 (gene encoding β-catenin). PCPs occur mainly in adults as solid tumours and frequently harbour somatic BRAFV600E mutations [1, 2].

21.2 Clinical Presentation

A wide range of symptoms may be present, depending upon the precise location of the tumour, and the diagnosis is often established 1 or more years after the initial appearance of symptoms.

M. Bondanelli (✉) · I. Gagliardi · M. R. Ambrosio
Section of Endocrinology & Internal Medicine, Dept of Medical Sciences, University of Ferrara, Ferrara, Italy
e-mail: marta.bondanelli@unife.it; irene.gagliardi@unife.it; mariarosaria.ambrosio@unife.it

E. Manzato
Formerly University of Ferrara, Chief Eating Disorders Unit, Private Hospital "Salus", Ferrara, Italy
e-mail: emilia.manzato@gmail.com

© Springer Nature Switzerland AG 2022
E. Manzato et al. (eds.), *Hidden and Lesser-known Disordered Eating Behaviors in Medical and Psychiatric Conditions*,
https://doi.org/10.1007/978-3-030-81174-7_21

Primary manifestations are visual impairment (62–84%) and endocrine deficits (52–87%) [3]. Endocrine abnormalities are caused by direct damage or disturbances to the hypothalamic-pituitary axes that affect deficiencies of growth hormone (GH), gonadotropin, thyroid-stimulating hormone (TSH), and adrenocorticotropic hormone (ACTH) in an estimated 75, 40, 25, and 25 percent of cases, respectively. Diabetes insipidus may be frequent when the pituitary stalk is involved, or it may be a complication of neurosurgery [2]. In children, growth failure is the most common presentation, caused by either hypothyroidism or GH deficiency [GHD]. Significant weight gain, predictive of hypothalamic obesity, may occur shortly before diagnosis of APC. In adults, sexual dysfunction is the most common endocrine manifestation, due to gonadotropin deficiency and/or hyperprolactinemia [2, 3] (Table 21.1). Moderate to severe daily headaches are present in 50% of patients at the time of diagnosis. Additional symptoms of intracranial pressure (nausea, vomiting, and lethargy) and hypothalamic symptoms, including psychiatric disturbances, may be present at diagnosis of adult CP [3].

21.3 Diagnosis

The diagnosis of CP is suggested by the presence of a mass, in the sellar/parasellar region, on magnetic resonance imaging (MRI) and/or computed tomography (CT). The most common localization is suprasellar, with an intrasellar portion; sometimes CP is exclusively suprasellar or intrasellar, and occasionally it extends into the anterior, middle, or posterior fossa. Calcification is seen in 60 to 80% of patients with CP, and one or more cysts are present in approximately 75%. The combination of solid, cystic, and calcified tumour components is an important radiological clue to the diagnosis of CP. MRI, before and after gadolinium, is the standard imaging for detection of CP, further imaged by native CT to detect calcifications [4].

All patients with CP must undergo endocrine testing for diagnosis of hypopituitarism, particularly adrenal and thyroid, as their defects need treatment before surgery (Table 21.2). Accurate neuro-ophthalmologic examination is also indicated to evaluate optic pathway compression and to establish a presurgical baseline.

21.4 Management

Historically, the optimal treatment of CPs has been controversial and included two basic approaches: aggressive surgery aimed to achieve complete resection at diagnosis versus a more conservative surgical approach associated with radiation therapy (RT) to treat residual disease.

Today, the best treatment for CP is considered which leads to the least long-term morbidity.

It may include surgery alone, irradiation alone, or, more commonly, a combination of the two. Intracystic treatments (chemotherapy, immunological therapy, or radioisotopes) are an alternative option in well-selected patients [1, 2, 4, 5].

Table 21.1 Main clinical manifestations of hypopituitarism

Hormonal defect	Signs and symptoms	Laboratory data
Corticotropin, ACTH	Acute: weakness, dizziness, nausea, vomiting, fever, cardiovascular collapse	Hyponatremia, anaemia, eosinophilia, hypoglycaemia
	Chronic: asthenia, pallor, anorexia, nausea, weight loss, hypotension, myalgia, absence of hyperpigmentation	Absence of hyperkalaemia
Thyrotropin, TSH	Children: growth retardation	
	Adults: fatigue, cold intolerance, constipation, dry skin, hair loss, weight gain, reduction of tendon reflexes, ideo-motor slowdown, reduction of memory	Anaemia High CPK
Gonadotropin (LH, FSH)	Children: delayed puberty	
	Men: loss of libido and impotence, reduced fertility, reduced muscle mass and strength, reduced bone mass density, anaemia, reduced hair growth, fine skin roughness, testicular hypotrophy	
	Women: oligo-amenorrhea, infertility, loss of libido, dyspareunia, fine skin roughness, breast atrophy, osteoporosis, atherosclerosis	
Growth hormone, GH	Children: growth retardation, short stature, increased adiposity	
	Adults: visceral adiposity, reduced muscle mass and strength, reduced exercise capacity, increased cardiovascular risk, reduced attention and memory, reduced well-being and quality of life	Dyslipidaemia
Prolactin, PRL	Inability to breastfeed	
Arginine vasopressin, AVP	Polyuria and polydipsia, nicturia	Low urinary osmolality, hypernatraemia

A wide range of endocrine or neurological complications are observed following treatment of CP, contributing to the increased mortality of these patients. Endocrine abnormalities (e.g., panhypopituitarism) can be exacerbated by treatment. Hypothalamic dysfunction can cause disabling obesity, disorders of temperature regulation, sleep disorders, or diabetes insipidus.

Common neurologic complications include visual and neurocognitive deficits, sleep disorders, and a disrupted circadian rhythm and behavioural problems.

Table 21.2 Screening test for diagnosis of hypopituitarism

1. **Corticotropin (ACTH) deficiency**: serum cortisol at 8 to 9 AM on two or more occasions [<3 mcg/dL (83 nmol/L) = cortisol deficiency; >15 mcg/dL (414 nmol/L) = cortisol sufficiency. Values persistently intermediate⇒ test of ACTH reserve. Peak cortisol levels <18.1 µg/dL (500 nmol/L) at 30 or 60 min after corticotropin stimulation test indicate adrenal insufficiency]
2. **Thyrotropin (TSH) deficiency**: serum free T4 below the laboratory reference range, with a low, normal, or mildly elevated TSH
3. **Gonadotropin deficiency**: Low serum total testosterone concentration on two or more occasions at 8 to 10 AM in males (free testosterone in obese), and luteinizing hormone (LH) not elevated (combined with normal serum prolactin). Low estradiol and not elevated follicle-stimulating hormone (FSH) in premenopausal women; low gonadotropin levels in postmenopausal
4. **Growth Hormone (GH) deficiency**: subnormal GH response GH stimulation test
5. **Central Diabetes Insipidus:** serum and urine osmolality in patients with polyuria

Moreover, vascular abnormalities and/or secondary intracranial malignancies can follow radiation of CP, especially in children [2, 6, 7].

Even if CP has shown benign histological characteristics and high survival rates, it may be associated with high morbidity and reduced quality of life, which appears to be related to several factors, including number of surgical interventions, histological type, degree of hypothalamic involvement, obesity, endocrine deficiencies, and neuropsychological disorders [7, 8]. Moreover, recurrence of CPs is a frequent problem, especially in patients treated with subtotal resection without subsequent RT, and it has a high impact on the long-term prognosis [9]. Therefore, an experienced multidisciplinary team is essential for the optimal treatment of both paediatric and adult patients with CPs.

21.5 Hypothalamic Obesity

Damage to the hypothalamus, either by tumour, surgical intervention, or radiation therapy, can result in a syndrome of hypothalamic obesity, which is typically a morbid obesity whose degree is strictly related to the extent of the hypothalamic damage [10–12].

The prevalence of obesity at diagnosis is 12–19% up to 70% following treatment of CP, with rapid weight gain during the first 6–12 months. Weight gain occurs despite adequate endocrine replacement of pituitary hormone deficiencies and is resistant to lifestyle interventions, therefore leading to severe obesity in up to 55% of CP patients [1, 10, 11, 13]. Obesity is associated with increased risks of related morbidity (metabolic syndrome, type 2 diabetes mellitus, cardiovascular disease, and nonalcoholic liver disease), reduced quality of life (QoL), and increased mortality [9, 14].

Hypothalamic obesity is predominantly caused by damage to the ventromedial hypothalamus (VMH) and arcuate nucleus, which regulate hunger, satiety, energy expenditure, and metabolism balance. Hypothalamic damage could cause an

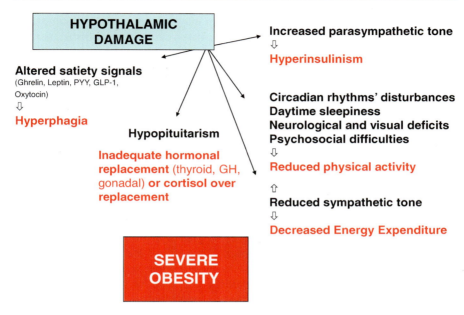

Fig. 21.1 Pathogenesis of hypothalamic obesity

imbalance of the autonomic nervous system consisting in decreased sympathetic activity, which is responsible for a lower total energy expenditure and increased parasympathetic activity, which results in hyperinsulinemia [2, 6, 11].

Other factors (Fig. 21.1) may contribute to decreased energy expenditure, such as circadian rhythms' disturbances, marked daytime sleepiness, and decreased physical activity, the latter due also to neurological and visual deficits and psychosocial difficulties. Neurobehavioural dysfunction (behavioural disturbances; impaired social, emotional, and neurocognitive functioning; and overall reduced QoL) are frequently present in CP patients [2, 11, 12]. An inadequate replacement of pituitary hormone defects may also contribute to obesity in CP patients [12, 15].

21.6 Eating Behaviour

Peripheral satiety and hormones, such as insulin, ghrelin, and leptin, play an essential role in the regulation of energy balance and signalling to hypothalamus. Recent reports suggest an important role for hyperinsulinemia in fat accumulation and obesity in CP patients, who are also leptin resistant [2, 16, 17]. Other studies demonstrated a reduced postprandial suppression of ghrelin and/or a reduced postprandial response for PYY in CP patients, suggesting a role of these factors in disturbed regulation of appetite and severe obesity [18, 19]. Moreover, reduced postprandial oxytocin level has been found to be associated with adverse eating behaviour and weight problems in CP patients [20]. Oxytocin is linked to eating behaviour and weight regulation, with anorexic effects, and it may influence social relationships. Therefore, it is today considered a promising therapeutic agent in obese patients with CP [12, 20]. In addition, excessive weight gain could be the result of deficient hypothalamic neural circuits communicating with corticolimbic and other brain regions to regulate appetite, thus leading to unbalanced eating [21].

Eating behaviour in CP patients with hypothalamic obesity is altered, but the specificity of these findings is controversial. Injury to the mediobasal hypothalamus causes hyperphagia and inappropriate food intake. Feeding behaviour is characterised by three processes (meal initiation, meal termination, and food choice) which are controlled by different parts of the brain that integrate central and peripheral signals. Meal initiation, primarily regulated by the hypothalamus, is the most disturbed process in CP patients. However, not all patients with CP develop hyperphagia. Several studies demonstrate equal or less caloric intake in both paediatric and adult patients with CP than that observed in the general population [2, 10, 18]. Eating behaviour appears to be related to the degree of hypothalamic damage.

Unfavourable eating behaviour has been observed in CP children with grade 2 hypothalamic damage (involving both anterior and posterior hypothalamic areas) associated with obesity. By contrast, children with anterior lesion (grade 1) presented with tendency towards high dietary restraints and to self-discipline which may contribute to reduced risk for hypothalamic obesity [20].

Eating disorders are characterised by disturbed eating behaviour and typical psychopathological features. The presence of obesity in CP could be linked to changes in appetite and in eating behaviour, particularly the onset of binge eating episode, that is, eating unusually large amounts of food in a discrete period [22]. We observed positive Binge Eating Scale in 8 out of 11 CP patients after surgery; however eating disorders persisted only in two patients at follow-up of 5 and 7 years [23].

Disturbed eating behaviour in CP cannot be inserted in eating disorders, because it does not result in significant impaired psychosocial functioning, and it is not accompanied by the typical psychopathological alterations. In fact, binge eating episodes are not accompanied by fear of gaining weight (as in anorexia nervosa), inappropriate compensatory behaviours (as in bulimia nervosa), or marked distress or shame regarding binge episodes (as in binge eating disorder).

In conclusion, hypothalamic damage caused by CP may produce inappropriate feelings of starvation or disturbed neuropsychologic behaviours that result in excessive food intake. Because the QoL of CP patients is greatly determined by the severity of obesity, urgent interventions are necessary.

21.7 Treatment of Obesity

All the causes of obesity in CP patients (hyperphagia, psychosocial disorders, sleep disturbances, decreased energy expenditure, hyperinsulinemia, and hypopituitarism) should be considered for an individual treatment algorithm of hypothalamic obesity based on lifestyle, diet, psychiatric support, and pharmacotherapeutic or surgical intervention [12].

Primarily, early detection and timely treatment of pituitary insufficiencies are necessary to avoid consequence of hypopituitarism. An adequate hormone replacement may help to prevent weight gain in CP patients. According to the current guidelines, glucocorticoid over-replacement should be avoided, with positive effects on BMI. Free T4 levels should be maintained in the middle to upper half of the reference range, although it is unknown how this beneficially affects body weight [12, 24, 25]. Testosterone replacement reduces fat mass and improves muscle mass and well-being in adult males [26]. GH therapy may be considered for children and adults with GHD and history of CP. GH replacement in adults is associated with amelioration in body composition, metabolic profile, and QoL [27, 28].

The lack of efficacy for dietary restriction and lifestyle modification among patients with CP is well known. In fact, the combination of decreased satiety and reduced energy expenditure requires lifelong compliance with dietary and regular physical activity. Moreover, many patients with CP also suffer from eating and behavioural disorders; therefore dietary compliance is not easily achievable. Additional psychosocial and psychiatric support may be required to treat specific psychosocial and/or psychiatric disorders, such as impulse control disorders, depression, anxiety, and severe food craving behaviours [2, 12, 18].

Methylphenidate, a drug approved for the treatment of attention-deficit/hyperactivity disorder, increases dopamine efficiency and reduces food reinforcement, which can reduce food intake and overcome physical hypoactivity. Therefore, it may be considered for children with hypothalamic obesity and hyperphagia after treatment of CP [29].

Oversecretion of insulin, due to autonomic nervous system imbalance in the hypothalamic, causes increased adipogenesis and intractable weight gain. It has been postulated that octreotide can control obesity in CP via the suppression of insulin secretion. However, data from literature are conflicting, and registered trials did not provide sufficient data [30].

Metformin is known to favour weight loss with various mechanisms, including increased leptin levels, insulin sensitivity, and physiological hypothalamic changes. However, there are limited reliable data regarding the ability of metformin to induce weight loss in obese CP patients [12].

Glucagon-like peptide 1 (GLP-1) and its analogues have provided promising weight loss in patients with diabetes mellitus and obesity, due to a direct action in the brain, especially in the hypothalamic nuclei and limbic system, as well as in the peripheral tissues and organs. GLP-1 analogues (exenatide or liraglutide) can induce weight loss and promote satiety also in CP patients with hyperphagia and obesity [2, 12].

Bariatric surgery is considered the most effective strategy for severe obesity in the general population, because it improves quality of life and reduces morbidity and mortality [31]. Thus, bariatric surgery has been attempted among patients with CP who experience greater risk, due to hormone deficiencies and associated neurologic disorders. Evidence for bariatric surgery is limited but offers promising results and may be considered for selected adults with morbid obesity and hyperphagia after treatment of CP [2, 12, 32–34].

References

1. Müller HL. Craniopharyngioma. Endocr Rev. 2014;35:513–43.
2. Müller HL, Merchant TE, Warmuth-Metz M, Martinez-Barbera JP, Puget S. Craniopharyngioma. Nat Rev Dis Primers. 2019;5:75.
3. Khan RB, Merchant TE, Boop FA, et al. Headaches in children with craniopharyngioma. J Child Neurol. 2013;28:1622.
4. Garnett MR, Puget S, Grill J, Sainte-Rose C. Craniopharyngioma. Orphanet J Rare Dis. 2007;2:18.
5. Honegger J, Tatagiba M. Craniopharyngioma surgery. Pituitary. 2008;11:361.
6. Lustig RH. Hypothalamic obesity after craniopharyngioma: mechanisms, diagnosis, and treatment. Front Endocrinol. 2011;2:1–8.
7. Li X, Wu W, Miao Q, He M, Zhang S, Zhang Z, Lu B, Yang Y, Shou X, Li Y, Wang Y, Ye H. Endocrine and metabolic outcomes after transcranial and endoscopic endonasal approaches for primary resection of craniopharyngiomas. World Neurosurg. 2019;121:e8–e14.
8. Olsson DS, Andersson E, Bryngelsson IL, et al. Excess mortality and morbidity in patients with craniopharyngioma, especially in patients with childhood onset: a population-based study in Sweden. J Clin Endocrinol Metab. 2015;100:467.
9. Sterkenburg AS, Hoffmann A, Gebhardt U, Warmuth-Metz M, Daubenbuchel AMM, Muller HL. Survival, hypothalamic obesity, and neuropsychological/psychosocial status after childhood-onset craniopharyngioma: newly reported long-term outcomes. Neuro Oncol. 2015;17:1029–38.
10. Rosenfeld A, Arrington D, Miller J, Olson M, Gieseking A, Etzl M, Harel B, Schembri A, Kaplan AA. Review of childhood and adolescent craniopharyngiomas with particular attention to hypothalamic obesity. Pediatr Neurol. 2014;50:4–10.
11. Müller HL. Consequences of craniopharyngioma surgery in children. J Clin Endocrinol Metab. 2011;96:1981–91.
12. van Iersel L, Brokke KE, Adan RAH, Bulthuis LCM, van den Akker ELT, van Santen HM. Pathophysiology and individualized treatment of hypothalamic obesity following craniopharyngioma and other suprasellar tumors: a systematic review. Endocr Rev. 2019;40:193–235.
13. Fouda MA, Zurakowski D, Scott RM, Marcus KJ, Manley PE, Ullrich NJ, Cohen LE, Goumnerova LC. Novel predictive scoring system for morbid hypothalamic obesity in patients with pediatric craniopharyngioma. Childs Nerv Syst. 2021;37:403–10.
14. Hidalgo ET, Orillac C, Kvint S, McQuinn MW, Dastagirzada Y, Phillips S, Wisoff JH. Quality of life, hypothalamic obesity, and sexual function in adulthood two decades after primary gross-total resection for childhood craniopharyngioma. Childs Nerv Syst. 2020;36:281–9.
15. Chemaitilly W, Armstrong GT, Gajjar A, Hudson MM. Hypothalamic-pituitary axis dysfunction in survivors of childhood cns tumors: importance of systematic follow-up and early endocrine consultation. J Clin Oncol. 2016;34:4315–9.
16. Fjalldal S, Follin C, Gabery S, Sundgren PC, Björkman-Burtscher IM, Lätt J, Mannfolk P, Nordström CH, Rylander L, Ekman B, Cheong R, Pålsson A, Petersén Å, Erfurth EM. Detailed assessment of hypothalamic damage in craniopharyngioma patients with obesity. Int J Obes (Lond). 2019;43:533–44.
17. Lustig RH. Autonomic dysfunction of the b-cell and the pathogenesis of obesity. Rev Endocr Metab Disord. 2003;4:23–32.
18. Müller HL. Craniopharyngioma and hypothalamic injury: latest insights into consequent eating disorders and obesity. Curr Opin Endocrinol Diabetes Obes. 2016;23:81–9.
19. Roth CL, Gebhardt U, Müller HL. Appetite-regulating hormone changes in patients with craniopharyngioma. Obesity (Silver Spring). 2011;19:36–42.
20. Daubenbüchel AM, Özyurt J, Boekhoff S, Warmuth-Metz M, Eveslage M, Müller HL. Eating behaviour and oxytocin in patients with childhood-onset craniopharyngioma and different grades of hypothalamic involvement. Pediatr Obes. 2019;e12527:14.

21. Roth CL. Hypothalamic obesity in patients with craniopharyngioma: profound changes of several weight regulatory circuits. Front Endocrinol (Lausanne). 2011;2:49.
22. Hrz KC, Müller HL, Waldeck R, Pudel V, Roth C. Obesity in patients with Craniopharyngioma: assessment of food intake and movement counts indicating physical activity. J Clin Endocrinol Metab. 2003;88:5227–31.
23. Onofri A, Ambrosio MR, Bondanelli M, Leoni M, Carli A, De Paola G, Manzato E, degli Uberti EC. Binge eating disorder in patients operated for craniopharyngioma. J Endocrinol Invest. 2006;29, Suppl.to n. 4.
24. Müller HL, Heinrich M, Bueb K, Etavard-Gorris N, Gebhardt U, Kolb R, Sörensen N. Perioperative dexamethasone treatment in childhood craniopharyngioma: influence on short-term and long-term weight gain. Exp Clin Endocrinol Diabetes. 2003;111:330–4.
25. Fleseriu M, Hashim IA, Karavitaki N, Melmed S, Murad MH, Salvatori R, Samuels MH. Hormonal replacement in hypopituitarism in adults: an endocrine society clinical practice guideline. J Clin Endocrinol Metab. 2016;101:3888–921.
26. Bhasin S, Brito JP, Cunningham GR, Hayes FJ, Hodis HN, Matsumoto AM, Snyder PJ, Swerdloff RS, Wu FC, Yialamas MA. Testosterone therapy in men with hypogonadism: an Endocrine Society clinical practice guideline. J Clin Endocrinol Metab. 2018;103:1715–44.
27. Heinks K, Boekhoff S, Hoffmann A, Warmuth-Metz M, Eveslage M, Peng J, Caluminus G, Müller HL. Quality of life and growth after childhood craniopharyngioma: results of the multinational trial KRANIOPHARYNGEOM 2007. Endocrine. 2018;59:364–72.
28. Boekhoff S, Bogusz A, Sterkenburg AS, Eveslage M, Muller HL. Long- term effects of growth hormone replacement therapy in childhood onset craniopharyngioma: results of the German craniopharyngioma registry (HIT- Endo). Eur J Endocrinol. 2018;179:331–41.
29. Elfers CT, Roth CL. Effects of methylphenidate on weight gain and food intake in hypothalamic obesity. Front Endocrinol (Lausanne). 2011;2:78.
30. Tzotzas T, Papazisis K, Perros P, Krassas GE. Use of somatostatin analogues in obesity. Drugs. 2008;68:1963–73.
31. Durrer Schutz D, Busetto L, Dicker D, Farpour-Lambert N, Pryke R, Toplak H, Widmer D, Yumuk V, Schutz Y. European practical and patient-centred guidelines for adult obesity management in primary care. Obes Facts. 2019;12:40–66.
32. Ni W, Shi X. Interventions for the treatment of craniopharyngioma-related hypothalamic obesity: a systematic review. World Neurosurg. 2018;118:e59–71.
33. Bretault M, Boillot A, Muzard L, Poitou C, Oppert JM, Barsamian C, Gatta B, Müller H, Weismann D, Rottembourg D, Inge T, Veyrie N, Carette C, Czernichow S. Clinical review: bariatric surgery following treatment for craniopharyngioma: a systematic review and individual-level data meta-analysis. J Clin Endocrinol Metab. 2013;98:2239–46.
34. Garrez I, Lapauw B, Nieuwenhove YV. Bariatric surgery for treatment of hypothalamic obesity after craniopharyngioma therapy: a matched case–control study. Obes Surg. 2020;30:2439–44.

Cyclic Vomiting Syndrome

22

Toshiyuki Hikita

22.1 Introduction

Cyclic vomiting syndrome (CVS) is a disorder characterized by recurrent, stereotypic episodes of incapacitating nausea, vomiting, and other symptoms, separated by intervals of comparative wellness [1]. J.R. Hayes' group found that mean ages at onset of symptoms and at diagnosis of children with cyclic vomiting pattern were, respectively, 5.7 and 8.0 years [2]. I.e., on average 2.3 years elapsed between onset and diagnosis, reflecting the difficulty of diagnosing CVS. Recurrent vomiting was first described in the literature by Gee in 1882 [3]. Clinically, CVS is considered a variant of migraine and in the third edition of the International Headache Classification (ICHD-3) [4] is assigned to the "Episodic syndromes that may be associated with migraine" subgroup. CVS is also classified as a functional gastrointestinal disorder in the ROME IV textbook (2016) [5].

22.2 Pathophysiology

CVS has been classified as a migraine variant as described in the preceding section, but its pathophysiology, prognosis, and natural history remain poorly understood. G. Russell's group reported overall CVS prevalence of 1.9%, with 20%, 29%, and 29% of patients diagnosed, respectively, with migraine, travel sickness, and atopic diseases [6]. In a study of 71 CVS patients by M. Matar's group, 79% experienced vomiting at times specific to the individual, 60% reported disturbance at night or symptoms on waking, and 19% experienced episodes at

T. Hikita (✉)
Department of Pediatrics, Teikyo University School of Medicine, Tokyo, Japan
e-mail: t-hikita@ra2.so-net.ne.jp

© Springer Nature Switzerland AG 2022
E. Manzato et al. (eds.), *Hidden and Lesser-known Disordered Eating Behaviors in Medical and Psychiatric Conditions*,
https://doi.org/10.1007/978-3-030-81174-7_22

characteristic times of the day [7]. CVS often responds to migraine-directed prophylaxis with beta-blockers, amitriptyline, or cyproheptadine [33]. Valproate has been utilized for treatment of pediatric migraine since 2005, and our group reported its effectiveness for CVS in 2009 [8]. Abnormally high levels during CVS attacks of adrenocorticotropic hormone (ACTH) and antidiuretic hormone (ADH), which are secreted from the anterior and posterior pituitary, have been reported; however, relationships between CVS symptoms and these hormones remain unclear. High stress levels induced by vomiting may raise ACTH and ADH levels, or alternatively high ACTH and ADH levels may trigger CVS. Attack duration was correlated with both ACTH and ADH levels, suggesting that high levels of these hormones prolong attack duration and may be useful markers for attack severity [9].

22.3 Epidemiology

Prevalence of CVS appears to range from roughly 0.3% to 2% [6, 10–13]. In a study of US children, van Tilburg et al. reported CVS prevalence of 0% in the <1 year and 3.4% in the 1–3 year age groups [10]. In a study of UK school children, Abu-Arafeh et al. reported 1.9% prevalence [6]. Saps et al. reported 0.3% prevalence in Colombian school children [12]. Devanarayana et al. reported 0.5% prevalence in 12- to 16-year-old children at a semi-urban school in Sri Lanka [13].

22.4 Diagnostic Criteria and Differential Diagnosis

Diagnostic criteria for CVS have been described by ICHD-3 [4], ROME IV [5], and the North American Society for Pediatric Gastroenterology Hepatology and Nutrition (NASPGHAN) [14]. There are slight differences among these three references. An important step in making a diagnosis of CVS is to rule out organic diseases. For example, the criteria presented in ICHD-3 are as follows: "**A.** At least five attacks of intense nausea and vomiting, fulfilling criteria B and C. **B.** Stereotypical in the individual patient and recurring with predictable periodicity. **C.** All of the following: 1. nausea and vomiting occur at least four times per hour; 2. attacks last for over 1 hour, up to 10 days; 3. attacks occur over 1 week apart. **D.** Complete freedom from symptoms between attacks. **E.** Not attributed to another disorder." It is always necessary to perform appropriate examinations before making a diagnosis of CVS. Differential diagnosis and useful examinations are described in Table 22.1. There is no specific examination for CVS; a combination of examinations as in Table 22.1 must be conducted.

Table 22.1 Differential diagnosis and useful examinations for CVS

Digestive disease: chronic appendicitis, abnormality (intestinal malrotation), mucosal disorder (ulcer, esophagitis, Crohn's disease), pancreatitis, hepatobiliary disease (cholelithiasis, choledochal cyst)
– Blood examination: blood count, ALT, γ-GTP, amylase, lipase
– Urinalysis: VMA, HVA
– Fecal examination: fecal culture
– Diagnostic imaging: abdominal ultrasonography, abdominal ultrasonography, esophagogastroduodenoscopy, upper GI series
Neurological disorder: brain tumor, intracranial hypertension, abdominal migraine, abdominal epilepsy
– Diagnostic imaging: brain MRI and/or CT, electroencephalogram
Otolaryngologic disorder: chronic sinusitis, vestibular disorder
– Diagnostic imaging: paranasal sinus CT
Urological diseases: kidney stones, hydronephrosis, etc.
– Diagnostic imaging: abdominal ultrasonography
– Urinalysis: uric acid, Ca/Cr ratio
Metabolic or endocrine disease: mitochondrial disease, urea cycle disorder, fatty acid metabolism disease, acute intermittent porphyria, diabetes mellitus, Addison disease, pheochromocytoma, hereditary angioedema
– Blood examination: electrolyte, blood glucose, catecholamine, blood gas, lactic acid, amino acid, ammonia, ACTH, ADH
– Urinalysis: ketone body, organic acid, carnitine, porphobilinogen
Other: Munchausen syndrome, anxiety, depression, pregnancy
– Blood examination: hCG
– Urinalysis: drug test
– Other: psychological consult

22.5 Clinical Features

Patients with CVS often have histories of nausea, abdominal pain, and headache; 44% of patients report migraine headache, and 48% have a family history of migraine, consistent with the ICHD-3 classification of CVS as an episodic syndrome that may be associated with migraine (see Table 22.2). Median age at onset in a study by Li et al. was 4.8 years, and median duration was >3.6 years [15]. In our 2016 study, median age at onset was 4 years, overall median duration was 5.42 years, and in most cases CVS resolved over time [9]. However, the long average duration (5.42 years) indicated a need for good treatment and prophylaxis of CVS patients. Dignan et al. reported that CVS resolved in 69% of their patients (18/26) but did not specify the observation period [16]. We observed resolution in 96% of patients (24/25) over a 5-year observation period [9]; i.e., most patients achieved full recovery over a long-term follow-up period.

Table 22.2 Clinical characteristics of CVS

Parameter	Characteristic
Male:female	17:14
Age at onset	3–177 (median 48) months
Symptoms	
Vomiting	4–30 (median 10) times/h at peak, bilious (16%), bloody (28%)
Systemic	Lethargy (35%), pallor (45%), fever (55%), salivation (16%)
Gastrointestinal	Nausea (90%), abdominal pain (74%), anorexia (39%), diarrhea (32%)
Neurologic	Headache (58%), photophobia (9.8%), phonophobia (3.2%), vertigo (12%)
Temporal pattern	
Duration	1–7 (median 3) days
Periodic	52% have regular intervals, generally 2–4 weeks
Stereotypical	100%
Precipitating events	Psychological stress (13%), infection (16%), exhaustion (9.7%), dietary (6.5%), joyful event (9.7%)
	One or more triggers identified (45%)
Natural history	42–310 (median 116.5) months ($n = 28$), 41% + progress to migraine headache ($n = 27$)
Family history of migraine	CVS (13%), migraine headache (42%)

22.6 Treatment

Mild cases of CVS can be effectively treated simply by oral rehydration or antiemetic drugs. Severe cases may require hospitalization and intravenous rehydration. In the most severe cases (long vomiting duration, very frequent attacks, and/or hospitalization for rehydration), abortive therapy and/or prophylactic therapy should be considered.

22.7 Abortive Therapy

To date, no randomized control study has been performed in regard to abortive therapy (i.e., treatment intended to stop a migraine once it starts) for CVS. Clinical studies have indicated that vomiting by CVS patients may be effectively suppressed by treatment with ondansetron (serotonin-3 receptor antagonist), sumatriptan (serotonin 1B/1D agonist), or aprepitant (neurokinin-1 receptor antagonist) [17–19].

22.8 Prophylactic Therapy

Prophylactic therapy (i.e., a medication taken daily to reduce frequency and severity of attacks) should be considered for CVS patients whose attacks occur more than once per month and/or are severe and disabling [19]. In randomized controlled trial studies, amitriptyline and cyproheptadine were equally effective [20], and amitriptyline was more effective than topiramate [21]. In other clinical trials, phenobarbital, valproic acid, propranolol, riboflavin, L-carnitine, flunarizine, and co-enzyme Q10 were effective in some CVS cases [8, 19, 22]. A study period of at least 2 or 3 months is necessary to evaluate the effectiveness of a particular prophylactic therapy.

22.9 Conclusion

Differential diagnosis of CVS is often difficult. Appropriate therapy is important in potentially severe CVS cases, and correct diagnosis and initiation of therapy should be made at an early stage of the disorder.

References

1. Li BU, Murray RD, Heitlinger LA, Robbins JL, Hayes JR. Is cyclic vomiting syndrome related to migraine? J Pediatr. 1999;134:567–72.
2. Li BU, Murray RD, Heitlinger LA, Robbins JL, Hayes JR. Heterogeneity of diagnoses presenting as cyclic vomiting. Pediatrics. 1998;102:583–7.
3. Gee S. On fitful or recurring vomiting. St Bartholomew's Hosp Rep. 1882;18:1–6.
4. Headache Classification Committee of the International Headache Society (IHS). The International Classification of headache disorders, 3rd edition. Cephalalgia. 2018;38:1–211.
5. Drossman DA, editor. Rome IV functional gastrointestinal disorders: disorders of gut-brain interaction. 4th ed. Raleigh, NC: The Rome Foundation; 2016.
6. Abu-Arafeh I, Russell G. Cyclical vomiting syndrome in children: a population-based study. J Pediatr Gastroenterol Nutr. 1995;21:454–8.
7. Fleisher DR, Matar M. The cyclic vomiting syndrome: a report of 71 cases and literature review. J Pediatr Gastroenterol Nutr. 1993;17:361–9.
8. Hikita T, Kodama H, Nakamoto N, Kaga F, Amakata K, Ogita K, Kaneko S, Fujii Y, Yanagawa Y. Effective prophylactic therapy for cyclic vomiting syndrome in children using valproate. Brain Dev. 2009;31:411–3.
9. Hikita T, Kodama H, Ogita K, Kaneko S, Nakamoto N, Mimaki M. Cyclic vomiting syndrome in infants and children: a clinical follow-up study. Pediatr Neurol. 2016;57:29–33.
10. van Tilburg MA, Hyman PE, Walker L, Rouster A, Palsson OS, Kim SM, Whitehead WE. Prevalence of functional gastrointestinal disorders in infants and toddlers. J Pediatr. 2015;166:684–9.
11. Fitzpatrick E, Bourke B, Drumm B, Rowland M. The incidence of cyclic vomiting syndrome in children: population-based study. Am J Gastroenterol. 2008;103:991–5; quiz 996.
12. Saps M, Nichols-Vinueza DX, Rosen JM, Velasco-Benitez CA. Prevalence of functional gastrointestinal disorders in Colombian school children. J Pediatr. 2014;164:542–545 e541.
13. Devanarayana NM, Adhikari C, Pannala W, Rajindrajith S. Prevalence of functional gastrointestinal diseases in a cohort of Sri Lankan adolescents: comparison between Rome II and Rome III criteria. J Trop Pediatr. 2011;57:34–9.
14. Li BU, Lefevre F, Chelimsky GG, Boles RG, Nelson SP, Lewis DW, Linder SL, Issenman RM, Rudolph CD, North American Society for Pediatric Gastroenterology H, Nutrition. North American Society for Pediatric Gastroenterology, Hepatology, and Nutrition consensus statement on the diagnosis and management of cyclic vomiting syndrome. J Pediatr Gastroenterol Nutr. 2008;47:379–93.

15. Li BU, Misiewicz L. Cyclic vomiting syndrome: a brain-gut disorder. Gastroenterol Clin North Am. 2003;32:997–1019.
16. Dignan F, Symon DN, AbuArafeh I, Russell G. The prognosis of cyclical vomiting syndrome. Arch Dis Child. 2001;84:55–7.
17. Moses J, Keilman A, Worley S, Radhakrishnan K, Rothner AD, Parikh S. Approach to the diagnosis and treatment of cyclic vomiting syndrome: a large single-center experience with 106 patients. Pediatr Neurol. 2014;50:569–73.
18. Hikita T, Kodama H, Kaneko S, Amakata K, Ogita K, Mochizuki D, Kaga F, Nakamoto N, Fujii Y, Kikuchi A. Sumatriptan as a treatment for cyclic vomiting syndrome: a clinical trial. Cephalalgia. 2011;31:504–7.
19. Gelfand AA. Episodic syndromes of childhood associated with migraine. Curr Opin Neurol. 2018;31:281–5.
20. Badihian N, Saneian H, Badihian S, Yaghini O. Prophylactic therapy of cyclic vomiting syndrome in children: comparison of amitriptyline and cyproheptadine: a randomized clinical trial. Am J Gastroenterol. 2018;113:135–40.
21. Bagherian Z, Yaghini O, Saneian H, Badihian S. Comparison of the efficacy of amitriptyline and topiramate in prophylaxis of cyclic vomiting syndrome. Iran J Child Neurol. 2019;13:37–44.
22. Gokhale R, Huttenlocher PR, Brady L, Kirschner BS. Use of barbiturates in the treatment of cyclic vomiting during childhood. J Pediatr Gastroenterol Nutr. 1997;25:64–7.

Current Knowledge on Eating Experiences and Behaviours in Cystic Fibrosis: Exploring the Challenges and Potential Opportunities for Interventions

Helen Egan and Michail Mantzios

Cystic fibrosis (CF) is an autosomal recessive inherited disorder affecting up to 100,000 people worldwide and is the most common genetic disease in Caucasian North European populations. In the European Union, 1 in 2000–3000 newborns have CF, and in the USA, the incidence is 1 in every 3500 births [1] and is caused by defects in a recessive gene, the cystic fibrosis transmembrane conductance regulator (CFTR). The resulting imbalance in fluids and salts increases the production of thick, sticky mucus and impairs the functioning of the respiratory tract, inhibiting the clearance of microorganisms leading to recurrent infections. Lung disease is progressive and is the most significant life-limiting complication of CF [2]. CF also impacts on digestive system organs (liver, pancreas and intestine) causing pancreatic ducts to become blocked, preventing the production of digestive enzymes, leading to the maldigestion and malabsorption of nutrients [3, 4]. Secondary conditions such as diabetes mellitus and chronic liver damage are common, and other complications also include pneumothorax, haemoptysis and osteoporosis [3, 5]. Over the past two decades, life expectancy for people with CF has increased in the UK from 18 to 47 years [6]. This increased life expectancy is a result of developments in treatments, and as medications to treat the basic defect in CFTR develop further, life expectancy is likely to continue to rise [2]. This timely advancement also brings new challenges for patients and clinicians alike as complications of CF are seen to increase with age.

CF remains a progressive disease, and daily treatments are focused on managing symptoms; for the respiratory system, these include physiotherapy, nebulised bronchodilators, intravenous and/or oral antibiotics, steroids and mucolytics. For the digestive system, enzymes and nutritional supplements are required, and for more than a third of adults with CF-related diabetes (CFRD), tablets or insulin are required

---

H. Egan · M. Mantzios (✉)
Department of Psychology, Birmingham City University, Birmingham, England
e-mail: Helen.Egan@bcu.ac.uk; Michael.Mantzios@bcu.ac.uk

© Springer Nature Switzerland AG 2022
E. Manzato et al. (eds.), *Hidden and Lesser-known Disordered Eating Behaviors in Medical and Psychiatric Conditions*,
https://doi.org/10.1007/978-3-030-81174-7_23

[7]. The symptoms resulting from this genetic disorder require complex medical management which is burdensome and time-consuming; treatments take up to 4 h each day, with frequent hospital stays even when a person is relatively well. It is extremely challenging for people to find the time to complete all treatments every day, particularly when having to prioritise prescribed treatments within a daily routine which may include school, work, family and social activities. In addition, the motivation to undertake all treatments may be reduced as the positive association between current treatment regimens and future health is not always salient [8] and health is likely to progressively deteriorate regardless of adherence efforts [9]. Treatment adherence is a major concern [10]; poor adherence causes an increase in outpatient visits and hospital admissions, creating incorrect conclusions about treatment efficacy.

The damaging effects of CF frequently result in a compromised nutritional status due to a number of factors. Most people with CF have an increased energy need, between 150 and 200% of usual requirements due to increased resting energy expenditure [11], and damage caused to the lungs makes breathing more difficult which increases energy requirements. Pancreatic insufficiency, affecting up to 90% of the CF population, leads to malabsorption of fat and a need to ingest more fatty food. Enzymes are needed at every meal and snack, but even with this medication, many experience a number of difficult digestive symptoms including greasy and bulky stools, frequent and difficult bowel movements, constipation, nausea, swollen painful abdomen, heart burn and loss of appetite, all of which make it difficult to meet and maintain energy requirements [12].

These symptoms impact strongly on eating behaviours and nutritional and weight status, and this is of vital importance because optimal nutritional status is closely linked to respiratory status. Weight and body mass index (BMI) are well established in the literature as being independent predictors of mortality in CF [13, 14]. The importance of optimal nutritional status for health and for quality of life [3] means that dietetic treatments, counselling and support constitute a major part of treatment, and in the UK dieticians are important members of paediatric and adult multidisciplinary teams. From birth there is a necessary focus on following a prescribed dietary regimen alongside all other treatments including regular weighing and monitoring of weight, having to eat an elevated amount of calories each day, eating particular (high fat) foods and drinking plenty of water. Trying to comply with the recommendations can prove to be a very difficult challenge for both children and adults, especially when one considers that lack of appetite is a main symptom for many people. Nutritional supplements and enteral tube feeding are often needed to achieve adequate energy intake, and malnutrition remains a significant problem within CF [15].

Such an intense focus on diet, weight and exercise for disease management inevitably impacts on the development of eating behaviours, and eating difficulties in childhood including poor appetite, longer mealtimes, slower pace of eating and food refusal are well documented [16]. There is limited evidence investigating eating behaviours within adolescent and adult CF populations; research focuses on the psychopathology of eating, with initial early findings suggesting that people with

CF may be at risk of developing eating disorders [17]. Later studies suggested that formal eating disorders such as anorexia nervosa, bulimia nervosa and binge eating were not more prevalent but that disturbed eating attitudes and behaviours were evident, specifically using exercise to influence shape and a higher influence of weight on self-evaluation [18]. Given the serious consequences of low body weight on morbidity and mortality, some authors called for regular screening for disturbed eating in people with CF.

There are a number of challenges with investigating disordered eating behaviours within CF and indeed in other chronic lifelong conditions. The focus on diet and eating as part of a treatment regimen necessitates a preoccupation with eating, and being highly attentive to eating and diet is considered good adherence. Therefore interpreting research relying on self-report measures is problematic, as it is subject to respondent bias as participants may answer in a way that denotes their compliance and adherence, and even if this is not the case, an elevated focus on eating and body weight may be considered adaptive for health rather than disordered.

In a recent study, experiences and practices on disturbed eating behaviours in CF were sought from health-care providers [19]; this methodology circumvents the issue of potential patient responder bias. Health-care providers reported that almost half of patients misused pancreatic enzymes (though this may be poor adherence rather than disordered eating) and engaged in food restriction behaviours, while almost a third engaged in binge eating and/or skipping meals. Authors highlighted the need for a CF-specific disordered eating screening tool, a standard protocol for disordered CF eating and more specific training for health providers around disordered eating.

There is a paucity of research in regard to eating experiences and behaviours for people with CF; the available literature focuses on eating disorders and disordered eating and does not reach any clear conclusions for all the reasons discussed above. The narrative that is clear is that rules around eating and diet are very much in the clinical domain, what and how they eat become less of a personal life choice for people with CF and rather it is dictated by CF, clinical teams, parents and relatives. Enteral tube feeding is one of the treatment options available when insufficient calorie intake is prolonged, and while this can be highly effective in improving wellbeing [12], it is perceived by some people with CF as an ever-present threat. Having to resort to enteral feeding was seen in a recent study to epitomise a failure to self-regulate eating and illustrated the lack of personal control and choice over eating and an inability to keep oneself alive [20].

A fuller understanding of the eating behaviours in people with CF is needed to identify the prevalence of problematic eating, but also how to better support eating behaviours to achieve the maintenance of a healthy weight and to align any interventions with good psychological wellbeing. Egan et al.'s [20] research on everyday eating experiences of people with CF highlighted clearly the amount of time and cognitive effort expended in self-regulating eating, from thinking about eating, preparing to eat and actually consuming food. In this qualitative interview, study participants described using a number of strategies to try and reduce the effort needed to eat. These strategies included avoiding food preparation by using take-away, eating out or having partners prepare food, eating easy-to-swallow foods such as yoghurt and soup and eating easily available foods that need no preparation (crisps and chocolate). Distraction and multitasking, such as eating while watching a film, were also used in order to eat sufficient calories. Collectively these strategies present a picture of avoidance and inattentive or distracted eating, which are the very opposite to what is usually considered adaptive and healthy eating, namely, mindful eating.

This research also identified a preoccupation with weight gain, body image and dietary health implications, and eating was frequently seen as another treatment to endure. Overall in this study, there was an overriding lack of pleasure in eating; even when weight was stable and eating was not particularly difficult, it was not pleasurable and still created anxiety. The anxiety felt was related to previous experiences of how quickly health can fluctuate, from being able to self-regulate eating when relatively well; a person with CF can quickly become very ill, experiencing reduced appetite and increased nausea at a time when they need to consume more calories to maintain weight. This results in weight loss which then exacerbates symptoms and can bring the (usually unwanted) prospect of enteral feeding into the treatment plan.

This triad of experiences, lack of pleasure in food and eating, anxiety around eating and the fluctuating nature of CF, strike at the core of attempts to understand the nuances between disordered eating attitudes and behaviours and usual eating behaviours for someone with CF. Interventions to support eating experiences and behaviours need to be adaptive to fluctuations in health status which alter nutritional needs, requiring a change in how a person regulates their eating according to the current clinical assessment of the individual. They also need to address the fundamental issue of how to eat well when there is no pleasure in eating. Given the lack of current evidence on eating in CF, it is necessary to look at the wider literature on eating, particularly around modifying eating behaviours, to help in the development of effective interventions that enable self-regulation in a chronic condition that is constantly at risk of fluctuating and requiring different interventions.

Self-regulation, which is a primary aim for people with CF, has been explored extensively in association with eating and is increasingly problematic across the Western world. Researchers have attempted to address the problems of obesity and related diseases, to enable lower calorific consumption, and therefore weight loss and maintenance, by regulating food consumption [21]. While the problems around self-regulation are evidential for much of the general population, findings also propose that the main issue for obesity is living in an 'obesogenic environment', whether it related to a macro- or micro- level approach of environmental influence to overconsume. At a macro-level, researchers have proposed public health initiatives of increasing the availability of smaller portions and alternatives to sugary soft drinks [22]. Research evidence at a micro-level shows that overconsumption is evident when serving oneself on a larger plate or sitting too close to a bowl of chocolates. It is suggested that the obesogenic environment bears the most accountability for the increasing numbers in obesity [23, 24]. Other research has focused on the occurrence of multi-tasking (such as watching TV while eating) and indicates that not being attentive to the food leads to inaccurate recalling of how much food was consumed and to higher consumption compared to people who are not paying attention to another activity while eating [25, 26].

All such research has been classified as standing under the umbrella of mindless eating and has been given much attention in tackling the obesity epidemic. While this research shows how mindless eating poses a problem to the general population, Mantzios, Egan and Patchell [27] proposed that there is potential to enhance calorific intake by utilising the research conducted with the general population and to enable people with CF to mindlessly enhance their calorific intake. In essence, they suggested that the cognitive and environmental factors that lead the general public to overconsume may be a method of clinical and nutritional counselling and advice to help people with CF consume more calories when needed.

Over the past 10 years, there has been an emerging evidence of over-nutrition in people with CF leading to being overweight and obese [28]. This is due to a number of clinical and treatment factors including earlier diagnosis of CF and of pancreatic insufficiency and improved medical therapies, especially, but not confined to, CFTR targeted therapies. In addition, dietary and eating behaviour advice to consume a higher fat diet than non-CF people that has been endorsed over a lifetime by health providers may not be so consistently relevant, as the Western diet and the obesogenic environment have increased intake of high fat foods in the general population. The applicability of mindless eating in response to under nutrition has been suggested, and a fuller exploration of how mindfulness and mindful eating may support weight regulation in other health scenarios for people with CF is indicated.

Kabat-Zinn [29] described mindfulness as experiencing the present moment, whether it is pleasant or unpleasant, with qualities of awareness and non-judgement. Similarly, mindful eating adopts the fundamentals of mindfulness practices and applies them to eating- and food- related experiences. Mindful eating has been effective in increasing the pleasure around eating, while decreasing fat and sugar consumption, grazing and motivations to eat that are not aligned to internal feelings of hunger and satiety [30–34]. Furthermore, while some researchers have made clear propositions around eating less and making more informed choices [35–37], others have instigated the usefulness of mindful eating when eating is problematic or disordered [38, 39]. Egan and Mantzios [40] proposed how mindful eating may form an additional tool for achieving optimal weight for people with CF and how it could propose an element of self-regulation around eating and food. Their assumption was that mindful eating assists self-regulation by reducing the automatic, affect and cognitive alignments when eating, which are primarily responsible for eating and weight difficulties. Currently, self-regulation may be achieved through combining current findings and the need for both mindless and mindful eating in the repertoire of eating practices for clinicians and people with CF.

Levels of anxiety and depression are similar between individuals with CF and the general population [41]; however the impact of even slightly increased levels is detrimental for a person with CF as they are linked to reduced lung function, quality of life and adherence. Anxiety, stress and depression are also associated with emotional, external and restrained eating [42]; however this is so far largely unexplored in the CF literature. In a recent study, Egan and Mantzios' findings [43] suggested that higher levels of emotional eating (i.e. eating in response to emotions) significantly predicted higher BMI in a sample of people with CF. While a higher BMI is often the aim and is desirable, an increase in levels of emotional eating is not desirable for holistic health and wellbeing.

Emotional eating is more problematic in changing as a health behaviour (when compared to environmental influences) and may form a platform that would lead to other problematic eating such as binge eating and grazing. When mindfulness and mindful eating were tested conditionally in assessing their impact on the relationship between emotional eating and BMI, it was found that both mindfulness and mindful eating moderated this relationship to the extent of making it non-significant [44]. This research proposes the potential of mindfulness and mindful eating in creating a better eating environment for people with CF.

Within the literature on eating in people with CF, there is clear evidence for problematic eating experiences and attitudes. A strong focus on eating, high levels of anxiety, reduced or non-existent pleasure in eating and a difficulty self-regulating healthy weight are all very apparent. Whether these factors constitute disordered eating or not is debatable. Certainly being highly aware and attentive to weight and diet may be considered adaptive for the physiological health of people with CF, but the anxiety and lack of pleasure in eating are detrimental to both physiological and psychological health and wellbeing. The pressing need is find holistic ways of supporting healthy eating behaviours which assist in managing co-morbid conditions such as CFRD and osteoarthritis, maintain optimal weight rather than simply focusing on losing or gaining weight and tackle the psychological and social barriers to pleasurable eating. Given the complex fluctuating symptoms and extensive burden of treatments for people with CF, this is a considerable challenge.

References

1. Elborn JS. Cystic fibrosis. Lancet. 2016;388(10,059):2519–31.
2. Brennan AL, Blackman SM. EnVisioning the future: endocrinology in cystic fibrosis. J Cyst Fibros. 2019;18(6):743–5.
3. Abbott J, Hart A, Morton A, Gee L, Conway S. Health-related quality of life in adults with cystic fibrosis: the role of coping. J Psychosom Res. 2008;64(2):149–57.
4. Sinaasappel M, Stern M, Littlewood J, Wolfe S, Steinkamp G, Heijerman HG, Robberecht E, Döring G. Nutrition in patients with cystic fibrosis: a European Consensus. J Cyst Fibros. 2002;1(2):51–75.
5. Couce MARTA, O'Brien TD, Moran A, Roche PC, Butler PC. Diabetes mellitus in cystic fibrosis is characterized by islet amyloidosis. J Clin Endocrinol Metabol. 1996;81(3):1267–72.
6. Ramsden D, Carr S. Cystic fibrosis trust annual report; 2018. http://www.cysticfibrosis.org.uk/the-work-we-do/uk-cf-registry/reporting-and-resources. Accessed 28 Aug 2018.
7. Marshall BC, Butler SM, Stoddard M, Moran AM, Liou TG, Morgan WJ. Epidemiology of cystic fibrosis-related diabetes. J Pediatr. 2005;146(5):681–7.
8. Keyte R, Egan H, Mantzios M. An exploration into knowledge, attitudes, and beliefs towards risky health behaviours in a paediatric cystic fibrosis population. Clin Med Insights. 2019;13:1179548419849427.
9. Kettler LJ, Sawyer SM, Winefield HR, Greville HW. Determinants of adherence in adults with cystic fibrosis. Thorax. 2002;57(5):459–64.

10. Horne R, Weinman J, Barber N, Elliott R, Morgan M, Cribb A, Kellar I. Concordance, adherence and compliance in medicine taking. London: NCCSDO. 2005;2005:40–6.
11. Stallings VA, Stark LJ, Robinson KA, Feranchak AP, Quinton H, on Growth CP, Subcommittee N. Ad Hoc Working Group. Evidence-based practice recommendations for nutrition-related management of children and adults with cystic fibrosis and pancreatic insufficiency: results of a systematic review. J Am Diet Assoc. 2008;108(5):832–9.
12. Shimmin D, Lowdon J, Remmington T. Enteral tube feeding for cystic fibrosis. Cochrane Database Syst Rev. 2019:7.
13. Meyer KC, Sharma A, Brown R, Weatherly M, Moya FR, Lewandoski J, Zimmerman JJ. Function and composition of pulmonary surfactant and surfactant-derived fatty acid profiles are altered in young adults with cystic fibrosis. Chest. 2000;118(1):164–74.
14. Stern M, Wiedemann B, Wenzlaff P. From registry to quality management: the German Cystic Fibrosis Quality Assessment project 1995–2006. Eur Respir J. 2008;31(1):29–35.
15. Dray X, Kanaan R, Bienvenu T, Desmazes-Dufeu N, Dusser D, Marteau P, Hubert D. Malnutrition in adults with cystic fibrosis. Eur J Clin Nutr. 2005;59(1):152.
16. Quick VM, Byrd-Bredbenner C, Neumark-Sztainer D. Chronic illness and disordered eating: a discussion of the literature. Adv Nutr. 2013;4(3):277–86. https://doi.org/10.3945/an.112.003608.
17. Pumariega AJ, Pursell J, Spock A, Jones JD. Eating disorders in adolescents with cystic fibrosis. J Am Acad Child Psychiatry. 1986;25(2):269–75.
18. Shearer JE, Bryon M. The nature and prevalence of eating disorders and eating disturbance in adolescents with cystic fibrosis. J Royal Soc Med. 2004;97:36–42.
19. Quick V, Chang G. Health care provider's experiences, practices, and recommendations for interventions and screening of cystic fibrosis patients with disordered eating: a qualitative analysis. Chronic Illn. 2019;10:1742395319881182.
20. Egan HH, Mantzios M, Nash EF, Barrett J, Regan AM. A qualitative study: mindful eating attitudes and behaviours in a cystic fibrosis population. J Cyst Fibros. 2017;16:S147.
21. World Health Organization. Diet, nutrition and the prevention of chronic diseases: report of a joint WHO/FAO expert consultation. Geneva: World Health Organization; 2003.
22. Osei-Assibey G, Dick S, Macdiarmid J, et al. The influence of the food environment on overweight and obesity in young children: a systematic review. BMJ Open. 2012;2:e001538.
23. Van Ittersum K, Wansink B. Plate size and color suggestibility: the Delboeuf Illusion's bias on serving and eating behavior. J Consum Res. 2011;39(2):215–28.
24. Van Kleef E, Shimizu M, Wansink B. Serving bowl selection biases the amount of food served. J Nutr Educ Behav. 2012;44(1):66–70.
25. Higgs S, Rutters F, Thomas JM, Naish K, Humphreys GW. Top down modulation of attention to food cues via working memory. Appetite. 2012;59(1):71–5.
26. Higgs S, Woodward M. Television watching during lunch increases afternoon snack intake of young women. Appetite. 2009;52(1):39–43.
27. Mantzios M, Egan H, Patchell C. Can existing knowledge on eating behaviors and obesity support people with cystic fibrosis who are nutritionally compromised? Front Psychol. 2016;7:1477.
28. Litvin M, Yoon JC, Casella JL, Blackman SM, Brennan AL. Energy balance and obesity in individuals with cystic fibrosis. J Cyst Fibros. 2019;18:S38–47.
29. Kabat-Zinn J. Full catastrophe living: the program of the stress reduction clinic at the University of Massachusetts Medical Center. New York: Delta.
30. Hong PY, Lishner DA, Han KH. Mindfulness and eating: an experiment examining the effect of mindful raisin eating on the enjoyment of sampled food. Mindfulness. 2014;5(1):80–7.
31. Keyte R, Egan H, Mantzios M. How does mindful eating without non-judgement, mindfulness and self-compassion relate to motivations to eat palatable foods in a student population? Nutr Health. 2019;28:7.
32. Mantzios M, Egan H. An exploratory examination of mindfulness, self-compassion, and mindful eating in relation to motivations to eat palatable foods and BMI. Health Psychol Rep. 2018;6

33. Mantzios M, Egan H, Bahia H, Hussain M, Keyte R. How does grazing relate to body mass index, self-compassion, mindfulness and mindful eating in a student population? Health Psychol Open. 2018;5(1):2055102918762701.
34. Mantzios M, Egan H, Hussain M, Keyte R, Bahia H. Mindfulness, self-compassion, and mindful eating in relation to fat and sugar consumption: an exploratory investigation. Eat Weight Disord. 2018;23(6):833–40.
35. Dutt S, Keyte R, Egan H, Hussain M, Mantzios M. Healthy and unhealthy eating amongst stressed students: considering the influence of mindfulness on eating choices and consumption. Health Psychol Report. 7(2):113–20.
36. Jordan CH, Wang W, Donatoni L, Meier BP. Mindful eating: trait and state mindfulness predict healthier eating behavior. Personal Individ Differ. 2014;68:107–11.
37. Miller CK, Kristeller JL, Headings A, Nagaraja H, Miser WF. Comparative effectiveness of a mindful eating intervention to a diabetes self-management intervention among adults with type 2 diabetes: a pilot study. J Acad Nutr Diet. 2012;112(11):1835–42.
38. Albers S. Using mindful eating to treat food restriction: a case study. Eat Disord. 2010;19(1):97–107.
39. Hepworth NS. A mindful eating group as an adjunct to individual treatment for eating disorders: a pilot study. Eat Disord. 2010;19(1):6–16.
40. Egan H, Mantzios M. Mindfulness and mindful eating: reflections on how individuals with cystic fibrosis may benefit. Eat Weight Disord. 2016;21(3):511–2.
41. Quittner AL, Goldbeck L, Abbott J, Duff A, Lambrecht P, Solé A, Tibosch MM, Brucefors AB, Yüksel H, Catastini P, Blackwell L. Prevalence of depression and anxiety in patients with cystic fibrosis and parent caregivers: results of The International Depression Epidemiological Study across nine countries. Thorax. 2014;69(12):1090–7.
42. Gan WY, Nasir MM, Zalilah MS, Hazizi AS. Disordered eating behaviors, depression, anxiety and stress among Malaysian University students. Coll Stud J. 2011;45(2):296–310.
43. Egan H, Keyte R, Nash EF, Barrett J, Regan A, Mantzios M. Exploring the moderating influence of mindfulness, mindful eating and self-compassion on the relationship of emotional eating and BMI in a cystic fibrosis population. J Cyst Fibros. 2019;18:S182.
44. Egan H, Keyte R, Nash EF, Barrett J, Regan A, Mantzios M. Mindfulness moderates the relationship between emotional eating and body mass index in a sample of people with cystic fibrosis. Eating and weight disorders-studies on anorexia, bulimia and obesity. 2021;26(5):1521–7.

Type 2 Diabetes and Eating Disorders

Walter Milano

Several clinical and epidemiological observations have been reported in literature indicating a more rising risk of developing eating disorders (ED) in patients with type 1 diabetes (T1DM) and type 2 diabetes (T2DM) than the overall population. There are more data about the relationship between type 1 diabetes and eating disorders than between people with type 2 diabetes and eating disorders. The presence of eating disorders in both the types of diabetes shall complicate and make the diabetes more instable. Not by chance these will be directly or indirectly responsible for other issues (like the disorder of metabolism) and even represent a remarkable risk factor for diabetes chronic issues.

Type 1 diabetes more often occurs in juvenile age because of a reduced insulin production in the pancreas and the beta-cell destruction, and it is characterised by an absolute lack of insulin, on autoimmune and idiopathic basis, supported by genetic and environmental factors. Type 2 diabetes more often occurs in old age because of defects resulting from the use of insulin by body cells and the interaction between predisposing genetic and environmental factors. Overweight and obesity shall be associated with type 2 diabetes in almost 80% of patients, and this prerogative has led to the connotation "diabesity", underlining the fact that the majority of patients with diabetes is either overweight or obese [1–4].

The interest of either T2DM or ED was born only during the 1990s, highlighting that the T2DM diagnosis occurs in juvenile age increasingly with overweight and obesity [5, 6] and it frequently presents clinical symptoms of eating behaviour disorders, in particular with the binge eating disorder (BED) [7].

W. Milano (✉)
Departmental Operational Eating Disorder Unit, Mental Health Department ASL Napoli 2 Nord, Napoli, Italy
e-mail: walterdonato.milano@aslnapoli2nord.it

© Springer Nature Switzerland AG 2022
E. Manzato et al. (eds.), *Hidden and Lesser-known Disordered Eating Behaviors in Medical and Psychiatric Conditions*,
https://doi.org/10.1007/978-3-030-81174-7_24

The most remarkable longitudinal predictor of eating disorder emergency in diabetes shall be the eating restriction, and the use of diets could be seen either as a risk factor of ED beginning or the first step of its clinical presentation. Handling diabetes, therefore, shall represent an implicit risk factor, linked to the focusing on food intake and restriction. This might set off an eating dysregulation with episodes of overeating and binge eating. Vulnerable patients could therefore intensify their efforts to control food intake and weight, being trapped in the diet circle, binging and trying to compensate weight control [8]. Although recent innovations on handling diabetes might help several patients adopt a more flexible food plan, carbohydrate control intake is still remarkable in meal plans of a diabetic patient and in the dose titration of drugs and insulin.

Food plan for diabetics shall be more flexible than the diet one, but it will be focused more on food and calories, suggesting food restrictions [8]. High levels of body unsatisfaction observed in overweight and obese patients with type 2 diabetes tend to increase their desire to be thin and be linked to severe depressive symptoms.

Among the several clinical manifestations, anorexia nervosa and bulimia nervosa are exceptional in patients with type 2 diabetes, since they generally occur in much younger age groups, while binge eating disorder (BED) might occur even in old age; thus, this disorder could be more frequently associated with type 2 diabetes too [7, 9, 10]. The mechanisms involved in the association between type 2 diabetes and ED are not completely clear. The risk factors mostly related to ED development in diabetes shall be high body mass index, weight gain, dissatisfaction with their bodies, desire of thinness and depressed attitude [6, 11–13].

The correlation between T2DM and BED has been frequently discovered in prevalence studies [14, 15]. Herpetz et al. [16] have conducted the first multicentric study to value ED prevalence in a sample of type 1 diabetic patients ($n = 341$) and type 2 diabetic patients ($n = 322$). Although the authors had found similar gaps of ED prevalence in the two samples, the distribution of ED categories differed one another. In T2DM group a higher prevalence of 12.6% was found in women (2.4% BN; 7.1% BED; 3% EDNOS) than a prevalence of 7.1% in men (1.3% BN; 4.5% BED; 1.3% EDNOS). In the group of type 1 diabetes mellitus, a prevalence of ED lifetime of 16.5% was found with a higher value of anorexia nervosa (AN) and bulimia nervosa (BN). In total, ED mostly associated with type 2 diabetes was BED, with a prevalence of 5.9%.

The association between ED and T2DM could vary, in several studies, from 2.5% to 40%, and the most frequent eating disorder is BED with a prevalence of 2.5%–25.6%. Moreover, the presence of BED seems to be directly related to the obesity value. Subjects with T2DM and a concurrent BED are generally younger with a higher body mass index (BMI) and more depressive sypmtoms [17]. Even Nicolau et al. [18] have recently underlined a positive correlation between eating psychopathology and BMI in a sample of T2DM patients.

Kenardy et al. [19] have reported the presence of binge crisis of 14% in 50 patients with recent diagnosis of T2DM and 4% in healthy controls.

Papelbaum [20] has recently found in a study conducted on 70 patients with T2DM, in which 77% women, average aged 52.9 + 6.8 and with an average BMI of

30.6 + 5.2 kg/m^2, a ED prevalence of 20%. Also in this study the most frequent condition found was the BED, reported in 7 out of 14 patients with ED (10%). BN has been diagnosed in three patients and four individuals who have shown an eating disorder unless otherwise specified (EDNOS), with subclinical BED. In this study it is also shown that patients with an ED had higher levels of obesity. Moreover, patients with ED presented a less control of insulin than patients with normal eating behaviour, not related specifically to age or duration of diabetes.

In a randomly and multicentric study named TODAY, published in 2011 [21], it was shown that 6% of 678 teenagers with type 2 diabetes presented diagnostic criteria for BED, while 20% was classified as a subclinical group. Moreover, there was a higher severity of depressive symptoms in young patients with BED.

Although uncontrolled eating disorder is quiet frequent, minor phenomena of losing control and hypereating, such as a frequency of binge crisis inferior to the one planned for a diagnosis of BED [5, 22, 23], are current in type 2 diabetes. Thus, uncontrolled eating disorder is the tip of the iceberg, whose submerged portion comprehends alterations of eating behaviour subthreshold that could interfere with the metabolic control. In fact, even modest alterations of eating behaviour, variously measured, correlate with the metabolic control in patients with type 2 diabetes [9]. For this reason, an accurate verification of eating behaviour, by a deep interview, is suggested for all patients with type 2 diabetes and with ponderal excess in which it is not possible to get an appropriate control of insulin easily [9].

Night eating syndrome (NES) could also occur in patients with T2DM [24–26]. In a systematic review of 10 studies, which included more than 7500 patients with T2DM, Abbott et al. [27] found, in 2018, a prevalence of BED of 1.2–8% and of 3.8–8.4% of NES. Patients with T2DM and BED had a higher BMI than patients with T2DM without BED in two studies reporting BMI. There weren't differences of value of glycated haemoglobin (HbA1c) among patients with and without BED in two studies measuring HbA1c. NES is characterised by night hyperphagia, insomnia and morning anorexia, and it affects almost 1% of overall population and till 6–16% in patients with obesity and from 2 to 20% in patients candidate for bariatric surgery [28]. BED and NES could have the same negative impact on metabolic values in patients with T2DM. It has been proved that a higher severity of binge eating is strictly related to a higher risk of metabolic problems, such as an increase of HbA1C, blood pressure and BMI [29].

Moreover, it has been found that only 1 day of high fat overeating could cause a significant increase of postprandal glucose of 17.1% and a reduction of insulin sensitivity of 28% [30]. Also sleep deprivation and reduced quality of sleep are characteristics of NES and risk factors for T2DM and obesity [31, 32]. Suffering from BED and NES could have implications on the treatment choice for patients with T2DM. For example, eating disorders could have an impact on bariatric surgery results, while bariatric surgery could have an impact on BED and NES [33–35].

The occurrence of eating disorders in people with diabetes increases the risk of severe diabetic complications, such as retinopathy, nephropathy and untimely death [36, 37]. Thus, it is extremely important to consider the occurrence of possible ED since the first signals of metabolic lack of control.

The first signal is the inconstant control of insulin: a high level of HbA1C should raise the suspicion not only of a reduced conformity to the diabetic treatment in general terms, but also of possible episodes of binge [23, 38]. Another signal is repeated hypoglycaemia; this could interest self-provoked vomit patients, who try to compensate their binge crisis, or patients who overtake insulin intentionally to compensate dessert overeating [39, 40]. On the other hand, recurrent ketoacidosis (associated with intentional deprivation or reduction of insulin intakes to lose weight) should raise as many concerns as irregularity of medical controls [41, 42]. Moreover, a higher attention should be paid to the occurrence of depressive symptoms, lack of self-confidence and typical clinical signals of eating disorder, like strict dietary restrictions or the opposite, like eating too much food, the use of laxatives, self-provoked vomit, intensive physical exercise or excessive attention to weight and body shape [9, 43].

The evidence, thus, of a substantial comorbidity between diabetes, both type 1 and type 2, and eating disorders, makes it necessary that health employees who work in the diabetology field have to pay attention to a likely ED diagnosis, because of the high occurrence of BED and NES in their patients. The treatment of eating disorder in patients with type 2 diabetes is still a field to be explored. ED includes a wide variety of behaviours and attitudes towards food [44]. Nutritional intervention for diabetic therapy could improve or paradoxically deteriorate the eating behaviour of these patients, causing, for example, current phenomena of weight loss, feelings of inadequacy, reduction of self-confidence and mood deflection. Depressive symptoms also deteriorate eating behaviour, creating a vicious circle. It is not possible to reply to the complexity of eating behaviour and its reasons, on therapeutical basis, with a merely prescriptive or directive approach, but in a multiprofessional way with a multidisciplinary team of therapists, including a diabetes specialist, a psychiatrist and a dietician, who provide the usage of behavioural techniques, procedures to strengthen patients' motivation and, above all, an appropriate patients' accountability, beside medical and nutritional approach. Further studies shall be needed to explore the impact of BED and NES in the managing of T2DM and the development of long-term diabetic complications. The effect of new anti-diabetes therapies that reduce appetite and the increasing use of low-calorie diets and bariatric surgery in the managing of T2DM could make more important the screening and the early diagnosis of these eating disorders.

References

1. International Diabetes Federation. IDF diabetes atlas. 8th ed; 2017. p. 155.
2. Mokdad AH, Ford ES, Bowman BA, Dietz WH, Vinicor F, Bales VS, Marks JS. Prevalence of obesity, diabetes, and obesity-related health risk factors, 2001. JAMA. 2003;289(1):76–9.
3. Butler AE, Janson J, Bonner-Weir S, Ritzel R, Rizza RA, Butler PC. Beta-cell deficit and increased beta-cell apoptosis in humans with type 2 diabetes. Diabete. 2003;52(1):102–10.
4. Kahn SE, Hull RL, Utzschneider KM. Mechanisms linking obesity to insulin resistance and type 2 diabetes. Nature. 2006;444(7121):840–6.

5. Herpertz S, Albus C, Lichtblau K, Köhle K, Mann K, Senf W. Relationship of weight and eating disorders in type 2 diabetic patients: a multicenter study. Int J Eat Disord. 2000;28(1):68–77.
6. Herpertz S, Albus C, Kielmann R, Hagemann-Patt H, Lichtblau K, Köhle K, Mann K, Senf WJ. Comorbidity of diabetes mellitus and eating disorders: a follow-up study. Psychosom Res. 2001;51(5):673–8.
7. García-Mayor RV, García-Soidán FJ. Eating disorders in type 2 diabetic people: brief review. Diabetes Metab Syndr. 2017;11(3):221–4.
8. Colton PA, Olmsted MP, Daneman D, Rydall AC, Rodin GM. Natural history and predictors of disturbed eating behaviour in girls with type 1 diabetes. Diabet Med. 2007;24(4):424–9.
9. Mannucci E. Disturbi del comportamento alimentare nel diabete il Diabete 18 (3) Settembre; 2006.
10. Crow S, Kendall D, Praus B, Thuras P. Binge eating and other psychopathology in patients with type II diabetes mellitus. Int J Eat Disord. 2001;30(2):222–6.
11. Raevuori A, Suokas J, Haukka J, et al. Highly increased risk of type 2 diabetes in patients with binge eating disorder and bulimia nervosa. Int J Eat Disord. 2015;48(6):555–62.
12. Thomas JG, Butryn ML, Stice E, Lowe MR. A prospective test of the relation between weight change and risk for bulimia nervosa. Int J Eat Disord. 2011;44(4):295–303.
13. Carroll P, Tiggemann M, Wade T. The role of body dissatisfaction and bingeing in the self-esteem of women with type II diabetes. J Behav Med. 1999;22(1):59–74.
14. Javaras KN, Pope HG, Lalonde JK, Roberts JL, Nillni YI, Laird NM, et al. Cooccurrence of binge eating disorder with psychiatric and medical disorders. J Clin Psychiatry. 2008;69(2):266–73.
15. Kessler RC, Berglund PA, Chiu WT, Deitz AC, Hudson JI, Shahly V, et al. The prevalence and correlates of binge eating disorder in the World Health Organization world mental health surveys. Biol Psychiatry. 2013;73(9):904–14.
16. Herpertz S, Wagener R, Albus C, Kocnar M, Wagner R, Best F. Diabetes mellitus and eating disorders: a multicenter study on the comorbidity of the two diseases. J Psychosom Res. 1998;44(3/4):503–15.
17. Pinhas-Hamiel O, Levy-Shraga Y. Eating disorders in adolescents with type 2 and type 1 diabetes. Curr Diab Rep. 2013;13(2):289–97.
18. Nicolau J, Simo R, Sanchís P, Ayala L, Fortuny R, Zubillaga I, et al. Eating disorders are frequent among type 2 diabetic patients and are associated with worse metabolic and psychological outcomes: results from a cross-sectional study in primary and secondary care settings. Acta Diabetol. 2015;52(6):1037–44.
19. Kenardy J, Mensch M, Bowen K, Pearson S. A comparison of eating behaviors in newly diagnosed NIDDM patients and case-matched control subjects. Diabetes Care. 1994;17(10):1197–9.
20. Papelbaum M, de Oliveira Moreira R, Coutinho WF, Kupfer R, Freitas S, Luz RR, Appolinario JC. Does binge-eating matter for glycemic control in type 2 diabetes patients? J Eat Disord. 2019;7:30.
21. TODAY Study Group, Wilfley D, Berkowitz R, Goebel-Fabbri A, Hirst K, Ievers-Landis C, et al. Binge eating, mood, and quality of life in youth with type 2 diabetes: baseline data from the today study. Diabetes Care. 2011;34(4):858–60.
22. Kenardy J, Mensch M, Bowen K, Green B, Walton J, Dalton D. Disordered eating behaviours in women with type 2 diabetes mellitus. Eat Behav. 2001;2:183–92.
23. Mannucci E, Tesi F, Ricca V, Pierazzuoli E, Barciulli E, Moretti S, Di Bernardo M, Travaglino R, Carrara S, Zucchi T, Placidi GF, Rotella CM. Eating behavior in obese patients with type 2 diabetes mellitus. Int J Obes Relat Metab Disord. 2002;26:848–53.
24. Gallant AR, Lundgren J, Drapeau V. The night-eating syndrome and obesity. Obes Rev. 2012;13(6):528–36.
25. Kessler RC, Berglund PA, Chiu WT, et al. The prevalence and correlates of binge eating disorder in the World Health Organization world mental health surveys. Biol Psychiatry. 2013;73(9):904–14.
26. de Zwaan M. Binge eating disorder and obesity. Int J Obes Relat Metab Disord. 2001;25(Suppl 1):S51–5.

27. Abbott S, Dindol N, Tahrani AA, Piya MK. Binge eating disorder and night eating syndrome in adults with type 2 diabetes: a systematic review. J Eat Disord. 2018;6:36.
28. De Zwaan M, Marschollek M, Allison KC. The night eating syndrome (NES) in bariatric surgery patients. Eur Eat Disord Rev. 2015;23:426–34.
29. Meneghini LF, Spadola J, Florez H. Prevalence and associations of binge eating disorder in a multiethnic population with type 2 diabetes. Diabetes Care. 2006;29(12):2760.
30. Parry S, Woods R, Hodson L, Hulston C. A single day of excessive dietary fat intake reduces whole-body insulin sensitivity: the metabolic consequence of binge eating. Nutrients. 2017;9(8):818.
31. Byberg S, Hansen A-LS, Christensen DL, et al. Sleep duration and sleep quality are associated differently with alterations of glucose homeostasis. Diabet Med. 2012;29(9):e354–60.
32. McNeil J, Doucet É, Chaput J-P. Inadequate sleep as a contributor to obesity and type 2 diabetes. Can J Diabetes. 2013;37(2):103–8.
33. Webb JB, Applegate KL, Grant JP. A comparative analysis of type 2 diabetes and binge eating disorder in a bariatric sample. Eat Behav. 2011;12(3):175–81.
34. Meany G, Conceição E, Mitchell JE. Binge eating, binge eating disorder and loss of control eating: effects on weight outcomes after bariatric surgery. Eur Eat Disord Rev. 2014;22(2):87–91.
35. Livhits M, Mercado C, Yermilov I, et al. Preoperative predictors of weight loss following bariatric surgery: systematic review. Obes Surg. 2012;22(1):70–89.
36. Goebel-Fabbri AE, Fikkan J, Franko DL, Pearson K, Anderson BJ, Weinger K. Insulin restriction and associated morbidity and mortality in women with type 1 diabetes. Diabetes Care. 2008;31(3):415–9.
37. Nielsen S, Emborg C, Mølbak AG. Mortality in concurrent type 1 diabetes and anorexia nervosa. Diabetes Care. 2002;25(2):309–12.
38. Petitti DB, Klingensmith GJ, Bell RA, Andrews JS, Dabelea D, Imperatore G, et al. Glycemic control in youth with diabetes: the SEARCH for diabetes in Youth Study. J Pediatr. 2009;155:668–72.
39. Schober E, Wagner G, Berger G, Gerber D, Mengl M, Sonnenstatter S, et al. Prevalence of intentional under—and overdosing of insulin in children and adolescents with type 1 diabetes. Pediatr Diabetes. 2011;12(7):627–31.
40. Racicka E, Bryńska A. Eating disorders in children and adolescents with type 1 and type 2 diabetes—prevalence, risk factors, warning signs. Psychiatr Pol. 2015;49(5):1017–24.
41. Goebel-Fabbri AE. Diabetes and eating disorders. J Diabetes Sci Technol. 2008;2(3):530–2.
42. Newton CA, Raskin P. Diabetic ketoacidosis in type 1 and type 2 diabetes mellitus: clinical and biochemical differences. Arch Intern Med. 2004;164(17):1925–1931.37.
43. Mannucci E, Tesi F, Ricca V, Pierazzuoli E, Barciulli E, Moretti S, et al. Eating behavior in obese patients with and without type 2 diabetes mellitus. Int J Obes Relat Metab Disord. 2002;26:848–53.
44. Walter M. I disturbi dell'alimentazione. Clinica e terapia. Giovanni Fioriti Editore; 2015.

Type 1 Diabetes and Disordered Eating Behavior

Rita Francisco

25.1 Introduction

Type 1 diabetes mellitus (T1DM) is a chronic condition in which the pancreas produces little or no insulin, and most cases of T1DM are diagnosed in childhood. The prevalence estimates indicate almost 500,000 children under 15 years of age suffer from T1DM worldwide [1]. Access to affordable treatment, including insulin, is critical to the survival of individuals living with diabetes. According to the World Health Organization [2], data on global trends in T1DM prevalence and incidence are not available, but many high-income countries have reported an annual increase in the incidence of T1DM in childhood of between 3% and 4%. T1DM is characterized by chronic hyperglycemia, which leads to macrovascular and microvascular complications [3] that may be prevented or delayed with current treatment recommendations. However, the risk of complications of T1DM (e.g., eye disease, kidney disease, nerve damage) and mortality increase when diabetes is comorbid with disordered eating behaviors (DEBs) or eating disorders (EDs) [4, 5] because EDs have the highest mortality rate of any mental illness [6].

Patients with T1DM are at heightened risk for developing comorbid DEBs or EDs, primarily due to daily disease management, which requires mandatory food monitoring and surveillance of the insulin-to-carbohydrate ratio [7–9], and other psychological difficulties, including depression, anxiety symptoms, or psychological distress [10–13]. A longitudinal study of girls with T1DM for 14 years (with a mean age of 11.8 years at time 1) revealed a probability of developing DEBs or an ED over this period of 79% and 60%, respectively [14]. Diverse studies reported a higher risk of 2–3 times in individuals with T1DM compared to healthy controls

R. Francisco (✉)
Universidade Católica Portuguesa, Católica Research Centre for Psychological, Family and Social Wellbeing (CRC-W), Lisboa, Portugal
e-mail: ritafrancisco@ucp.pt

(e.g., [15, 16]). The estimated prevalence of DEBs in T1DM individuals is 25–50% in women and 9–27% in men, with variations depending on the sample, age range, and measures used [13, 17–20]. Despite males and females are equally affected by T1DM, the highest occurrence of DEBs and EDs is observed in females and young adults [13]. A meta-analysis of controlled studies on the prevalence of EDs in T1DM revealed no increased prevalence of anorexia nervosa compared to the general population, but there was an increase in the prevalence for bulimia nervosa and eating disorder not otherwise specified (EDNOS) in this group of patients [21].

25.2 Disordered Eating and Eating Disorders Among Type 1 Diabetes Patients

Living with T1DM requires major lifestyle changes and demanding daily disease management from an early age, including insulin administration and dietary intake monitoring (e.g., carbohydrate counting), exercise, and the frequent monitoring of blood glucose levels, to reduce the risk of short- and long-term complications [22]. Weight gain is a common side effect as glycemic control improves, which leads to frequent weight concerns and body dissatisfaction [4] that may increase the risk of restrictive and overeating DEBs. Previous studies demonstrated that poor metabolic control, as measured by HbA1c as an indicator of long-term blood glucose levels, especially in females [16, 18, 23], and high body mass index [22, 24] are strongly associated with DEBs. In addition to the typical behaviors associated with DEBs in the general population (e.g., excessive dieting, excessive exercise, binge eating, purging behaviors), a common and serious DEB in individuals with T1DM is intentional insulin restriction or omission, which is not currently appropriately reflected in the fifth edition of the *Diagnostic and Statistical Manual of Mental Disorders* [4]. This specific condition—when prescribed insulin doses are omitted or altered with the sole goal of achieving weight loss and the purging of calories occurs via glucosuria (glucose excreted through the urine)—have been referred to as "diabulimia" [25–27]. Diverse studies reported that a significant percentage of people with T1DM intentionally omit insulin, from 7.3% of young adults [8] to approximately 30% in women who participated in longitudinal studies [5, 14]. Deliberate insulin omission is a widely recognized cause of recurrent diabetic ketoacidosis in adolescents and young adults with T1DM [12, 24], which is a life-threatening emergency in which the body is unable to use glucose as an energy source and breaks down fatty acids as an alternative energy source [25]. T1DM patients who omit insulin exhibit significantly increased rates of diabetes complications (e.g., nephropathy and foot problems) and earlier death than those who use insulin appropriately [5].

It is of particular importance to reflect in a systemic and integrated way on the process of the development of DEBs and EDs in patients with T1DM. The development of T1DM in preadolescence or adolescence seems to place girls at risk for the subsequent development of DEBs or EDs because of the hormonal changes and gains in weight and fat mass associated with the transition from childhood to adolescence [28]. In addition to dealing with the typical demands of adolescence (e.g., accepting body changes, integration in peer groups, becoming more independent of the family), patients with T1DM must also cope with the demands of this chronic metabolic disease (e.g., hospital stays, blood glucose self-control, injections, maintaining a strict diet) and the emotional and social demands of adjustment. All of these aspects are a constant challenge to the well-being of the adolescent and may trigger DEBs and/or EDs [22, 29].

Qualitative studies using the "voices" of patients provided rich insights into why people with T1DM are at increased risk for disordered eating. For example, adolescents with T1DM identified some main causative factors for their eating problems, such as body image dissatisfaction (because "it is more important to be beautiful than to take care of diabetes"), low compliance with insulin intake and food control, or fear of weight gain and judgment by family and friends [30]. Young adults also referred to the greater difficulty in losing weight since their diagnosis with diabetes, which contributes to higher body dissatisfaction and the tendency to stop taking insulin in order to lose weight [8].

Some models have been developed to encompass the development and maintenance of disordered eating in T1DM (e.g., [22, 31]). Recently, De Paoli and Rogers [4] proposed a transdiagnostic model of disordered eating in T1DM based on a systematic literature review and previous models. According to these authors, perfectionism and low self-esteem (complicated by feeling different due to diabetes) predispose an individual to dysfunctional self-evaluation (such as overconcern with eating, weight, and shape), as in the general population. The pressure of disease management exacerbates the body concerns of an individual with T1DM, because of the learned importance of eating, exercise, and the effects of insulin (including weight gain). If strict behaviors (e.g., dieting) are used to cope with the uncertainties and frustration of T1DM, these behaviors may develop into DEBs, such as restricting, binging, and/or purging (including insulin restriction). Poor affect regulation, perceived low blood glucose, and disinhibited eating contribute to the maintenance of insulin restriction. Besides the health complications related to ED (e.g., loss of bone density, hypotension), patients with T1DM suffer additional health effects, such as the effects arising from hypo- or hyperglycemia, which may be very deleterious. The confrontation with these short- and medium-term diabetes-related complications, including the fear of weight gain and poor glycemic control, feeds back into the overevaluation of shape, weight, and eating, and the cycle continues [4].

Given the frequency and severity of comorbid T1DM and DEBs and EDs, as well as their strong association with long-term medical complications in patients with T1DM, significant attention must be given to screening, early detection, and subsequent treatment efforts (e.g., [5, 14]).

25.3 Screening and Assessment

The identification of DEBs and the diagnosis of an ED in the general population and patients with T1DM are difficult. Different screening methods produce different results for DEBs in this population because these patients present specific DEBs related to their disease (e.g., insulin omission), which are not reflected in traditional measures of EDs, such as EAT-26, EDE-Q, or SCOFF. However, the special focus on healthy eating, carbohydrate counting, and insulin timing required for the management of T1DM can lead to an overfocus on body weight and shape, implying a risk of false positives when these questionnaires are used [32, 33]. Therefore, the Diabetes Eating Problem Survey—Revised (DEPS-R) was developed as a disordered eating screening tool specifically for people with diabetes and presents good psychometric properties in children, adolescents, and adults with T1DM (e.g., [32, 34]). The DEPS-R is a 16-item diabetes-specific self-report measure for DEBs organized into three factors: maladaptive eating, preoccupation with thinness, and concept of maintaining high blood glucose values to lose weight. It may be completed in less than 10 min during a routine clinical encounter [34].

Evidence exists that patients with DEBs or EDs frequently hide or avoid exposing their disordered eating behaviors and attitudes, and this tendency is especially true for adolescents. Therefore, an adequate strategy for performing an accurate evaluation of adolescents with T1DM who may exhibit DEBs is to also consider a parent-report evaluation, who may contribute to the prompt detection of DEBs and timely intervention [15].

25.4 Treatment and Recovery

T1DM patients with EDs show worse outcomes with conventional outpatient treatment for EDs and have a higher likelihood of dropping out of treatment, and their EDs are more likely to relapse after recovery [14, 27]. Some specific aspects of the T1DM treatment itself may conflict with ED treatment. On the one hand, T1DM requires learning how to control glucose levels through the monitoring of weight, shape, and eating and insulin administration. On the other hand, in order to recover from an ED, patients are encouraged to stop calorie counting, be flexible in their eating behaviors, and moderate their high standards and perfectionism [22]. It is essential to ensure that all needs, including adherence to insulin administration and normalization of eating behaviors, are met during treatment and recovery. Multidisciplinary teams and joint work between diabetes and mental health teams are needed from childhood [9, 22, 28, 33, 35, 36]. Family members and other agencies, such as school or youth workers, should also be considered when defining individual treatment plans because of the importance of communication and collaboration between the systems involved and support from all sources [33]. A recent systematic review of the efficacy of interventions for people with T1DM and DEBs found that inpatient therapy with multiple components (e.g., cognitive-behavioral therapy, psychoeducation, and family therapy) was the most effective treatment because of the intensity and complexity of treating this dual diagnosis [36].

Some authors consider the lack of motivation for changing the principle obstacle in treating these patients, possibly related to the low levels of consciousness of the illness [27, 28]. However, it is important to note that "recovery is built on the triad of struggle, strength, and support," as stated by Goebel-Fabbri [9] based on interviews with 25 women who recovered from insulin restriction for weight control. For this reason, using a motivational interview with emphasis on affirmations and avoiding conflict are particularly valuable when treating patients with T1DM and EDs [22]. On the other hand, empathetic and non-judgmental support from family and friends, mental health providers, and diabetes clinicians positively impacts treatment and recovery [8, 9, 37].

25.5 Conclusion

The diagnosis of T1DM results in major lifestyle changes and a demanding daily disease management beginning in an early period of development. Emotional issues related to having this illness and disease management are characterized by some routines that may favor potentially unhealthy eating patterns, which leaves these individuals at risk for the development of eating disorders. Intentional insulin omission for the purpose of reducing or preventing weight gain is a disordered eating behavior unique to this population with serious health consequences. Disordered eating screening tools specifically developed for people with diabetes are essential for accurate evaluation, prompt detection, and timely intervention, which require multidisciplinary teams and joint work between diabetes and mental health teams.

References

1. Patterson C, Guariguata L, Dahlquist G, Soltész G, Ogle G, Silink M. Diabetes in the young—a global view and worldwide estimates of numbers of children with type 1 diabetes. Diabetes Res Clin Pract. 2014;103(2):161–75.
2. World Health Organization (WHO). Classification of diabetes mellitus 2019. Geneva: World Health Organization; 2019.
3. Ismail K. Eating disorders and diabetes. Psychiatry. 2008;7(4):179–82.
4. De Paoli T, Rogers PJ. Disordered eating and insulin restriction in type 1 diabetes: a systematic review and testable model. Eat Disord. 2018;26(4):343–60.
5. Goebel-Fabbri AE, Fikkan J, Franko DL, Pearson K, Anderson BJ, Weinger K. Insulin restriction and associated morbidity and mortality in women with type 1 diabetes. Diabetes Care. 2008;31(3):415–9.
6. Arcelus J, Mitchell AJ, Wales J, Nielsen S. Mortality rates in patients with anorexia nervosa and other eating disorders: a meta-analysis of 36 studies. Arch Gen Psychiatry. 2011;68(7):724–31.
7. Rancourt D, Foster N, Bollepalli S, Fitterman-Harris HF, Powers MA, Clements M, et al. Test of the modified dual pathway model of eating disorders in individuals with type 1 diabetes. Int J Eat Disord. 2019:1–13.
8. Falcão MA, Francisco R. Diabetes, eating disorders and body image in young adults: an exploratory study about "diabulimia". Eat Weight Disord. 2017;22(4):675–82.
9. Goebel-Fabbri A. Prevention and recovery from eating disorders in type 1 diabetes: injecting hope. New York: Routledge; 2017.
10. Reynolds KA, Helgeson VS. Children with diabetes compared to peers: depressed? Distressed? A meta-analytic review. Ann Behav Med. 2011;42(1):29–41.
11. Bächle C, Lange K, Stahl-Pehe A, Castillo K, Scheuing N, Holl RW, et al. Symptoms of eating disorders and depression in emerging adults with early-onset, long-duration type 1 diabetes and their association with metabolic control. PLoS One. 2015;10(6):1–16.

12. Berger G, Waldhoer T, Barrientos I, Kunkel D, Rami-Merhar BM, Schober E, et al. Association of insulin-manipulation and psychiatric disorders: a systematic epidemiological evaluation of adolescents with type 1 diabetes in Austria. Pediatr Diabetes. 2019;20(1):127–36.
13. Wisting L, Skrivarhaug T, Dahl-Jørgensen K, Rø Ø. Prevalence of disturbed eating behavior and associated symptoms of anxiety and depression among adult males and females with type 1 diabetes. J Eat Disord. 2018;6(1):1–10.
14. Colton PA, Olmsted MP, Daneman D, Farquhar JC, Wong H, Muskat S, et al. Eating disorders in girls and women with type 1 diabetes: a longitudinal study of prevalence, onset, remission, and recurrence. Diabetes Care. 2015;38(7):1212–7.
15. Troncone A, Cascella C, Chianese A, Zanfardino A, Confetto S, Piscopo A, et al. Parental assessment of disordered eating behaviors in their children with type 1 diabetes: a controlled study. J Psychosom Res. 2019;119:20–5. https://doi.org/10.1016/j.jpsychores.2019.02.003.
16. Young V, Eiser C, Johnson B, Brierley S, Epton T, Elliott J, et al. Eating problems in adolescents with Type1 diabetes: a systematic review with meta-analysis. Diabet Med. 2013;30:189–98.
17. Araia E, Hendrieckx C, Skinner T, Pouwer F, Speight J, King RM. Gender differences in disordered eating behaviors and body dissatisfaction among adolescents with type 1 diabetes: results from diabetes MILES youth—Australia. Int J Eat Disord. 2017;50(10):1183–93.
18. Cherubini V, Skrami E, Iannilli A, Cesaretti A, Paparusso AM, Alessandrelli MC, et al. Disordered eating behaviors in adolescents with type 1 diabetes: a cross-sectional population-based study in Italy. Int J Eat Disord. 2018;51(8):890–8.
19. Doyle EA, Quinn SM, Ambrosino JM, Weyman K, Tamborlane WV, Jastreboff AM. Disordered eating behaviors in emerging adults with Type 1 diabetes: a common problem for both men and women, J Pediatr Heal Care. 2017;31(3):327–33. https://doi.org/10.1016/j.pedhc.2016.10.004.
20. Wisting L, Frøisland DH, Skrivarhaug T, Dahl-Jørgensen K, Rø Ø. Disturbed eating behavior and omission of insulin in adolescents receiving intensified insulin treatment: a nationwide population-based study. Diabetes Care. 2013;36(11):3382–7.
21. Mannucci E, Rotella F, Ricca V, Moretti S, Placidi GF, Rotella CM. Eating disorders in patients with Type 1 diabetes: a meta-analysis. J Endocrinol Invest. 2005;28(5):417–9.
22. Treasure J, Kan C, Stephenson L, Warren E, Smith E, Heller S, et al. Developing a theoretical maintenance model for disordered eating in Type 1 diabetes. Diabet Med. 2015;32(12):1541–5.
23. Wisting L, Bang L, Natvig H, Skrivarhaug T, Dahl-Jørgensen K, Lask B, et al. Metabolic control and illness perceptions in adolescents with Type 1 Diabetes. J Diabetes Res. 2016;501:456340.
24. Nip ASY, Reboussin BA, Dabelea D, Bellatorre A, Mayer-Davis EJ, Kahkoska AR, et al. Disordered eating behaviors in youth and young adults with Type 1 or Type 2 Diabetes receiving insulin therapy: the SEARCH for Diabetes in Youth Study. Diabetes Care. 2019:dc182420.
25. Davidson J. Diabulimia: how eating disorders can affect adolescents with diabetes. Nurs Stand. 2015;29(2):44–9.
26. Torjesen I. Diabulimia: the world's most dangerous eating disorder. BMJ. 2019;364:l982. https://doi.org/10.1136/bmj.l982.
27. Custal N, Arcelus J, Agüera Z, Bove FI, Wales J, Granero R, et al. Treatment outcome of patients with comorbid type 1 diabetes and eating disorders. BMC Psychiatry [Internet]. 2014;14:140. http://www.biomedcentral.com/1471-244X/14/140
28. Pinhas-Hamiel O. Eating disorders in adolescents with type 1 diabetes: challenges in diagnosis and treatment. World J Diabetes. 2015;6(3):517.
29. Grylli V, Wagner G, Hafferl-Gattermayer A, Schober E, Karwautz A. Disturbed eating attitudes, coping styles, and subjective quality of life in adolescents with Type 1 diabetes. J Psychosom Res. 2005;59(2):65–72.
30. Sien P, Jamaludin N, Samrin S, NS S, Ismail R, Zaini AA, et al. Causative factors of eating problems among adolescents with type 1 diabetes mellitus: a qualitative study. J Health Psychol. 2020;25:1310–8.
31. Peterson CM, Fischer S, Young-Hyman D. Topical review: a comprehensive risk model for disordered eating in youth with type 1 diabetes. J Pediatr Psychol. 2015;40(4):385–90.

32. Wisting L, Wonderlich J, Skrivarhaug T, Dahl-Jørgensen K, Rø Ø. Psychometric properties and factor structure of the diabetes eating problem survey—revised (DEPS-R) among adult males and females with type 1 diabetes. J Eat Disord. 2019;7(2):1–7.
33. Candler T, Murphy R, Pigott A, Gregory JW. Fifteen-minute consultation: Diabulimia and disordered eating in childhood diabetes. Arch Dis Child Educ Pract Ed. 2018;103:118–23.
34. Markowitz JT, Butler DA, Volkening LK, Antisdel JE, Anderson BJ, Laffel LMB. Brief screening tool for disordered eating in diabetes: internal consistency and external validity in a contemporary sample of pediatric patients with type 1 diabetes. Diabetes Care. 2010;33(3):495–500.
35. Macdonald P, Kan C, Stadler M, De Bernier GL, Hadjimichalis A, Le Coguic AS, et al. Eating disorders in people with Type 1 diabetes: experiential perspectives of both clients and healthcare professionals. Diabet Med. 2018;35(2):223–31.
36. Clery P, Stahl D, Ismail K, Treasure J, Kan C. Systematic review and meta-analysis of the efficacy of interventions for people with Type 1 diabetes mellitus and disordered eating. Diabet Med. 2017;34(12):1667–75.
37. Hastings A, McNamara N, Allan J, Marriott M. The importance of social identities in the management of and recovery from 'Diabulimia': a qualitative exploration. Addict Behav Rep. 2016;4:78–86. https://doi.org/10.1016/j.abrep.2016.10.003.

Food Allergies

26

Elaine Kathleen Tyndall and Fabrizio Jacoangeli

26.1 Introduction: Food Allergies and Eating Disorder, A Confusing Mix

Understanding the pathophysiology of food allergies is essential when dealing on a daily basis with patients suffering from eating disorders (ED), as there are a number of symptoms and manifestations that may appear similar in both allergies and so-called food intolerances, of non-allergic and non-immune nature, [1] in the form of abdominal colic with diarrhoea, vomiting and other symptoms such as eructation. It is clear that the presence of symptoms such as these can lead to aberrant dietary behaviour including food aversion and refusal or real phobias regarding specific foods, particularly in early and later childhood as well as during puberty.

Moreover, malnutrition itself, which causes thinning of the intestinal wall and modification of the microbial flora in proximity to the mucosa, may provoke a condition of altered tolerance towards certain foods, which may mimic those symptoms of true food allergens.

The most common response in the presence of all these disorders is the elimination of the food or foods considered to be responsible for the symptoms and malnutrition. However, this intervention is often futile and in 50% of cases does not prove effective precisely because no recognizable IGE or cell-mediated mechanism is at play [2].

E. K. Tyndall (✉)
Department of Internal and Correctional Medicine, Sandro Pertini Hospital Rome, Rome, Italy
e-mail: elaine.tyndall@aslroma2.it

F. Jacoangeli
Department of Internal Medicine, Tor Vergata University Rome, Rome, Italy
e-mail: jcnfrz00@uniroma2.it

© Springer Nature Switzerland AG 2022
E. Manzato et al. (eds.), *Hidden and Lesser-known Disordered Eating Behaviors in Medical and Psychiatric Conditions*,
https://doi.org/10.1007/978-3-030-81174-7_26

If this situation persists, the subject risks both physical consequences directly linked to lack of specific micro- and macronutrients [3] and indeed the development of a true eating disorder (ED).

ED are mental illnesses including anorexia nervosa, bulimia nervosa orthorexia [4] or avoidant/restrictive food intake disorder (ARFID) described in the DSM-V [5] that usually first present in childhood. Deficiency of specific foods that have a regulatory effect on the central nervous system (CNS) such as vitamin D, calcium, magnesium or B vitamins can induce alterations in mood and depression [6–9].

In turn, the drugs used in the treatment of food allergies can affect appetite control through inhibition of histamine H1, H2, H3 and H4 receptors by antihistamines [10] or can act on weight, water retention and body composition in the case of prolonged use of anti-inflammatory steroids [11]. When these therapies are administered during periods in which young patients are typically more at risk of developing an eating disorder (puberty and adolescence), they contribute to increasing the likelihood that a true eating disorder takes hold. As anorexia nervosa (AN) tends to present even at a young age, this risk must be taken seriously and dealt with early on [12].

The National Institute of Allergy and Infectious Diseases (NIAID) defines food allergy as "an adverse health effect arising from a specific immune response that occurs reproducibly on exposure to a given food" that involves around 240–500 million people worldwide with a very significant impact on the quality of life of affected people, in large part children.

26.2 Epidemiology

The prevalence of food allergy appears to be increasing, and self-reported food allergy often exceeds clinically proven cases. The overall lifetime prevalence of self-reported food allergy in European countries has been estimated as 17.6%, with a point prevalence of 5.9% for self-reported food allergy (FA) compared to 10.1% of subjects with positive serum IgE to a specific food allergen (which falls to 2.7% when positive IgE is considered together with symptoms elicited by clinical history taking), 2.7% for positive skin prick test (SPT) to at least one food and 0.9% if the food allergy was confirmed by an oral food challenge [13–16].

26.3 Pathogenesis and Classification

Food allergies occur due to a breakdown in the normal processes of immune tolerance towards food antigens, usually proteins or protein-bound haptens such as nickel. The presentation of food antigens by CD 103+ dendritic cells in the gastrointestinal tract or CD 11b+ dendritic cells and Langerhans cells in the skin normally induces T regulatory cells, which regulate immune tolerance, but they increased expression of inflammatory mediators such as interleukins 4, 9, 13 and 33 and may subvert this process, provoking instead the activation of T helper 2 cells and the immune response [17].

Food allergy may be further classified according to whether the reaction is known to be Ig-E mediated, non Ig-E mediated or mixed. Ig-E-mediated allergies manifest within minutes to hours of ingestion of the offending food, with more rapid onset generally associated with greater clinical severity. Examples of Ig-E-mediated reactions include [11, 17–24]:

- Anaphylactic shock: anaphylactic shock is defined as a "severe, life-threatening generalized or systemic hypersensitivity reaction", which rapidly compromises respiratory and circulatory function. Cutaneous and mucosal manifestations are present in over 80% of cases.
    - Skin and mucosal tissue involvement (e.g. urticaria; oedema of the lips, tongue, uvula; pruritus; and flushing)
    - Hypotension or manifestations of related end-organ dysfunction (syncope, incontinence, hypotonia)
    OR
    - Two of skin and mucosal involvement, respiratory compromise, hypotension and associated symptoms or persistent gastrointestinal manifestations such as vomiting and cramping
    OR
    - Hypotension defined as systolic blood pressure of less than 90 mmHg in adults, lower than 70 mmHg in infants or lower than the age-specific cut-offs in children (<70 + (age in years × 2) or less than 30% of the patient's baseline
  Anaphylaxis can be provoked by any number of allergens, but the most frequently implicated foods include peanuts and other tree nuts, fish and shellfish, milk and eggs, as well as sesame seeds and other seeds, spinach and avocado.
- Oral allergy syndrome (food pollen syndrome): pruritus and oedema of the oral cavity on exposure to raw fruits and vegetables, of brief duration (minutes) which rarely progresses beyond the mouth (approximately 7% of cases) or anaphylaxis (1–2%).
- Latex allergy: IgE-mediated allergy to natural rubber latex can provoke serious respiratory and mucocutaneous reactions, extending to anaphylaxis. Up to 50% of latex allergy sufferers also experience cross-reactions to fruit, such as avocado, banana, tomato, kiwi and chestnuts that may provoke allergic reactions in latex-sensitized individuals.
- Alpha-gal allergy: antibodies (IgG, IgM, IgA) to galactose-alpha-1,3-galactose (alpha-gal) are implicated in delayed (3–6 h) hypersensitivity reactions to red meat (beef, pork, goat, sheep and other mammals), dairy products, gelatin in sweets and colloid solutions and porcine digestive enzymes, as well as organs and heart valves used in transplant medicine. Sensitization may occur through transmission of alpha-gal from tick bites, particularly of the species *Amblyomma americanum*.

- Respiratory symptoms (asthma, rhinitis): isolated respiratory symptoms are rare and more frequently observed in infants and children, triggered by inhalation of aerosolized food protein (milk, egg). In adults, respiratory Ig-E-mediated food allergies can be associated with occupational exposure, for example, inhalation of wheat allergens such as omega-5-gliadin in Baker's asthma (also egg, fish, milk). Respiratory reactions are more commonly observed in subjects with poorly controlled underlying respiratory allergies, and such reactions may precede full-blown anaphylaxis.
- Immediate GI hypersensitivity/gastrointestinal symptoms: rapid onset of nausea, vomiting, severe abdominal pain and/or diarrhoea following ingestion of the responsible food allergen, usually in the context of an anaphylactic reaction.
- Food-dependent, exercise-induced anaphylaxis: severe hypersensitivity reactions which exclusively present when physical exercise is performed shortly after consumption of a food to which the patient is allergic, particularly wheat.

Mixed IgE- and cell-mediated allergies include atopic dermatitis and eosinophilic gastrointestinal diseases (EGID). EGID include eosinophilic esophagitis (EoE) and gastroenteritis (EE) and can affect both children and adults. Symptoms of EoE include gastroesophageal reflux, dysphagia, vomiting and food impaction, and diarrhoea, abdominal pain, bloating and malabsorption leading occasionally to intestinal strictures, occlusion and ascites in EE. The majority of patients with EGID have an associated allergic condition including atopic dermatitis, urticaria, food and drug allergy, asthma and hay fever. The differential diagnoses of EGID include celiac disease, connective tissue and autoimmune disease, infection, Crohn's disease, hypereosinophilic syndrome and drug sensitivity.

26.4 Nickel

Nickel is an ubiquitous environmental element found in the soil, water, air and atmosphere and is an increasingly common cause of contact dermatitis, affecting up to 20% of the population worldwide. Nickel allergy tends to be persistent and is more common in women, generally peaking in the third decade of life, although any age group may be affected. A small percentage (between 1 and 5%) of nickel allergy sufferers have been reported to experience more widespread cutaneous or extra-cutaneous manifestations on contact with or ingestion of nickel, termed the systemic nickel allergy syndrome (SNAS). Symptoms may include eczema, urticaria and vasculitic-type rashes as well as respiratory symptoms (asthma, rhinitis), myalgia, arthralgia, headache and gastrointestinal symptoms (heartburn, nausea, diarrhoea, abdominal pain, meteorism, constipation, vomiting). SNAS should only be suspected in subjects who have tested positive to nickel patch testing [25–28].

26.5 Diagnosis of Food Allergies

According to the EAACI and WAO guidelines [17, 29, 30], the correct diagnosis of food allergy must follow a logical sequence of clinical evaluation and testing. The first, and arguably the most important, step in establishing a diagnosis of food allergy is taking an accurate clinical history. It is important to attempt to elicit the following information in order to better direct further testing, treatment and prevention strategies:

1. Ask the patient to accurately describe the symptoms, rapidity of onset from the time of exposure to the suspected allergens and how quickly symptoms resolved and any treatment they received. Identify serious or life-threatening reactions requiring more urgent and intensive evaluation and management.
2. Inquire as to which food may have triggered the allergen, and the reproducibility of the reaction on further exposure to the suspected allergen may support the diagnosis.
3. Timing of symptom onset:
   (a) IgE-mediated reactions which arise within 2 h and usually within minutes of exposure and may be followed by a "late phase" of continuous or prolonged symptoms
   (b) Mixed and non-IgE-mediated reactions, which usually occur between 8 and 28 h after exposure
4. Inquire as to the quantity and route of exposure (contact with the skin, inhalation, ingestion) of the allergen. Ask whether foods were raw or cooked/processed.
5. Inquire about pre-disposing factors such as personal or family history of atopy and presence of co-factors immediately preceding or following the allergic episode such as participation in physical exercise or ingestion of alcohol or drugs (e.g. NSAIDS, ACE inhibitors).
6. Ask whether the patient suffers from any other allergies which may lead to cross-reactivity including latex, pollen or other foods and whether foods which may cross-react with the allergen in question are tolerated. Ascertain whether foods which may contain a small amount of the allergen are tolerated (e.g. multigrain bread in suspected soy allergy).
7. Evaluate nutritional status and dietary intake, whether foods from other main food groups are tolerated and if the patient has or is currently following an elimination diet and whether that has proved helpful.
8. Exclude alternative diagnoses including malabsorption due to lactose intolerance, celiac disease or pancreatic insufficiency.
9. Eating and anxiety disorders may also present to health services as food allergy, which may be elicited through careful, non-confrontational history taking, from speaking to the family or with the aid of specific self- or healthcare professional-administered questionnaires. Involvement of a multidisciplinary team is often required in order to investigate alternative or comorbid illnesses.

Initial diagnostic investigations for food allergy include the skin prick test (SPT) and specific serum IgE test (sIgE). Positive results represent sensitization to a food, which does not always equate to clinical manifestations. As such, the allergens chosen for testing must be selected on the basis of clinical history, patient and population characteristics and geographical location. Strength of reaction may vary with age (less in young children and the elderly), site (forearm or upper back) and sex of the patient, as well as the allergen extracts used, lancet type and interpersonal variability in reading test results. Sensitivity may vary from 70 to 100%; however specificity is lower (40–70%). As such, these tests should only be administered and interpreted by experienced professionals who are also trained in dealing with potential adverse reactions.

Once the presence of sensitization has been established, a focused elimination diet may be attempted for a period of 2–4 weeks in IgE-related allergy and potentially longer for non-IgE-mediated reactions.

26.6 Management of Food Allergies

Acute management of anaphylaxis and severe allergic reactions have been outlined above and are amply dealt with in the guidelines [17].

Following a valid diagnosis of a food allergy, advice on which foods and food products to avoid and adequate substitution of the food with alternative dietary sources and/or supplements may be necessary (see the FARE website https://www.foodallergy.org/common-allergens/wheat-allergy) [31].

A number of patient aspects and warning signs should alert the physician or carer to the possibility of increased nutritional risk, including:

- Body mass index (BMI) <18.5 kg/m^2 or more than 2 standard deviations below the age and height population standards
- Presence of feeding difficulties, avoidant/restrictive food intake or an eating disorder like anorexia nervosa or orthorexia nervosa
- Observance of specific diets for cultural or religious reasons, vegan diets and vegetarian diets
- Presence of comorbid conditions and dietary restrictions due to chronic diseases such as diabetes, renal and hepatic disease and cardiovascular disease
- Presence of multiple food allergies (particularly milk together with wheat allergy) and extensive elimination diets for eosinophilic esophagitis

Expert dietary advice involving the family when appropriate, regular follow-up in collaboration with the multi-disciplinary team and nutrient supplementation where necessary are required to prevent malnutrition and to address psychosocial issues and erroneous beliefs and practices arising from the diagnosis of an allergy or multiple allergies.

General guidelines for managing food allergies are as follows:

1. Diagnostic criteria for allergies must be strictly applied.
2. Patients at risk of severe allergic reactions should be provided with an adrenaline injector and, together with family members/significant others, must be instructed on how to intervene in case of emergency. Expert advice should be sought as regards to prescription of antihistamines, short-acting inhalatory beta-agonists and glucocorticosteroids, as well as immune therapy (which has not been approved for food allergy).
3. Foods avoided should be strictly limited to proven allergens (particularly in the case of potentially cross-reactive allergens which in general should not be eliminated unless proven to cause allergy). Dietary counselling should be available to all patients, and an adequate diet plan should be agreed in order to avoid nutritional deficiencies. Follow-up and reassurance are essential in order to prevent excessively restrictive behaviours, particularly in eating disordered patients.
4. Sensitivity towards costs and logistical issues is key in establishing a collaborative relationship with patients and families/carers in order to increase safety and balance vigilance with quality of life. Targeted counselling may be required and should be offered.
5. Training must be undertaken, and adequate facilities should be available to deal with serious complications including anaphylactic shock. Strict collaboration with an allergy expert is essential.

26.7 Food Allergies and Eating Disorders

Psychiatric disorders have been more frequently observed in patients with perceived food allergies, although data is contrasting [32, 33]. Risk of developing an eating disorder may begin in early childhood. Young children with food allergies often engage in maladaptive feeding behaviours, such as food refusal, avoidance of extensive food groups and new foods even if these do not provoke true allergic reactions and throwing tantrums at mealtimes. They may not acquire motor and cognitive feeding skills normally, nor learn the pleasureable sensory and social aspects of eating [34]

An interesting study recently published by Barbara Wróblewska et al. [35] in which the biopsychosocial implications of food allergies were studied in the prevalence of eating disorders in a group of 90 patients with food allergies confirmed by the presence of typical clinical manifestations and elevated specific IGE > 0.7 kUA/L versus 90 control patients has highlighted some very interesting data:

1. A tendency to the development of DCA in allergic patients was greater in females than in males ($p = 0.173$) and in particular in two age groups: in patients aged <6 years ($p = 0.0041$) and in those between 15 and 18 years ($p = 0.0027$).

2. Early nourishment by exclusive breastfeeding was significantly more frequent in the control group than in allergic subjects, and eating disorders were present in about 10% of allergic subjects with exclusive maternal breastfeeding compared to 5.8% of non-allergic controls.
3. The predominant therapeutic approach observed was the elimination diet (ELD) in 65% and 74% of cases in the recruitment phase and the 5-year follow-up, respectively, and there was a strong correlation between the tendency to develop a DCA and the therapeutic method chosen for the treatment of allergy, particularly when the choice of foods to exclude was not guided by professionals but self-managed. Self-implemented diet was very strongly correlated with ED ($r=0.8012; p=0.005$) and with reduced body weight parameters ($r=0.724; 0.005$).
4. As regards the multivariate logistic regression model, it was shown that three combined factors influenced the prevalence of ED: the diagnostic method used for the diagnosis, the dominant symptoms and the type of therapy implemented.
5. In the two groups, allergy + ED and non-allergy + ED, there was an excessive concern about body weight and eating behaviour and also an important element of dissatisfaction with one's body image, all this combined with a tendency to manage eating behaviour independently and in a contradictory manner as regards to the diagnosis made by an allergy specialist.

Fitzgerald et al. have reported increased frequency of eating disordered behaviour in adults with a perceived food allergy or intolerance, which parallel the features of the avoidant/restrictive food intake disorder (ARFID) described in the DSM-V [5]. As such, certain foods were avoided not only due to fear of provoking symptoms but also as a result of aversion to sensory aspects of the food, including texture, smell and taste, as well as functional dysphagia, and in many cases dietary patterns adopted led to weight loss and quality of life issues. Moreover, irritable bowel syndrome is frequently associated with psychopathologies including depression and anxiety [36], and these symptoms may be perceived as allergy or intolerance to certain foods. Functional gastrointestinal disorders as defined by the Rome III criteria are observed in over 80% of patients with eating disorders, with symptoms such as heartburn, post-prandial distress, nausea, irritable bowel syndrome and anorectal symptoms commonly described [37]. This may lead to avoidance of certain food groups, particularly gluten and dairy, due to perceived intolerance. Indeed, fasting and extreme exercising may worsen these symptoms, leading to a vicious cycle of restriction and avoidance. Refeeding and reintroduction of previously prohibited foods may cause varying degrees of gastrointestinal discomfort, and intensive counselling and reassurance are often required to support the patient through this process. Professional supervision in an appropriate clinical setting is advisable particularly if co-existing allergy cannot be excluded [38].

26.8 Conclusions

Many different types of food allergies exist, causing an array of symptoms and physical consequences, of differing severity.

Experiencing a food allergy or perceived intolerance can easily have repercussions on eating habits which, let us remember, represent the human behaviour that guarantees our personal survival, while sexual behaviour guarantees the survival of the species.

On the other hand, those who suffer from an eating disorder as a primary pathology can easily believe, or have people in their family believe, that an allergy or food intolerance is at the root of their problem, creating confusion and possible conflict in the management approach at a healthcare level.

It is, therefore, always necessary to abide by validated diagnostic criteria and methods at our disposal in order to clarify the diagnosis. This may also imply the occasional inclusion of a specialist expert in food allergies in a treatment team for eating disorders.

References

1. Pawankar R, Holgate ST, Canonica GW, Lockey RF, Blaiss MS. White book on allergy update. World Allergy Organization, section 2.6 "Food Allergy": Milwaukee Press; 2013.
2. Okada Y, Yamashita T, Kumagai H, Morikawa Y, Akasawa A. Accurate determination of childhood food allergy prevalence and correction of unnecessary avoidance. Allergy Asthma Immunol Res. 2017;9(4):322–8.
3. Fiocchi A, Bahna SL, Berg A, Von BK, Bozzola M, Compalati E, et al. World Allergy Organization (WAO) diagnosis and rationale for action against Cow's milk allergy (DRACMA) guidelines. Pediatr Allergy Immunol. 2010;21:1–125.
4. Young E, Stoneham MD, Petruckevitch A, Barton J, Rona R. A population study of food intolerance. Lancet. 1994;343(8906):1127–30.
5. Fitzgerald M, Frankum B. Food avoidance and restriction in adults: a cross-sectional pilot study comparing patients from an immunology clinic to a general practice. J Eat Disord. 2017;5:30.
6. Kosky NSM, Lacey JH. Bulimia nervosa and food allergy: a case report. Int J Eat Disord. 1993;14(1):117–9.
7. Ricca V, Mannucci E, Calabrò A, Bernardo MD, Cabras PL, Rotella CM. Anorexia nervosa and celiac disease: two case reports. Int J Eat Disord. 2000;27:119–22.
8. Yucel B, Ozbey N, Demir K, Polat A, Yager J. Eating disorders and celiac disease: a case report. Int J Eat Disord. 2006;39:530–2. https://doi.org/10.1002/eat.20294.
9. Wilczynska-Kwiatek A, Bargiel-Matusiewicz K, Lapinski L. Asthma, allergy, mood disorders, and nutrition. Eur J Med Res. 2009;14(Suppl 4):248–54.
10. Mollet A, Meier S, Riediger T, Lutz TA. Histamine H 1 receptors mediate the anorectic action of the pancreatic hormone amylin. Peptides. 2003;24:155–8.
11. Boyce JA, Assa'ad A, Burks AW, Jones SM, Sampson HA, Wood RA, et al. Guidelines for the diagnosis and management of food allergy in the United States: report of the NIAID-sponsored expert panel. J Allergy Clin Immunol. 2010;126(6 0):S1–58.
12. Herpertz-Dahlmann B, Dahmen B. Children in need-diagnostics, epidemiology, treatment and outcome of early onset anorexia nervosa. Nutrients. 2019;11(8):pii: E1932. https://doi.org/10.3390/nu11081932.

13. Sampson HA, et al. Food allergy: a practice parameter update—2014. J Allergy Clin Immunol. 2014;134(5):1016–1025.e43.
14. Verrill L, Bruns R, Luccioli S. Prevalence of self-reported food allergy in U.S. adults: 2001, 2006, and 2010. Allergy Asthma Proc. 2015;36:458–67.
15. Sicherer SH, Sampson HA. Food allergy: a review and update on epidemiology, pathogenesis, diagnosis, prevention, and management. J Allergy Clin Immunol. 2018;141(1):41–58.
16. Pali-Schöll I, Jensen-Jarolim E. Gender aspects in food allergy. Curr Opin Allergy Clin Immunol. 2019;19(3):249–55.
17. Muraro A, Werfel T, Hoffmann-Sommergruber K, et al. EAACI Food Allergy and Anaphylaxis Guidelines Group. EAACI food allergy and anaphylaxis guidelines: diagnosis and management of food allergy. Allergy. 2014;69(8):1008–25.
18. Muraro A, Roberts G, Worm M, et al. EAACI Food Allergy and Anaphylaxis Guidelines Group. Anaphylaxis: guidelines from the European Academy of Allergy and Clinical Immunology. Allergy. 2014;69(8):1026–45.
19. American Academy of Allergy Asthma and Immunology 2019. Oral Allergy Syndrome (OAS) or Pollen Fruit Syndrome (PFS). https://www.aaaai.org/conditions-and-treatments/library/allergy-library/outdoor-food-allergies-relate
20. Blanco C, Sánchez-García F, Torres-Galván MJ, Dumpierrez AG, Almeida L, Figueroa J, Ortega N, Castillo R, Gallego MD, Carrillo T. Genetic basis of the latex-fruit syndrome: association with HLA class II alleles in a Spanish population. J Allergy Clin Immunol. 2004;114(5):1070–6.
21. Hilger C, Fischer J, Wölbing F, et al. Role and mechanism of galactose-alpha-1,3-galactose in the elicitation of delayed anaphylactic reactions to red meat. Curr Allergy Asthma Rep. 2019;19:3.
22. Silverberg NB, Lee-Wong M, Yosipovitch G. Diet and atopic dermatitis. Cutis. 2016;97(3):227–32.
23. Pineton de Chambrun G, Dufour G, Tassy B, et al. Diagnosis, natural history and treatment of eosinophilic enteritis: a review. Curr Gastroenterol Rep. 2018;20(8):37.
24. Ishihara S, Kinoshita Y, Schoepfer A. Eosinophilic esophagitis, Eosinophilic gastroenteritis, and Eosinophilic colitis: common mechanisms and differences between east and west. Inflamm Intest Dis. 2016;1(2):63–9.
25. Pizzutelli S. Systemic nickel hypersensitivity and diet: myth or reality? Eur Ann Allergy Clin Immunol. 2011;43(1):5–18.
26. Goldenberg A, Jacob SE. Update on systemic nickel allergy syndrome and diet. Eur Ann Allergy Clin Immunol. 2015;47(1):25–6.
27. Ricciardi L, Arena A, Arena E. Systemic nickel allergy syndrome: epidemiological data from four Italian allergy units. Int J Immunopathol Pharmacol. 2014;27(1):131–6.
28. Pizzutelli S. Reply to: update on systemic nickel allergy syndrome and diet. Eur Ann Allergy Clin Immunol. 2015;47(1):27–32.
29. Johansson SG, Bieber T, Dahl R, et al. Revised nomenclature for allergy for global use: report of the Nomenclature Review Committee of the World Allergy Organization. J Allergy Clin Immunol. 2004;113:832–6.
30. Nowak-Wegrzyn A. Food allergy to proteins. Nestle Nutr Workshop Ser Pediatr Program. 2007;59:17–31; discussion 31-6.
31. Tips for avoiding your allergen. Food Allergy Research and Education (FARE); 2019. www.foodallergy.org
32. Peveler R, Mayou R, Young E, et al. Psychiatric aspects of food-related physical symptoms: a community study. J Psychosom Res. 1996;41(2):149–59.
33. Shanahan L, Zucker N, Copeland WE. Are children and adolescents with food allergies at increased risk for psychopathology? J Psychosom Res. 2014;77(6):468–73.
34. Haas AM. Feeding disorders in food allergic children. Curr Allergy Asthma Rep. 2010;10(4):258–64.

35. Wróblewska B, Szyc AM, Markiewicz LH, et al. Increased prevalence of eating disorders as a biopsychosocial implication of food allergy. PLoS One. 2018;13(6):e0198607.
36. Fadgyas-Stanculete M, Buga AM, Popa-Wagner A, et al. The relationship between irritable bowel syndrome and psychiatric disorders: from molecular changes to clinical manifestations. J Mol Psychiatry. 2014;2(4)
37. Wang X, Luscombe GM, Boyd C, et al. Functional gastrointestinal disorders in eating disorder patients: altered distribution and predictors using ROME III compared to ROME II criteria. World J Gastroenterol. 2014;20(43):16,293–9.
38. Kniskern MA, Anand M. Intolerance versus avoidance: identifying true food allergies. Academy of Nutrition and Dietetics Food and Nutrition Conference Expo, Chicago, Illinois; October 21–24, 2017.

Hirschsprung Disease and Eating Disorders

Anna I. Guerdjikova, Francisco Romo-Nava, and Susan L. McElroy

27.1 Hirschsprung Disease: History, Etiology, and Clinical Presentation

The first recorded observation of what is now known as Hirschsprung disease (HD) is credited to Frederick Ruysch, with his autopsy report publication entitled "Enormis intestini coli dilatation" from 1691 [1]. Two centuries later, in 1888, the Danish pediatrician Harald Hirschsprung first described two infant boys who were not relatives and who died from chronic severe constipation leading to dilatation and hypertrophy of the colon [2]. At the time of his observation, Dr. Hirschsprung erroneously believed that the proximal dilated bowel was diseased. More than half a century later, it was recognized that the absence of intramural ganglion cells of the myenteric (Auerbach) and submucosal (Meissner) plexuses downstream of the dilated part of the colon was the culprit. The lack of ganglion cells, which are replaced by hypertrophied nerve trunks, results in a chronically contracted state of the colon preventing the passage of stools and causing intestinal obstruction and constipation, the most common clinical findings in HD. In 1948, the first surgical intervention for HD was invented by Swenson and Bill [3]. This reduced infant mortality and enhanced survival of HD patients into adulthood, helping uncover the familial transmission of the disease.

HD is a congenital illness which occurs in about 1 in 5000 births. It is a sex-modified multifactorial malformation that occurs as an isolated trait in 70% of patients and with an overall occurrence risk in siblings of the proband of 4% [4]. In affected families, the reported overall incidence is 7.6%, increasing to 15–21% in total colonic aganglionosis and to 50% in the rare total intestinal aganglionosis. Commonly, HD is associated with other congenital and chromosomal anomalies. For example, individuals with Down syndrome have a 100-fold higher risk of developing HD than the average population [5]. It has been shown that mutations of the coding RET gene account for 7–25% of sporadic cases and 40–60% of familial cases. The cause of HD is most commonly attributed to defective craniocaudal migration of neuroblasts originating from the neural crest during the first 12 weeks of gestation, leading to functional intestinal obstruction. HD is more common in males, with an overall male to female ratio of 4:1. Up to 94% of individuals with HD are diagnosed before the age of 5 years. In typical HD diagnosed shortly after birth, aganglionosis starts from the anal valve, spreads proximally, and involves only the rectum and sigmoid colon. In rare cases, individuals may be undiagnosed until adulthood, often because the colonic region above the obstructed segment assumes a compensatory role and the mild symptoms do no prompt immediate intervention. Some patients can manage their chronic constipation with cathartic agents for many years. However, the dilated proximal colonic segment may decompensate secondary to the distal obstruction, and adult patients may experience rapidly worsening constipation or even acute obstruction. Suction rectal biopsy and full-thickness rectal biopsy are the gold standards in diagnosing HD, and the disease is treated using various operative techniques, the essence being surgical resection of the bowel to remove or bypass regions where the enteric nervous system is missing [6].

The first case of adult HD was reported in 1916 by Dr. Hubbard [7]. "Adult HD" is presently diagnosed when the patient is 10 years of age or older; to date, no more than 500 such cases have been described in the literature [5]. The true incidence of HD in adulthood is unknown, because the illness is often undiagnosed or misdiagnosed in the adult population. The typical adult patient with HD has a history of long-standing constipation, abdominal discomfort, distension, and abdominal pain since early childhood. The patients report chronic use of cathartics, suppositories, and enemas to relief constipation. Fecal incontinence is rarely a feature of the adult HD presentation.

27.2 Eating Disorders and Nonspecific Gastrointestinal Symptoms

A plethora of nonspecific gastrointestinal (GI) complains, which can be characteristic for HD, also commonly occur in eating disorders (EDs) [8]. GI symptoms are often the consequence of disordered eating behavior and malnutrition, but comorbid GI disorders are not unusual [9]. Low appetite, feelings of significant fullness after meals, pain in the upper abdomen, dysphagia, bloating, nausea, constipation, and abdominal distention are all common GI symptoms associated with the significant weight loss characteristic of anorexia nervosa (AN). Bloating can be the presenting symptom for gastroparesis (delayed emptying of the stomach), which can be severe and worsened by high-fiber diets, but is reversible upon weight restoration.

Constipation and obstructive defecation syndrome are very common in AN with over 80% of patients with AN struggling with defecatory disorders [10]. Etiologically, drastically reduced caloric intake leads to reflex hypofunctioning of the colon and slowing of colonic transit, which allows more water absorption from the colon, worsening constipation.

Laxative abuse is not uncommon in ED patients [11]. In bulimia nervosa (BN), prolonged laxative use may produce reflex constipation. Long-term stimulant laxative abuse may cause permanent damage to the colon nerve cells and impair colonic motility. In the most severe cases, habituation to stimulant laxatives leads to a dilated, atonic colon, incapable of normal colonic peristalsis and refractory constipation (often called cathartic colon syndrome) [12]. Constipation is a common digestive complaint with a prevalence of up to 15% in the general population [13] and especially common in ED patients. The differential diagnosis of constipation in adults is wide ranging and can be related to colorectal motility or be secondary to a variety of factors, including neurogenic disorders, metabolic abnormalities, myopathies, mechanical obstructions, or various medications. Finally, persistent avoidance of certain foods due to their taste, texture, or smell, lack of interest in food, or fear of choking or vomiting is characteristic for another ED, namely, avoidant restrictive food intake disorder (ARFID), which most commonly is diagnosed in children [14].

27.3 Eating Disorders and HD

Despite the symptomatic overlap between HD and EDs, as outlined above, true diagnostic overlap appears to be rare. To our knowledge, no systematic reports to date have described EDs in HD or vice versa. We were able to locate one anecdotal report of a child who developed ARFID-like symptoms after HD surgery. Despite the successful operative intervention and the lack of objective reasons to avoid food, he was unable to restart eating solid food and experienced persistent gagging, coughing, and anxiety, necessitating prolonged consumption of liquid foods [15]. Another case report described a 3-year-old with HD and pica who developed a bezoar and secretory diarrhea related to ingestion of silk surgical tape. He had had successful surgery for his HD over a year before the bezoar formation, and it was deemed unlikely that the HD-related motor abnormality caused the bezoar [16]. Of note, there is currently one prospective trial exploring neuropsychological development and functional outcome in school-aged children with HD [17]. The study is being conducted in France and utilizes the Strengths and Difficulties Questionnaire, a tool known to have low sensitivity for identifying EDs [18].

27.4 Clinical Considerations Regarding the Symptomatic Overlap Between HD and ED

In the pediatric population, the relationship between HD and EDs, particularly ARFID, can be bidirectional—children undergoing surgery for HD can develop ARFID symptoms during recovery, and some children with milder HD, not diagnosed and treated at birth, can present with classic ARFID symptoms of weight loss, lack of appetite, and constipation. In children who underwent surgery for HD, the two most common postsurgical defecation dysfunctions sequelae are obstructive symptoms and fecal incontinence. Obstructive symptoms can vary from abdominal pain and distension to bloating, vomiting, and severe constipation requiring ongoing enemas or laxative therapy. Untreated, those complications might lead to reduced appetite, aversion to certain foods, weight loss, and other ARFID-like symptoms. In milder cases, the diagnosis of HD can be missed during infancy, and the child can present with classic ARFID symptoms of lack of appetite, persistent abdominal pain, and chronic constipation. In such cases, collecting very thorough family and developmental history is critical for differential diagnosis. Evidence suggestive for HD include the following symptoms: failure to pass meconium in the first 48 h of life; persistent lack of appetite with failure to thrive, especially developing after weaning of breast milk for exclusively nursed infants; gross abdominal distention; obstructive defecation syndrome; and dependence on enemas without significant encopresis [19]. Referral for rectal biopsy might be warranted if these symptoms do not resolve with intensive therapy, including laxatives, dietary changes, and behavior modification. In adolescents, chronic GI issues stemming from mild undiagnosed HD can lead to significant weight loss potentially further "unlocking" an eating disorder; thus careful monitoring of weight trends and eating behaviors in children and adolescents with ongoing abdominal complains can be instrumental in not missing an ED diagnosis. Restrictive eating behavior may also be present after HD surgical treatment in adolescents and warrants continued monitoring [20]. Similarly, in adults, chronic constipation and abdominal discomfort from undiagnosed milder HD might be a risk factor for reduced food intake and further development of ED symptoms. Patients experiencing significant weight loss and constipation that do not resolve with weight restoration along with adequate hydration, fiber in low doses, and polyethylene glycol products might benefit from a complete GI workup, especially when there is a history of chronic constipation since early childhood. In adult patients presenting with normal weight and chronic constipation, collecting history and carefully assessing the timing of presenting symptoms and the motivation for chronic laxative use can be instrumental for correct diagnosis.

27.5 Summary

In conclusion, although the association between HD and ED has not been studied systematically, there is a notable symptomatic overlap between the two conditions. Thus, in a patient presenting for ED treatment, history of chronic constipation since early childhood continuously managed with laxatives might raise suspicion for short segment or zonal HD, particularly when the constipation does not resolve with improved nutrition. Conversely, patients who had surgery for HD as infants or later in life but continue to suffer from various degrees of lifelong GI complications [21] should be monitored for disordered eating. Careful monitoring of eating behavior and working with a multidisciplinary team of specialists, including a surgeon, a gastroenterologist, and a psychologist, can be instrumental in caring for these patients into adulthood.

References

1. F R. Observatinum anatomic-chirurgicarum centuria. Amsterdam: Henricum etViduramTheodri Boom; 1691.
2. Hirschsprung H. Stuhltragheit neugeborener in folge von dilatation und hypertrophie des colons. Jahrb Kinderheilkd. 1888;27:1–7.
3. Swenson O, Bill AH Jr. Resection of rectum and rectosigmoid with preservation of the sphincter for benign spastic lesions producing megacolon; an experimental study. Surgery. 1948;24(2):212–20.
4. Amiel J, Lyonnet S. Hirschsprung disease, associated syndromes, and genetics: a review. J Med Genet. 2001;38(11):729–39.
5. Doodnath R, Puri P. A systematic review and meta-analysis of Hirschsprung's disease presenting after childhood. Pediatr Surg Int. 2010;26(11):1107–10.
6. Das K, Mohanty S. Hirschsprung disease—current diagnosis and management. Indian J Pediatr. 2017;84(8):618–23.
7. Hubbard JC. Megacolon: Hirschsprung's disease-report of a case in an adult. Ann Surg. 1916;63(3):349–52.
8. Hetterich L, Mack I, Giel KE, Zipfel S, Stengel A. An update on gastrointestinal disturbances in eating disorders. Mol Cell Endocrinol. 2018;
9. Sato Y, Fukudo S. Gastrointestinal symptoms and disorders in patients with eating disorders. Clin J Gastroenterol. 2015;8(5):255–63.
10. Sileri P, Franceschilli L, De Lorenzo A, et al. Defecatory disorders in anorexia nervosa: a clinical study. Tech Coloproctol. 2014;18(5):439–44.
11. Roerig JL, Steffen KJ, Mitchell JE, Zunker C. Laxative abuse: epidemiology, diagnosis and management. Drugs. 2010;70(12):1487–503.
12. Mehler PS, Rylander M. Bulimia Nervosa—medical complications. J Eat Disord. 2015;3:12.
13. Black CJ, Ford AC. Chronic idiopathic constipation in adults: epidemiology, pathophysiology, diagnosis and clinical management. Med J Aust. 2018;209(2):86–91.
14. A.P.A. DSM-5: Feeding and eating disorders. http://www.dsm5.org/proposedrevision/Pages/FeedingandEatingDisorders.aspx. Accessed 5 July 2012.
15. Barry E. A Place to go when a child really refuses food; 2019. https://www.nytimes.com/2007/08/23/nyregion/23eating.html. Published 2017. Accessed 11 Dec 2019.
16. Nowicki MJ, Miller RC. Secretory diarrhea owing to a tape bezoar in a child with Hirschsprung's disease. J Pediatr Surg. 2003;38(11):1670–2.
17. NCT03406741 CgI. Neuropsychological development and functional outcome sin children with Hirschsprung disease at school age (Hirschsprung). Published 2019. Accessed 12 Feb 2019; 2019.
18. Goodman R, Ford T, Simmons H, Gatward R, Meltzer H. Using the Strengths and Difficulties Questionnaire (SDQ) to screen for child psychiatric disorders in a community sample. Br J Psychiatry. 2000;177:534–9.
19. Calkins CM. Hirschsprung disease beyond infancy. Clin Colon Rectal Surg. 2018;31(2):51–60.
20. Tran VQ, Mahler T, Dassonville M, et al. Long-term outcomes and quality of life in patients after soave pull-through operation for hirschsprung's disease: an observational retrospective study. Eur J Pediatr Surg. 2018;28(5):445–54.
21. Wester T, Granstrom AL. Hirschsprung disease-Bowel function beyond childhood. Semin Pediatr Surg. 2017;26(5):322–7.

Hypermobility Spectrum Disorders/ Ehlers–Danlos Syndrome and Disordered Eating Behavior

28

Carolina Baeza-Velasco, Paola Espinoza, Antonio Bulbena, Andrea Bulbena-Cabré, Maude Seneque, and Sebastien Guillaume

28.1 Joint Hypermobility-Related Disorders

Joint hypermobility (JH), which is defined as an distensibility of the joints beyond normal limits in passive and active movements, is a common somatic trait in the general population (prevalence ranging from 10% to 40% [1]. However, JH is also the hallmark of a group of diseases affecting connective tissue matrix proteins: the "hereditary disorders of connective tissue" (HDCT). HDCT are characterized by generalized fragility resulted from the distortion of the biochemical structure of proteins fibrous (e.g., collagens, elastins, fibrillins, tenascins) in turn induced by genetic aberrations [2]. The Ehlers-Danlos syndromes (EDS) are part of HDCT along with Marfan syndrome and osteogenesis imperfecta among others. In

---

C. Baeza-Velasco (✉)
Laboratoire de Psychopathologie et Processus de Santé, Institut de Psychologie, University of Paris, LPPS, Boulogne-Billancourt, France

Department of Emergency Psychiatry and Acute Care, CHU Montpellier, Montpellier, France
e-mail: carolina.baeza-velasco@u-paris.fr

P. Espinoza · A. Bulbena
Autonomous University of Barcelona, Barcelona, Spain
e-mail: paola.espinoza@uab.cat; 16359@parcdesalutmar.cat

A. Bulbena-Cabré
Icahn School of Medicine at Mount Sinai, New York, USA
e-mail: andrea.bulbena-cabre@mssm.edu

M. Seneque · S. Guillaume
Department of Emergency Psychiatry and Acute Care, CHU Montpellier, Montpellier, France

IGT, University of Montpellier, CNRS, INSERM, Montpellier, France
e-mail: m-seneque@chu-montpellier.fr; s-guillaume@chu-montpellier.fr

© Springer Nature Switzerland AG 2022
E. Manzato et al. (eds.), *Hidden and Lesser-known Disordered Eating Behaviors in Medical and Psychiatric Conditions*,
https://doi.org/10.1007/978-3-030-81174-7_28

addition to JH, common features of EDS are skin abnormalities and fragility and dysfunction of vessels and internal organs [3]. Thirteen subtypes of EDS have been described in the last classification dating from 2017 [4]. The genetic defect has been identified in all subtypes, except in the most common form which is the hypermobile EDS (hEDS). Thus, hEDS diagnosis remains clinical and represents 80%–90% of those EDS cases [5].

The 2017 EDS classification also highlights that JH should be understood as a continuum called "hypermobility spectrum disorders" (HSD), which ranges from asymptomatic JH to hEDS passing through intermediate phenotypes (i.e., symptomatic JH does not fulfill criteria for hEDS) [6]. An example of these intermediate phenotypes is the diagnosis category so called "joint hypermobility syndrome" [7], which before the apparition of the 2017 classification was considered as overlapping with hEDS. However, since the 2017 criteria are stricter, people fulfilling criteria for joint hypermobility syndrome are now considered in the HSD.

People suffering from HSD and hEDS present symptoms (many painful) of multisystemic nature, which can be explained by the wide distribution of collagen in the body. These include osteoarticular (e.g., arthralgia, recurrent joint dislocations, mild scoliosis, temporomandibular joint dysfunction, epicondylitis) and non-articular problems (e.g., gastrointestinal, mucocutaneous, cardiovascular, dental, urogynecological, ocular, and neuropsychiatric) [8]. Several of these symptoms may negatively impact the eating behaviors of those affected as well as their nutritional status [9] as we will comment further.

28.2 Weight/Nutritional Problems and Disordered Eating Behaviors in HSD and EDS

Although studies in this domain are scarce, there is increasing evidence suggesting that weight/nutritional problems and disordered eating behaviors occur in HSD and EDS more often than expected by chance. Table 28.1 summarized the available literature in this respect.

Four studies have explored nutritional/weight alterations and JH in children. These reported a greater proportion of JH and skin abnormalities in children with impaired fetal growth compared to controls [10], a negative correlation between the Beighton score [11] (the measure most used to evaluate JH) and BMI [12, 13], as well as an association between JH and malnutrition and musculoskeletal symptoms [14].

Altered BMI in JH and EDS also includes overweight as reported in two studies. Sanjay et al. [12] found that 57.14% of hypermobile Indian children were underweight while 19.15% were at risk of being overweight and 16.67% were overweight. On the other hand, a high proportion of altered BMI was also observed in a study in 80 adult patients with hEDS [15]: 42.5% presented overweight/obesity, while 15% was underweight.

Two studies compared JH in patients with eating disorders (ED). Goh et al. [16] reported that JH was significantly more common among anorexic subjects (63%)

Table 28.1 Studies about weight/nutritional problems and/or disordered eating behaviors in HSD and EDS

Authors	Country	Sample	Results
DeFelice et al. (2007) [10]	Italy	77 children, aged 9.45 ± 2.08 y/o with antenatally diagnosed intrauterine growth restriction and small-for-gestational-age birth	Significantly increased proportions of JH and skin softness in the intrauterine growth restriction-variant children as compared with controls subjects
Hasija et al. (2008) [14]	India	829 children, 3 and 19 y/o, lower economic strata	58.7% with BS ≥ 4/9. Positive BS in 61.5% children with 3° and 4° malnutrition and 36.8% with normal nutrition or 1°/2° of malnutrition. Moderate and severe malnutrition were associated with JH ($p < 0.05$)
Sanjay et al. (2013) [12]	India	420 healthy children aged 6–12 y/o	57.14% of hypermobile children present underweight, 35.93% normal weight, 19.15% risk overweight, and 16.67% overweight. Negative correlation between JH and BMI
Barçak et al. (2015) [13]	Turkey	Children aged 11–18 y/o, 52.2% girls	JH frequency = 9.1%. Highly negative correlation between BMI and BS ($p < 0.05$)
Baeza-Velasco et al. (2018) [15]	France	80 outpatients (90% women) with hEDS; 18 and 61 y/o (37.1 ± 11.5)	42.5% were overweight/obese and 15% were underweight
Hershenfeld et al. (2015) [23]	Canada	106 patients with EDS (classic and hypermobility type. 35.2 ± 13.9 age, 84.9 % female	Psychiatric disorders in 42.5% of the sample. Anxiety (23.6%), depression (25.5 %), AN (1.9%). High frequency of psychiatric disorders and an association with pain symptoms in EDS
Goh et al. (2013) [16]	Australia	Patients with AN ($n = 30$; 24.4 ± 1.4 y/o), first-degree relatives (29; 44.7 ± 2.9) and control group (16; 38.6 ± 3.7)	JH in patients (63%), relatives (34%), and controls (13%). High prevalence of intestinal symptoms, orthostatic intolerance, and JH in AN. First-degree relatives also have these complaints
Eccles (2016) [17]	UK	416 patients attending adult psychiatric services. 52% female. 18–65 y/o; 38.9 ± 0.61	Eating disorder = 7 (1.9%); on which 5 (71.4%) were hypermobile and 2 (28.6%) were non-hypermobile OR (95%CI) 10.48(2.04–53.96)
Bulbena-Cabré et al. (2017) [18]	Spain	117 nonclinical youngsters, 16.96 ± 0.87 y/o. 71.7% female	JHS in 33.3% of the sample. These participants had gastrointestinal problems (21.30%) and significantly higher percentages of anorexia ($p = 0.023$) and bulimia ($p = 0.012$) symptoms compared to those without JHS

(continued)

Table 28.1 (continued)

Authors	Country	Sample	Results
Zarate et al. (2010) [21]	UK	129 new unselected tertiary referrals (97 female, age range 16–78 y/o) to a neurogastroenterology clinic. Clinical case = female; 25 year; BMI 17	49% of patients have JH. Gastroesophageal reflux symptoms ($p = 0.005$) and abdominal bloating ($P = 0.05$) were particularly frequent among these patients. Clinical case: myriad of GI symptoms limited her food intake. Weight loss attributed to AN, denied by the patient. Diagnosis of JHS
Lee et al. (2018) [20]	Sweden	Clinical case = female 23 y/o; BMI 17–19.7. Diagnosis AN at 12 y/o	Numerous food allergies. Diffuse pains, bloating, nausea, involuntary vomiting, dysphagia, and weight loss. AN going into remission. Diagnosed with hEDS
Purkaple & Miidleman (2017) [22]	USA	Clinical case: male 18 y/o; BMI 16.79	Reflux, low stomach acid, forgetting to eat meals routinely, 12-lb weight loss coupled, diagnosis of malnutrition. Diagnosed with hEDS
Baeza-Velasco et al. (2015) [9]	France	Clinical case 1 = female 26 y/o; BMI 11–19. Diagnosis of AN in adolescence Clinical case 2 = female 23 y/o; BMI=12.9–15.8. Diagnosis of AN at 12 y/o	Case 1 = myriad of GI symptoms induced eating avoidance. Assessment negative for current AN. Diagnosed with JHS/hEDS Case 2 = myriad of GI symptoms. Painful eating. Diagnosed with JHS/hEDS at 15 y/o. Assessment negative for current AN

JH Joint hypermobility, *JHS* Joint hypermobility syndrome, *BS* Beighton score for JH, *BMI* Body mass index, *GJH* Generalized joint hypermobility, *EDS* Ehlers-Danlos syndromes, *AN* Anorexia nervosa, *GI* Gastrointestinal, *y/o* Years old

than in the relative (34%) and the healthy control group (13%). However with few subjects, Eccles [17] replicated these results, that is, a higher proportion of people with ED among psychiatric patients with JH compared to those non-hypermobile. In the same vein, we assessed JH with the Beighton score and related problems in a group of patients with ED followed at the University Hospital of Montpellier. Until the date this manuscript is written, 24 patients (83.3% anorexia nervosa) were evaluated in which 12 (50%) have ≥4 points out of 9 which is the more used cutoff for generalized JH. Compared to non-hypermobile patients, those with JH have suffered in a greater extent repeated dislocations of the knee or shoulder (12.5% vs. 41.6%; $X^2 = 8.2$; $p = 0.008$). In addition, a trend to significance was observed on joint pain (20.8% vs. 41.6%; $X^2 = 4.2$; $p = 0.063$) and frequent hemorrhages (e.g., nose, gums) (4.1% vs. 25%; $X^2 = 4.6$; $p = 0.063$), being the hypermobile group which has a greater proportion of subjects presenting these problems related to fragility of tissues.

Otherwise, Bulbena-Cabré et al. [18] compared scores on body awareness, bulimia, and anorexia assessed with the Body Perception Questionnaire [19] between non-hypermobile and hypermobile non-clinical youngsters. The last group has significantly higher scores on these dimensions than their counterpart.

Five clinical cases have been published illustrating underweight and eating problems in patients with hEDS [9, 20–22]. Only the study by Hershenfield et al. [23] explored anorexia nervosa in EDS patients with different subtypes. They found a prevalence of 1.9% in this group. From our side, in a comparison between patients with hEDS ($n = 36$) and rheumatoid arthritis ($n = 40$) and healthy subjects ($n = 51$) with respect to the prevalence of psychiatric disorders assessed with the Mini-International Neuropsychiatric Interview (MINI 5.0.0) [24], we observed that 16.7% of the hEDS sample reported having suffered from an ED at some time during their life, while the rheumatoid arthritis group reported 2.5% and healthy subjects 5.9%. However, the difference between groups did not reach statistical significance (Baeza-Velasco et al. unpublished).

28.3 Explaining the Link Between Weight Problems, Disordered Eating Behaviors, and HSD/EDS

Evidence concerning the link between weight and nutritional problems, disordered eating behaviors, and HSD/EDS is preliminary. Consequently, the mechanisms underlying such as connection remain poorly understood. A plausible explanation is that people in the hypermobility spectrum present problems susceptible to negatively impact eating behaviors and weight [9] as illustrated in Fig. 28.1. These problems are temporomandibular joint pain and disturbances [25] that alter patterns of mastication, gastrointestinal problems (e.g., dysphagia, gastro-esophageal reflux, bloating, constipation/diarrhea, abdominal pain), and dental problems [26] that may induce a painful eating. In this sense, the study by Berglund and Björck [27], which explored oral quality of life in patients with EDS using the Oral Health Impact Profile [28], observed that the most statistically significant differences between the subjects with EDS and the comparison group were found for items 3, 4, and 8: "I have had pain in the mouth," "I have had discomfort when eating," and "I have been forced to interrupt meals," respectively. In addition, the fragility of oral mucosa may reduce acceptability of some foods according to temperature and/or texture and altered chemosensory perceptions such as hyperosmia [25] that also may contribute to food selectivity. Moreover, enhanced interoception, hyperalgesia, and somatosensory amplification observed in these patients contribute to increase the perception of pain/discomfort when eating [9]. Finally, the proprioception impairment [25] probably influence eating behavior since it might alter body scheme and consequently the body image. Thus, a vicious circle may be developed by people with these characteristics leading to avoid eating if this is perceived as painful or even ED in complex cases [9].

Moreover, altered BMI pattern observed in HSD/EDS seems to be seen at both ends, that is, under- and overweight. Since pain is frequent in HSD and EDS, especially in hEDS where pain is often chronic, overweight can come from sedentarity induced by chronic pain in a subgroup of patients.

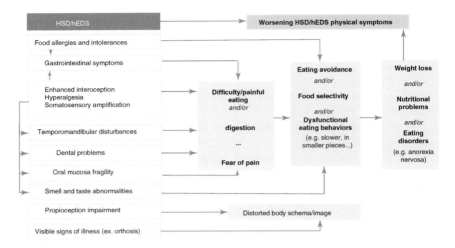

Fig. 28.1 Diagram illustrating possible relationships between some features or common co-occurring problems in HSD/hEDSmight contributing to eating difficulty and weight loss [9]

28.4 Conclusion

Although preliminary, available data suggests a connection between HSD and EDS and weight, nutritional, and altered eating behaviors that should be explored in more depth in future studies. From a clinical perspective, awareness of this association should motive, in the presence of JH, further explorations not only in the physical domain but also in the psychological/behavioral such as disordered eating behaviors. Alike, patients addressed to mental health services suspected of ED should benefit from physical explorations including hypermobility-related problems in order to have a more comprehensive picture of each patient and adapt treatments accordingly.

References

1. Hakim A, Grahame R. A simple questionnaire to detect hypermobility: an adjunct to the assessment of patients with diffuse musculoskeletal pain. Int J Clin Pract. 2003;57(3):163–6.
2. Grahame R. Hypermobility and the heritable disorders of the connective tissue. In: Keer R, Grahame R, editors. Hypermobility syndrome, recognition and management for physiotherapist. New York: Bitterworth Heinemann; 2003. p. 15–25.
3. Callewaert B, Malfait F, Loeys B, De Paepe A. Ehlers-Danlos syndromes and Marfan syndrome. Best Pract Res Clin Rheumatol. 2008;22(1):165–89.
4. Malfait F, Belmont J, Berglund B, Belmont J, Berglund B, Black J, et al. The 2017 international classification on the Ehlers–Danlos syndromes. Am J Med Genet C Semin Med Genet. 2017;175(1):8–26.
5. Tinkle B, Castori M, Berglund B, Cohen H, Grahame R, Kazkaz H, Levy H. Hypermobile Ehlers-Danlos syndrome (a.k.a. Ehlers-Danlos syndrome Type III and Ehlers-Danlos syn-

drome hypermobility type): Clinical description and natural history. Am J Med Gen Part C. 2017;175:48–69.
6. Castori M, Tinkle B, Levy H, Grahame R, Malfait F, Hakim A. A framework for the classification of joint hypermobility related conditions. Am J Med Genet C Semin Med Genet. 2017;175(1):148–57.
7. Grahame R, Bird HA, Child A. The revised (Brighton 1998) criteria for the diagnosis of benign joint hypermobility syndrome (BJHS). J Rheumatol. 2000;27(7):1777–9.
8. Colombi M, Dordoni C, Chiarelli N, Ritelli M. Differential diagnosis and diagnostic flow chart of joint hypermobility syndrome/Ehlers-Danlos syndrome hypermobility type compared to other heritable connective tissue disorders. Am J Med Genet C Semin Med Genet. 2015;169C(1):6–22.
9. Baeza-Velasco C, Van den Bossche T, Grossin D, Hamonet C. Eating difficulties and significant weight loss in Joint Hypermobility Syndrome/Ehlers-Danlos Syndrome, Hypermobility Type. Eat Weight Disord. 2016;21:175–83.
10. De Felice C, Tassi R, De Capua B, Jaubert F, Gentile M, Quartulli L, Tonni G, Constantini D, Strambi M, Latini G. A new phenotypical variant of intrauterine growth restriction? Pediatrics. 2007;119:e938–90.
11. Beighton P, Salomon L, Soskolne C. Articular mobility in an African population. Ann Rheum Dis. 1973;32(5):413–8.
12. Sanjay P, Bagalkoti PS, Kubasadgoudar R. Study of correlation between hypermobility and body mass index in children aged 6-12 years. Indian J Physiother Occup Ther. 2013;7:247–9.
13. Barçac OF, Karkucak M, Çapkin E, Karagüzel G, Dilber B, Dedeoglu SS. Prevalence of generalized joint hypermobility and fibromyalgia syndrome in the children population of Trabzon: a Turkish study. Turk J Phys Med Rehabil. 2015;61:6–11.
14. Hasija RP, Khubchandani RP, Shenoi S. Joint hypermobility in Indian children. Clin Exp Rheumatol. 2008;26:146–50.
15. Baeza-Velasco C, Bourdon C, Montalescot L, de Cazotte C, Pailhez G, Bulbena A, Hamonet C. Low- and high-anxious hypermobile Ehlers-Danlos syndrome patients: comparison of psychosocial and health variables. Rheumatol Int. 2018;38(5):871–8.
16. Min G, Olver J, Huang CH, Millard M, O'Callaghan CH. Prevalence and familial patterns of gastrointestinal symptoms, joint hypermobility and diurnal blood pressure variations in patients with anorexia nervosa. J Eat Disord. 2013;1(Suppl 1):O45.
17. Eccles J. Hypermobility and autonomic hyperactivity: relevance for the expression of psychiatric symptoms. (Thesis) University of Brighton and University of Sussex; February 2016.
18. Bulbena-Cabré A, Pailhez G, Cabrera A, Baeza-Velasco C, Porges S, Bulbena A. Body perception in a sample of nonclinical youngster with joint hypermobility. Ansiedad y Estrés. 2017;23:99–103.
19. Porges S. Body perception questionnaire. Laboratory of development assessment. University of Maryland. 1993.
20. Lee M, Strand M. Ehlers-Danlos syndrome in a young woman with anorexia nervosa and complex somatic symptoms. Int J Eat Disord. 2018;51:281–4.
21. Zarate N, Farmer AD, Grahame R, Mohammed SD, Knowles CH, Scott SM, Aziz Q, et al. Unexplained gastrointestinal symptoms and joint hypermobility: is connective tissue the missing link? Neurogastroenterol Motil. 2010;22:252–e78.
22. Purkaple B, Middleman A. On pins and needles: complex pain and malnutrition. Clin Pediatr. 2017;56(6):589–92.
23. Hershenfeld SA, Wasim S, McNiven V, Parikh M, Majewski P, Faghfoury H, So J. Psychiatric disorders in Ehlers-Danlos syndrome are frequent, diverse and strongly associated with pain. Rheumatol Int. 2016;36:341–8.
24. Sheehan DV, Lecubrier Y, Sheehan KH, Amorim P, Janavs J, Weiller E, et al. The MINI-International Neuropsychiatric Interview (M.I.N.I.): the development and validation of a structured diagnostic psychiatric interview for DSM-IV and ICD-10. J Clin Psychiatry. 1998;20(Suppl):22–33.

25. De Coster PJ, Van den Berghe LI, Martens LC. Generalized joint hypermobility and temporomandibular disorders: inherited connective tissue disease as a model with maximum expression. J Orofac Pain. 2005;19:47–57.
26. Hamonet C, Gompel A, Raffray Y, Zeitoun JD, Delarue M, Vlamynck E, Haidar R, Mazaltarine G. Multiple pains in Ehlers-Danlos syndrome. Description and proposal of a therapy protocol. Douleur. 2014;15:264–77.
27. Berglund B, Björck E. Women with Ehlers-Danlos syndrome experience low oral health-related quality of life. J Orofac Pain. 2012;26(4):307–14.
28. Slade GD. Derivation and validation of a short-form oral health impact profile. Community Dent Oral Epidemiol. 1997;25(4):284–90.

Kleine–Levin Syndrome and Eating and Weight Disorders

29

Antonio F. Radicioni, Chiara Tarantino, and Matteo Spaziani

29.1 Introduction

Kleine-Levin syndrome (KLS) is a rare neuropsychiatric disorder with a relapsing-remitting course characterized by recurrent episodes of hypersomnia and cognitive and behavioral changes. The first detailed report of multiple cases of recurrent hypersomnia was reported by Kleine in 1925 [1]. In 1936, Levin described seven cases of people with hypersomnia and morbid hunger [2]. In 1962, Critchley named the condition Kleine-Levin syndrome, based on his patients and the previous reports by Kleine and Levin [3]. Subsequent reports by Hoffman and Critchley identified the characteristic features of this condition: male predominance, onset during adolescence, pathological hunger, and the tendency of the syndrome to disappear spontaneously.

The exact cause of KLS is unknown. However, given its features, it may involve a dysfunction of the mesencephalic-hypothalamic-limbic system, and according to some authors, there may be an infection. This hypothesis is favored by evidence that KLS often arises as a result of an inflammatory state [4, 5]. For this reason, several studies have looked for associations with human leukocyte antigens, but some associations that seemed significant were not confirmed by subsequent studies [6]. Specific or probable genetic disorders were more frequent in KLS patients than in controls, including Klinefelter syndrome, mental retardation, autism, and idiopathic developmental delay [4].

A. F. Radicioni (✉) · C. Tarantino · M. Spaziani
Centre for Rare Diseases, Policlinico Umberto I, Department of Experimental Medicine, Section of Medical Pathophysiology, Food Science and Endocrinology, Sapienza University of Rome, Rome, Italy
e-mail: antonio.radicioni@uniroma1.it; chiara.tarantino@uniroma1.it; matteo.spaziani@uniroma1.it

The prevalence of KLS is estimated to be 1–5 per million [4]. It mainly affects males, with a male/female ratio of 3:1, but affected females have a longer course [7]. Although the familial risk is low (1% per first-degree relative), 5% of all cases are reported in relatives, suggesting an 800–4000-fold increase in risk [8]. The syndrome usually presents in adolescence (80% of cases), but symptoms can start at any age from childhood to adulthood. Regardless of the age of onset, episodes during adulthood are less severe and less sudden [4].

In a study of 186 patients, other neurological or psychiatric disorders were present before the onset of KLS and persisted among 10% of those patients, who were all significantly older and experienced more frequent and longer episodes and periods of incapacity than patients without such comorbidities [7].

Onset in childhood or adulthood is associated with a longer duration than adolescent onset. When the onset is in adolescence, the episodes often gradually diminish after the age of 30. In any case, episodes become less frequent with age and may even disappear (spontaneous remission). Childhood onset is associated with more frequent episodes than adolescent or adult onset [4].

29.2 Clinical Features and Diagnostic Criteria

KLS is classified as recurrent hypersomnia, although it has a number of clinical features. The diagnosis of KLS is usually delayed for several years after the presentation of the first episode, as the symptoms are initially attributed to other sleep disorders. The first episode is often mistaken for an infection, and KLS is typically only diagnosed after several episodes [5]. During the first episode, patients often go to the emergency room, where the common major causes of acute confusion and rapid changes in behavior are excluded. Alcohol or drug use is then investigated, and an MRI/CT study is carried out to exclude other causes, such as cancer, injury, inflammation, and vascular conditions.

Episodes may last from a few days to several weeks, usually with a sudden onset and interruption.

The typical triad of symptoms is sleep disorder, hyperphagia, and behavioral disorders, especially hypersexuality (above all in males). Numerous recent studies have established that hypersomnia is the constant symptom, with hyperphagia and hypersexuality found in no more than half of cases. For this reason they are no longer included in the 2005 revision of the mandatory diagnostic criteria. Most patients also exhibit apathy and derealization [4].

The diagnostic criteria for KLS are: [9, 10]

- At least two recurrent episodes of excessive drowsiness lasting from 2 days to 5 weeks.
- Episodes recur at least once every 18 months.
- Vigilance, cognitive functions, and behavior return to normal between episodes.
- The hypersomnia cannot be explained by other sleep disorders, neurological disorders, medication, or substance abuse.

- In addition, at least one of the following must be present during episodes:
  - Cognitive dysfunction
  - Altered perception
  - Eating disorder
  - Disinhibited behavior

Between episodes there are long asymptomatic periods of normal sleep, cognition, mood, and behavior. For this reason the disease is considered benign. Episodes may recur 6 months or a year later and tend to become shorter and more spaced out over time, until they finally disappear.

29.3 Clinical Typology (Mild, Moderate, and Severe Forms) [11]

Mild: 1 week 2–3 times a year
  Moderate: monthly episodes of 7–10 days or longer episodes at longer intervals
  Severe: 40–80 episodes in rapid succession

29.4 Symptoms

29.4.1 Hypersomnia

Patients experience sudden extreme fatigue and an irresistible need to sleep. They typically sleep for an average of 18 h a day or more during the early stages of an episode [12]. Sleep may occur night or day without a clear circadian rhythm. Patients are contactable during episodes and can be awakened, but this makes them aggressive and irritable, and they remain lethargic and apathetic [7].

After several episodes, patients may sleep less but remain inactive and prefer to stay in the dark and away from other people. At the end of an episode, brief insomnia is observed in about two-thirds of patients, sometimes associated with logorrhea and euphoria for 1–3 days. Several studies have reported that sleep patterns and alertness return to normal between episodes.

29.4.2 Cognitive Changes

Almost all patients complain of difficulty in communication (conversation and reading), concentration, decision-making, and memory. They often become unable to perform several tasks at once, have difficulty in motor coordination, and lose track of time. Confusion is generally mild, and patients remain able to count and answer complex questions, but much more slowly than between episodes. Most patients have anterograde amnesia of episodes and are disoriented in time and space [13].

29.4.3 Derealization, Hallucinations, and Delusions

The perception of the environment is altered in almost all patients, leading to derealization. This is the most specific symptom of KLS. Patients experience a feeling of unreality with altered perception of themselves and their environment. They report feeling as if they are inside a dream or a bubble, with changes in and reduced function of all their senses [13].

One-third of patients report threatening or disturbing hallucinations and delusions of short duration. Most perception disorders are mild, but even when more severe, they usually last from a few hours to a few days and stop spontaneously [13].

29.4.4 Eating Disorders

Around three-quarters of patients show eating disorders during episodes. The most typical is ingestion of large amounts of food; in one study patients showed an increase in body weight of 3.2–13.6 kg (7–30 lb.) (most patients gain weight during episodes). A minority of patients (5%) had a total aversion to food during some episodes, but ate more in others [7]. Some patients reduce their food intake, and these patients generally sleep more during episodes than those with hyperphagia [4].

Several authors have noted the compulsive rather than bulimic nature of the eating disorder, as patients did not self-induce vomiting or assume other compensatory behaviors to control their weight. Food craving and hyperphagia were the most critical elements. Some patients went so far as to steal food from shops or from other patients' plates, searched for food in dustbins, or even used both hands to shovel food in their mouth [14]. Patients with hyperphagia are also uninhibited toward specific tastes (e.g., sweet, salty, or sour) that may not be typical of their usual diet. Affected individuals usually do not recognize that they are particularly hungry but will still consume all available food without considering its condition, quality, or appearance or their personal preferences. Behavior toward food is often repetitive or compulsive.

To summarize, food craving and megaphagia are the most critical elements of KLS-associated eating disorders.

29.4.5 Mood Disorders

Flattened or depressed moods (with rare cases of suicide attempts) are reported in about half of patients and are more frequent in men than in women. They generally last a short time and often occur near the end of an episode. Some teenagers desperately fear that they will never get better, and some may wonder if they will die or say that they want to die if it does not stop [10].

Almost all patients experience irritability, especially if sleep, sexual behavior, or searching for food is prohibited. Anxiety can be accentuated during episodes. Some patients show fear or panic if left alone in unusual places, such as the hospital, or if they have to go outside or meet people [13].

Some patients report long-term mood swings and difficulty adapting to the disorder. This suggests that some patients never fully return to normal between episodes.

29.4.6 Hypersexuality

About half of patients suffer from hypersexuality during episodes. This symptom affects boys more than girls and frequently manifests itself as substantially increased masturbation or propositions toward sexual partners or other people of both sexes. Inappropriate sexual behavior can also occur, including exposing or touching genitals or masturbating in the presence of parents and doctors, using extreme sexual language or touching other people inappropriately [4, 15].

29.4.7 Social Impact

The unpredictable and sudden nature of the episodes means that they have adverse professional and social effects. For example, they may occur at school or during university exams (as they may be triggered by sleep deprivation or stress). Abnormal behavior (e.g., hypersexuality) can cause embarrassment and may even be dangerous.

29.5 Clinical Examination and Testing

Typically, there are no neurological signs on physical examination. Tests aim to exclude EEG epilepsy, focal brain lesions (imaging), meningitis, and encephalitis (by CSF analysis). Most tests are conducted while an episode is in progress [7]. One-quarter of subjects have a normal EEG during the episodes, but 70% show a non-specific and widespread slowdown in EEG activity [7]. No abnormalities are found on CT and MRI [4]. Functional imaging studies show a decrease in temporal lobe, frontal lobe, and thalamic activity during episodes. Functional MRI reveals that memory loss is correlated with reduced activity in the intermediate and adjacent dorsomedial prefrontal cortex and simultaneously increased activity in the medial and anterior thalamus (suggesting increased compensatory effort in controlling memory storage) compared to results in healthy volunteers [16]. The acute onset of cognitive impairment, apathy and derealization, altered perception, uninhibited behavior, anxiety, visual hallucinations, and delusions suggests that the associative cortex is affected.

29.6 Therapy

The objective of treatment is to stop hypersomnia and prevent subsequent episodes. Psychostimulant drugs such as amphetamines, methylphenidate, or pemoline are used to control episodes of drowsiness. Lithium salts [17] or carbamazepine in combination with antidepressants has been used as preventive therapy. A recent meta-analysis by the Cochrane group concluded that there is no evidence to indicate that pharmacological treatment for KLS is effective and safe [18].

References

1. Kleine W. Periodische Schlafsucht. Eur Neurol. 1925:285–304. https://doi.org/10.1159/000190426.
2. Levin M. Periodic somnolence and morbid hunger: a new syndrome. Brain. 1936; https://doi.org/10.1093/brain/59.4.494.
3. Critchley M. Periodic hypersomnia and megaphagia in adolescent males. Brain. 1962; https://doi.org/10.1093/brain/85.4.627.
4. Arnulf I, Lin L, Gadoth N, et al. Kleine-Levin syndrome: a systematic study of 108 patients. Ann Neurol. 2008; https://doi.org/10.1002/ana.21333.
5. Huang Y-S, Guilleminault C, Lin K-L, Hwang F-M, Liu F-Y, Kung Y-P. Relationship between Kleine-Levin syndrome and upper respiratory infection in Taiwan. Sleep. 2012; https://doi.org/10.5665/sleep.1600.
6. Arnulf I, Lecendreux M, Franco P, Dauvilliers Y. Kleine-Levin syndrome: state of the art. Rev Neurol (Paris). 2008; https://doi.org/10.1016/j.neurol.2008.04.020.
7. Arnulf I, Zeitzer JM, File J, Farber N, Mignot E. Kleine-Levin syndrome: a systematic review of 186 cases in the literature. Brain. 2005; https://doi.org/10.1093/brain/awh620.
8. Peraita-Adrados R, Vicario JL, Tafti M, García de León M, Billiard M. Monozygotic twins affected with Kleine-Levin syndrome. Sleep. 2012; https://doi.org/10.5665/sleep.1808.
9. Sateia MJ. International classification of sleep disorders-third edition highlights and modifications. Chest. 2014; https://doi.org/10.1378/chest.14-0970.
10. Miglis MG, Guilleminault C. Kleine-Levin syndrome. Curr Neurol Neurosci Rep. 2016; https://doi.org/10.1007/s11910-016-0653-6.
11. Aasm. International classification of sleep disorders: diagnostic and coding manual. (ICSD-2).; 2005.
12. Arnulf I, Rico TJ, Mignot E. Diagnosis, disease course, and management of patients with Kleine-Levin syndrome. Lancet Neurol. 2012; https://doi.org/10.1016/S1474-4422(12)70187-4.
13. Arnulf I, Groos E, Dodet P. Kleine–Levin syndrome: a neuropsychiatric disorder. Rev Neurol (Paris). 2018; https://doi.org/10.1016/j.neurol.2018.03.005.
14. Duffy JP, Davison K. A female case of the Kleine-Levin syndrome. Br J Psychiatry. 1968; https://doi.org/10.1192/bjp.114.506.77.
15. Schenck CH, Amulf I, Mahowald MW. Sleep and sex: What can go wrong? A review of the literature on sleep related disorders and abnormal sexual behaviors and experiences. Sleep. 2007; https://doi.org/10.1093/sleep/30.6.683.
16. Engström M, Vigren P, Karlsson T, Landtblom AM. Working memory in 8 Kleine-Levin syndrome patients: an fMRI study. Sleep. 2009; https://doi.org/10.1093/sleep/32.5.681.
17. Abe K. Lithium prophylaxis of periodic hypersomnia. Br J Psychiatry. 1977; https://doi.org/10.1192/bjp.130.3.312.
18. de Oliveira MM, Conti C, Prado GF. Pharmacological treatment for Kleine-Levin syndrome. Cochrane Database Syst Rev. 2016; https://doi.org/10.1002/14651858.CD006685.pub4.

Klinefelter Syndrome and Eating and Weight Disorders

30

Antonio F. Radicioni and Matteo Spaziani

30.1 Introduction

Klinefelter syndrome (KS) was first described in 1942 as a condition characterized by gynecomastia; small, firm testes; hyalinization of the seminiferous tubules; and subsequent azoospermia [1]. It is the most common sex chromosome disorder in males, with an estimated prevalence of 1 case per 660 newborns [2, 3]. It is commonly defined as the presence of one extra X chromosome in a male phenotype, resulting in a 47,XXY karyotype [4]. This extra X chromosome is the consequence of a non-disjunction mechanism normally taking place during the first or second maternal meiotic division or the first paternal meiotic division. A non-disjunction event is also possible, but is less common (3–10%), after zygote development, causing forms of mosaicism (mainly 46,XY/47,XXY) [5].

The classic KS phenotype is characterized by tall stature; small, firm testes; gynecomastia; large hips; scanty body hair; and visceral obesity. There may also be another, paucisymptomatic, phenotype with fewer clinical features [6].

The lack of clear signs is the most likely explanation for the underdiagnosis of KS [7]. In any case, its clinical presentation changes with age. In infancy, chromosomal evaluations may be performed due to hypospadias, small phallus, cryptorchidism, or developmental delay [9]. School-aged children may present language delay, learning disabilities, or behavioral problems. Older children and adolescents may be diagnosed during an endocrine evaluation for incomplete pubertal development with eunuchoid body habitus, gynecomastia, and small testes. Adults are often

---

A. F. Radicioni (✉) · M. Spaziani
Centre for Rare Diseases, Policlinico Umberto I, Department of Experimental Medicine, Section of Medical Pathophysiology, Food Science and Endocrinology, Sapienza University of Rome, Rome, Italy
e-mail: antonio.radicioni@uniroma1.it; matteo.spaziani@uniroma1.it

© Springer Nature Switzerland AG 2022
E. Manzato et al. (eds.), *Hidden and Lesser-known Disordered Eating Behaviors in Medical and Psychiatric Conditions*,
https://doi.org/10.1007/978-3-030-81174-7_30

evaluated for infertility, breast malignancy, decreased libido, sexual or ejaculatory disorders, metabolic syndrome, or osteoporosis [8].

30.2 Clinical Features and Diagnostic Criteria

After birth, babies with KS pass through mini-puberty as normal. This period of temporary hypothalamus-pituitary-gonadal (HPG) axis activation lasts from the first month of life to about the ninth month. During this period Sertoli and Leydig cell function in KS babies is normal, but there may be early impairment of the HPG axis, with higher gonadotropin levels and hence higher gonadal hormone concentrations. The most likely explanation of this aspect could be a higher pituitary pacing setting or a change in compartmental cross-talking in the gonads.

In contrast with other forms of hypogonadism, the normal or sub-normal pre-pubertal testosterone levels mean that KS boys undergo puberty at the normal time or even precociously, with the appearance of the classic sexual secondary characteristics (growth of pubic hair, morphology, and enlargement of the penis and testes). However, testicular growth tends to stop precociously during the intermediate phase of puberty (Tanner stage G3), with the testicles reaching an average maximum volume of 4–5 mL against a normal volume of 8–10 mL. The occurrence of true hypogonadism with pubertal delay is not common in this period [9].

During the late phases of the puberty, there is an increase in FSH and LH and the typical onset of hypergonadotropic hypogonadism associated with a gradual degeneration of germ cells. This reaches its peak between mid-puberty and adulthood, by which time the testes have undergone extensive seminiferous tubule hyalinization and Leydig and Sertoli cell hyperplasia [10]. This phase is associated with azoospermia or, more rarely, cryptozoospermia.

Individuals with KS are typically tall, with an increased arm span and an imbalance between the trunk and lower limbs (which are longer than the trunk). However, other clinical aspects may also characterize the syndrome, including a tendency for visceral obesity, dyslipidemia, hypertension and diabetes mellitus, and hence metabolic syndrome [11]. Its association with cardiovascular, bone, and immune disorders is another important implication [12].

Several studies have suggested that individuals with KS are at greater risk of developing various psychiatric disorders, including depression and schizophrenia. In a 2014 Swedish study comparing 860 Klinefelter patients and 86,000 matched controls, the KS patients had an almost four times higher risk of schizophrenia and bipolar disorder and about a six times higher risk of autism spectrum disorder [13].

Another study investigated the link between salivary testosterone concentration and social anxiety and social cognitive skills in 20 KS subjects aged 8–19 years, comparing them with 25 age-matched controls [14]. Lower levels of salivary testosterone in the KS group were strongly associated with higher levels of social anxiety. This correlation was independent of age and pubertal development, demonstrating the importance of androgen status on psychological risk in KS subjects. In contrast, salivary testosterone levels were not correlated with social cognitive skills [14].

There is virtually no literature about bulimia nervosa and binge eating disorder in KS subjects, while the literature data on anorexia nervosa amounts to a few case reports [15–17], with no original articles or systematic reviews. Evaluation of these case reports leads to the conclusion that anorexia nervosa has no direct pathophysiological links with the clinical and psychological aspects of KS. However, clinicians may wish to investigate the possibility of KS in boys and young men who present with anorexia nervosa, as it may be associated with the other features of KS.

30.3 Genetic Aspects

In relation to the genetic aspects of KS, the extra X chromosome has an interesting role in fat storage and hence in weight and body composition variations. There is a unanimous consensus that gonadal hormones play a substantial role in regulating fat storage, affecting processes from food intake and adipocyte differentiation to energy expenditure [18–20]. Some mouse studies show that the presence of two X chromosomes promotes fat storage more than a single X chromosome [21, 22]. It could therefore be predicted that KS men would have greater fat storage than normal karyotype men. In fact, many studies have highlighted increased truncal and abdominal fat in KS subjects compared to normal or hypogonadal XY individuals [23–25].

Animal studies enable the different influences of androgen status and genetic weight on adiposity and its distribution to be determined. This is not the case in human studies, where the main problem is to establish the exact contribution of reduced androgen levels in KS subjects as a driver of increased adiposity. However, studies of pre-pubertal KS boys revealed that there is already an increase in body fat over XY males, suggesting a genetic contribution even in the absence of the major differences in androgen levels that take place following puberty [26, 27].

A KS mouse model has been used to determine the effect on adiposity of the extra X chromosome and the respective contributions of the genetic status and androgen status [28]. Fat mass was determined both before and after gonadectomy and subsequent testosterone replacement to achieve similar levels in both XY and XXY mice. KS mice with or without normalized testosterone levels showed higher body fat and hence higher weight than normal karyotype mice, demonstrating that the number of X chromosomes has a distinct role that is unrelated to androgen status. It can therefore be concluded that the extra X chromosome is an important determinant of body weight, fat storage, and food intake in KS subjects.

30.4 Conclusions

In conclusion, KS is a condition that directly influences body composition and consequently body weight through the direct role of the extra X chromosome. Interindividual differences can be explained by the syndrome's great variability, which is mainly due to different expression of the genes of the extra X chromosome and the different degrees of androgen receptor deactivation. It is therefore possible to find

KS subjects of normal weight with a less dangerous fat distribution and a reduced cardiovascular risk factor. Body weight variations in KS do not seem to be associated with eating disorders per se, although some psychiatric disorders are described in KS. Anorexia nervosa seems to be the most common eating disorder, although there is very little literature evidence in this area.

References

1. Klinefelter HF, Refenstein EC, Albright F. Syndrome characterized by gynaecomastia, aspermatogenesis without a Leydigism and increased excretion of follicle-stimulating hormone. J Clin Endocrinol Metab. 1942:615–27.
2. Morris JK, Alberman E, Scott C, Jacobs P. Is the prevalence of Klinefelter syndrome increasing? Eur J Hum Genet. 2008;16:163–70.
3. Radicioni AF, De Marco E, Gianfrilli D, Granato S, Gandini L, Isidori AM, et al. Strategies and advantages of early diagnosis in Klinefelter's syndrome. Mol Hum Reprod. 2010;16:434–40.
4. Bojesen A, Juul S, Gravholt CH. Prenatal and postnatal prevalence of Klinefelter syndrome: a national registry study. J Clin Endocrinol Metab. 2003;88(2):622–6.
5. Forti G, Corona G, Vignozzi L, Krausz C, Maggi M. Klinefelter's syndrome: a clinical and therapeutic update. Sex Dev Gene Mol Biol Evol Endocrinol Embryol Pathol Sex Determ Differ. 2010;4(4–5):249–58.
6. Simpson JL, de la Cruz F, Swerdloff RS, Samango-Sprouse C, et al. Klinefelter syndrome: expanding the phenotype and identifying new research directions. Genet Med Off J Am College Med Genet. 2003;5(6):460–8.
7. Abramsky L, Chapple J. 47,XXY (Klinefelter syndrome) and 47,XYY: estimated rates of and indication for postnatal diagnosis with implications for prenatal counselling. Prenat Diagn. 1997;17:363–8.
8. Salzano A, D'Assante R, Heaney LM, Monaco F, Rengo G, Valente P, et al. Klinefelter syndrome, insulin resistance, metabolic syndrome, and diabetes: review of literature and clinical perspectives. Endocrine. 2018;61(2):194–203.
9. Radicioni AF, Ferlin A, Balercia G, Pasquali D, Vignozzi L, Maggi M, Foresta C, Lenzi A. Consensus statement on diagnosis and clinical management of Klinefelter syndrome. J Endocrinol Invest. 2010;33(11):839–50.
10. Aksglaede L, Skakkebaek NE, Almstrup K, Juul A. Clinical and biological parameters in 166 boys, adolescents and adults with nonmosaic Klinefelter syndrome: a Copenhagen experience. Acta paediatr (Oslo, Norway: 1992). 2011;100(6):793–806.
11. Bojesen A, Host C, Gravholt CH. Klinefelter's syndrome, type 2 diabetes and the metabolic syndrome: the impact of body composition. Mol Hum Reprod. 2010;16(6):396–401.
12. Shiraishi K, Matsuyama H. Klinefelter syndrome: from pediatrics to geriatrics. Reprod Med Biol. 2018;18(2):140–50.
13. Cederlöf M, Ohlsson Gotby A, Larsson H, Serlachius E, Boman M, Långström N, Landén M, Lichtenstein P. Klinefelter syndrome and risk of psychosis, autism and ADHD. J Psychiatr Res. 2014;48(1):128–30.
14. van Rijn S. Salivary testosterone in relation to social cognition and social anxiety in children and adolescents with 47,XXY (Klinefelter syndrome). PLoS One. 2018;13(7):e0200882.
15. el-Badri SM, Lewis MA. Anorexia nervosa associated with Klinefelter's syndrome. Compr Psychiatry. 1991;32(4):317–9.
16. Szabo CP. A case of male anorexia with Klinefelter's syndrome, 22 years later—case report. Br J Psychiatry. 2008;193(5):388.
17. Gritti A, Salerno F, Pisano S, Formicola F, Melis D, Franzese A. A case of Klinefelter syndrome, mosaicism (46,XY/47,XXY), associated with anorexia nervosa. Eat Weight Disord. 2011;16(1):e69–71.

18. Mauvais-Jarvis F, Clegg DJ, Hevener AL. The role of estrogens in control of energy balance and glucose homeostasis. Endocr Rev. 2013;34:309–38.
19. Arnold AP. A general theory of sexual differentiation. J Neurosci Res. 2017;95:291–300.
20. Asarian L, Geary N. Sex differences in the physiology of eating. AJP Regul Integr Comp Physiol. 2013;305:R1215–67.
21. Arnold AP, Reue K, Eghbali M, Vilain E, Chen X, Ghahramani N, Itoh Y, Li J, Link JC, Ngun T, Williams-Burris SM. The importance of having two X chromosomes. Philos Trans R Soc B Biol Sci. 2016;371:20150113.
22. Arnold AP. Mouse models for evaluating sex chromosome effects that cause sex differences in non-gonadal tissues. J Neuroendocrinol. 2009;21:377–86.
23. Aksglaede L, Molgaard C, Skakkebaek NE, Juul A. Normal bone mineral content but unfavourable muscle/fat ratio in Klinefelter syndrome. Arch Dis Child. 2008;93:30–4.
24. Gravholt CH, Jensen AS, Høst C, Bojesen A. Body composition, metabolic syndrome and type 2 diabetes in Klinefelter syndrome. Acta Paediatr. 2011;100:871–7.
25. Bojesen A, Kristensen K, Birkebaek NH, Fedder J, Mosekilde L, Bennett P, Laurberg P, Frystyk J, Flyvbjerg A, Christiansen JS, Gravholt CH. The metabolic syndrome is frequent in Klinefelter's syndrome and is associated with abdominal obesity and hypogonadism. Diabetes Care. 2006;29:1591–8.
26. Ishikawa T, Yamaguchi K, Kondo Y, Takenaka A, Fujisawa M. Metabolic syndrome in men with Klinefelter's syndrome. Urology. 2008;71:1109–13.
27. Bardsley MZ, Falkner B, Kowal K, Ross JL. Insulin resistance and metabolic syndrome in prepubertal boys with Klinefelter syndrome. Acta Paediatr. 2011;100:866–70.
28. Chen X, Williams-Burris SM, McClusky R, Ngun TC, Ghahramani N, Barseghyan H, Reue K, Vilain E, Arnold AP. The sex chromosome trisomy mouse model of XXY and XYY: metabolism and motor performance. Biol Sex Differ. 2013;4:15.

Parkinson's Disease and Eating and Weight Disorders

31

Massimo Cuzzolaro and Nazario Melchionda

31.1 Historical Notes

Parkinson's disease (PD) is a progressive systemic neurodegenerative disease.

The eponym refers to the English physician James Parkinson (1755–1824) who, in 1817, published the first description of the disease. He called it "shaking palsy" (paralysis agitans) and spoke of a neurological syndrome characterized by:

> "involuntary tremulous motion, with lessened muscular power (…) with a propensity to bend the trunk forward, and to pass from a walking to a running pace" [1] (Chap. 1, p. 1)

About nutrition in this disease, Parkinson especially noted the difficulties in chewing and swallowing solid food with possible results in undernutrition. One patient fed very little and almost only milk:

Nazario Melchionda was deceased at the time of publication.

The chapter is dedicated to the memory of Nazario Melchionda (1939–2020), dear colleague and friend.

M. Cuzzolaro (✉)
University of Roma Sapienza, Roma, Italy
e-mail: massimo.cuzzolaro@gmail.com

N. Melchionda (Deceased)
University of Bologna Alma Mater, Bologna, Italy

© Springer Nature Switzerland AG 2022
E. Manzato et al. (eds.), *Hidden and Lesser-known Disordered Eating Behaviors in Medical and Psychiatric Conditions*,
https://doi.org/10.1007/978-3-030-81174-7_31

"he is not only no longer able to feed himself, but when the food is conveyed to the mouth, so much are the actions of the muscles of the tongue, pharynx, &c. impeded by impaired action and perpetual agitation, that the food is with difficulty retained in the mouth until masticated; and then as difficultly swallowed." [1] (Chap. 1, p. 8)

"He took very little nourishment, could chew and swallow no solids, and even found great pain in getting down liquids. Milk was almost his only food" [1] (Chap. IV, p. 40)

The first drugs used in PD were anticholinergic agents active in the central nervous system, starting with belladonna alkaloids. They have been the basic therapy for almost a century.

In the 1960s, studies by Arvid Carlsson and collaborators have linked PD to a dopamine neurotransmitter deficit due to the gradual loss of dopaminergic neurons, mainly within the nigrostriatal pathway [2].

Following that discovery, for over half a century, l-dopa (levodopa or l-3,4-dihydroxyphenylalanine, $C_9H_{11}NO_4$) has become the leading pharmacological remedy for Parkinson's motor symptoms [3]. L-dopa is a molecule capable of overcoming the blood-brain barrier and being converted to dopamine ($C_8H_{11}NO_2$) by the dopa-decarboxylase enzyme.

At the end of the twentieth century, another important step was discovering alpha-synuclein, a presynaptic neuronal protein present in PD and other neurological diseases called synucleinopathies [4, 5].

As far as genetics is concerned, numerous genetic factors have been identified that increase the risk of developing the disease, as well as some rare monogenic forms of parkinsonism caused by a mutation in a gene, either dominant or recessive [6].

These monogenic forms are held collectively responsible for 5%–10% of cases of PD [7]. For example, mutations in the LRRK2 gene (also called Park8) are a cause of autosomal dominant PD, a genetic form responsible, in Italy, for 1–2% of sporadic cases of PD and 4–5% of family cases [8].

In recent decades, increasing attention has been paid to PD non-motor symptoms and dopaminergic treatment's side effects.

This line includes studies on impulse control disorders (ICDs) and, in particular, those on feeding and eating disorders and body weight abnormalities in people with PD. It has been seen that, compared to James Parkinson's observations on undernutrition, after the introduction of dopaminergic therapy, the onset of eating disorders, overweight, and obesity has become much more frequent. We have recently written:

"The study of ICDs in PD patients offers a heuristic opportunity to explore the role of different dopaminergic projections and dopamine receptors in impulse control difficulties and, in particular, in binge eating, food craving, and food addiction that are still controversial concepts with uncertain implications for etiology and treatment. Many clinical questions arise. Is binge eating disorder (BED) different in PD? Could BED-oriented cognitive-behavioral therapy be useful also in BED with PD? How could we prevent disordered eating behaviors and weight gain in PD?" [9] (p. 384)

31.2 Epidemiology, Course, and Survival

The number of PD patients is continuously growing due to the increased world population and life expectancy. In 1990–2016 the raw prevalence rates increased by 74.3%, those standardized by age by 21.7% [10].

The maximum prevalence is between 85 and 89 years old [10].

The incidence increases with age, and the highest falls in the 70–79 age group [11]. However, there are middle-onset PD (50–69 years) and young-onset PD (before 50 years).

PD affects both sexes, with a slight male prevalence increasing after age 60. The male-to-female ratio is 1.4:1 [10].

The increase in prevalence is due to the increase in older adults, longer illness duration, and probably environmental factors such as pesticides, solvents, metals, and air pollution [10, 12, 13].

The relationship between diet, microbiota, and PD is controversial [14]. For a long time, several studies argue that a healthy diet—for example, the Mediterranean diet—can be a protective factor [15–17]. Perhaps abnormalities in gut microbiota may contribute to the pathogenesis of PD [18, 19].

Some reports support a possible protective effect of physical activity, smoking, coffee, and black tea consumption [13, 20, 21].

Plasma caffeine levels were lower in PD subjects versus unaffected controls. Levels were even lower in PD patients carrying the LRRK2 gene mutation predisposing to the disease [22].

Nevertheless, this cross-sectional study is not enough to prove that caffeine consumption decreases the risk of developing PD. Besides, the results may also indicate that people predisposed to PD tend to drink less coffee.

Regarding the prognosis, a subdivision into three subtypes has been proposed [23]. The tripartition is based on the time lapse between diagnosis, worsening of symptoms and disabilities (first milestones: continuous falls, wheelchair dependence, dementia, accommodation in a residential/nursing home), and death. Table 31.1 sums up the division into three possible phenotypes.

This proposal is still under discussion, but it is crucial to keep in mind that PD phenotypic presentation and prognosis are very variable and a mild, slowly progressing course is frequent [24].

Death can be due to disease-related causes such as pneumonia *ab ingestis* and falls. However, for the most part, people with PD die from the same causes as their peers.

Table 31.1 Parkinson's disease: years from diagnosis

Subtype	First milestone	Survival
Mild motor-predominant (49%)	14.3 ± 5.7	20.2 ± 7.8
Intermediate (35%)	8.23 ± 5.3	13.2 ± 6.7
Diffuse malignant (16%)	3.5 ± 3.2	8.1 ± 5.4

31.3 Motor and Non-motor Symptoms

The typical representation of a PD patient has long been the picture drawn in the nineteenth century by James Parkinson [1] and then by William Richard Gowers [25]: a man, elderly, bent forward, trembling, debilitated, and substantially disabled.

This image must be corrected. It does not consider the numerous female cases, those that begin before the age of 50–60 years, the initial manifestations, and non-motor symptoms. Moreover, this stereotype does not recognize the significant variability in the course of PD and contributes to social stigma and internalized stigma (self-fulfilled prophecies) with increased damage to the quality of life [24].

The main motor symptoms are resting tremor, reduction of facial mimicry, rigidity, bradykinesia, foot dystonia, gait issues, and postural instability.

Non-motor symptoms are hyposmia, hypophonia, fatigue, sleep-wake cycle disturbances with daytime sleepiness and nighttime insomnia, orthostatic hypotension and blood pressure instability, sialorrhea, swallowing disorders, delayed gastric emptying, constipation, frequent and urgent urination, erectile dysfunction, cognitive disorders, and psychopathological symptoms (see Sect. 31.4).

Non-motor symptoms mostly appear as disease and treatment progress. Sometimes, however, they precede the appearance of motor disorders. In all cases, they contribute heavily to the deterioration of quality of life, disability, and disease burden for patients and caregivers.

PD and other neurodegenerative diseases can be associated with REM (rapid eye movement) sleep behavior disorder. REM sleep is normally associated with motor atony. Instead, there are very vivid and unpleasant dreams in REM sleep behavior disorder accompanied by vocal sounds and sudden and violent arm and leg movements. REM sleep behavior disorder can be, together with hyposmia, a prodromal symptom. Late-onset (over 50 years of age) leg restlessness can be an early manifestation of PD, as well [26].

It is unclear which non-motor symptoms depend on dopaminergic deficits, other neurotransmitter systems, or dopamine replacement therapy [27].

In the more advanced stages and malignant and rapidly progressing PD forms, both motor and non-motor symptoms are more severe and disabling, with or without tremor.

31.4 Psychiatric Comorbidity

Cognitive disorders may initially affect attention and executive and visual-spatial functions. They may be mild impairments, but in several cases, dementia is progressively established.

The cumulative probability of dementia after 10 years of PD was 46% [28].

In cases treated with subthalamic nucleus deep brain stimulation (DBS), incidence and prevalence of dementia were not higher than the rates reported in the general PD population [29].

Anxious and depressive symptoms are frequent, especially with advancing age. A study reported anxiety disorders in two-thirds of PD cases and depression in one-third [30].

The presence of obsessive-compulsive symptoms (in particular, hoarding) was also more frequent in elderly patients with PD (31%) than in a control group (21%) [31].

Personality changes and psychotic symptoms, especially visual hallucinations and delusions, can occur. Hallucinations often accompany cognitive decline [32], particularly that of executive functions [33].

Treatment with levodopa and dopamine agonists is implicated in the development of psychotic symptoms in people with PD. However, the interaction between the neurotransmitter dysfunction intrinsic to the disease and drugs is still unknown [34].

For several years, it has been reported that in people with PD taking antiparkinson drugs (dopamine replacement therapy), impulsive-compulsive spectrum disorders (ICSDs) and behavioral addictions (BA) are also often observed [35–39].

ICSDs appear in 40% of people with PD and dopamine replacement therapy [40]. Early-onset of PD seems to be associated with an increased risk of ICSDs and BA [41].

A list of the main ones in alphabetical order is as follows:

– Binge eating
– Compulsive buying
– Compulsive overeating
– Food addiction
– Medication abuse (in particular, overuse of dopamine agents or "dopamine dysregulation syndrome")
– Obsessive hobby
– Pathological gambling
– Punding (the term was coined to describe purposeless, stereotyped behaviors such as repetitive examining and handling objects or compelling attraction for activities such as cleaning) [42]
– Selective and non-selective food cravings
– Sex addiction
– Walkabout (need to wander aimlessly)

The neuro-anatomic circuits involved in ICSDs can be altered by Parkinson's disease itself and by exogenous influences, including drugs active on the central nervous system.

Treatment with dopaminergic drugs is believed to weaken the ability to control the compulsive repetition of rewarding behaviors.

In PD patients, long-term dopaminergic treatment over-stimulates, in particular, dopamine D2/D3 receptors and induces downregulation [43]. Not only L-DOPA but even more dopamine agonists—such as bromocriptine, pramipexole, rotigotine, and ropinirole—are linked to the development of ICSDs [44].

Many data support the hypothesis that addiction-like behaviors, ICSDs, and compulsive overeating are due to dopamine replacement therapy rather than PD alone [43].

However, not all patients with PD in dopaminergic treatment develop ICSDs. Predisposition [45] and, in particular, personality play an essential role [46].

Weintraub and collaborators found that about 20% of patients diagnosed with PD but not yet in therapy reported some ICSDs [47]. The percentage was not higher than that found in a control group. Therefore, PD itself does not seem to increase the risk of developing ICSDs significantly.

It is necessary to wonder whether those who have some premorbid impulse control disorders are at greater risk of developing others or worsening when starting dopaminergic therapy.

Some authors have noted in PD patients that dopaminergic therapy increases motivation for artistic activities and creativity. Related behaviors may look like compulsive, but the quality of life appears to have improved [48–51].

In conclusion, ICSDs in PD patients should be considered multifactorial phenomena involving drug-, patient-, and disease-related factors [52].

31.5 Eating and Weight Disorders

Is obesity a risk factor for the development of PD? The data are discordant.

A Finnish cohort study said yes [53]. However, more recently, a Swedish survey found the opposite [54]. In the same year, South Korean research published data according to which the metabolic syndrome—usually associated with abdominal obesity—increases the risk of developing PD [55].

As for the course, obesity has been associated with a faster progression of motor symptoms and disability, especially in patients with early-onset PD [56].

A balanced diet and healthy body weight are necessary to maintain PD people's overall health and muscle strength. Cognitive functions are also likely to benefit from a proper diet (e.g., Mediterranean diet), adopted from the early stages of the disease [57].

Eating disorders are frequent in PD patients and body weight tends to vary during the disease.

Decreases in caloric intake and unintentional weight loss have been observed frequently. As James Parkinson had already observed [1], dysphagia and tremor in the upper extremities contribute to undernutrition [58, 59].

A multicenter case-control study found that the mean BMI was significantly lower in PD patients ((22.0 ± 3.4 kg/m^2 vs. 25.4 ± 4.3 kg/m^2). Visual hallucinations and motor complications (dyskinesia) were associated with low BMI [60].

It has been reported, understandably, the risk of sarcopenia, related to the worsening of functional capacity and nutritional status [61].

On the other hand, many other PD patients develop obesity. The improvement of motor symptoms obtained with surgical and pharmacological therapies plays a role.

After surgery (subthalamic nucleus deep brain stimulation), many patients (men and women) present an increase in fat mass and become overweight/obese [62, 63].

As for dopaminergic drugs, they contribute to obesity by improving motor symptoms and promoting disinhibition of eating behavior [9, 37].

Disordered eating behaviors are common in PD, but little studied and little known [37].

They are mostly classified as impulse control disorders and occur as compulsive grazing, overeating, selective or non-selective food cravings, and binge eating disorder (BED).

In 2007, a review article reported compulsive eating among the frequent reward-based behaviors observed in PD patients treated with dopaminergic drugs [64].

A few years later, a large multicenter study found that compulsive eating was present in 3.4% of cases, but there was no dose-response relationship between L-dopa or dopamine agonist dose and odds ratio for the onset of the symptom [65].

In a sample of 3090 PD patients, Weintraub et al. found BED in 4.3% of cases [44]. Some researchers found a much higher prevalence for impulse control disorders less strictly defined than BED and called "compulsive eating" (14.3%) [66] and "eating behavior disorder" (7.2%) [36].

Ingrid de Chazeron and collaborators recently studied a sample of PD patients in dopaminergic therapy (age 68 ± 10 years; males 53%) who reported changes in their dietary habits following PD diagnosis [37]. The main results are the following:

- Anorexia nervosa (AN): no cases
- Bulimia nervosa (BN): no cases
- BED full criteria: 4%
- NES: 6%
- Addictive-like eating behaviors without BED: 39%
- Food cravings (sweets) more than once a week: 43%
- The habit of eating outside meal times and/or during the night: 69%
- Inappropriate compensatory behaviors:
  – Fasting or excessive exercise ($\geq$ 2 times/week): 10%
  – Laxatives: 6%
  – Self-induced vomiting: 2%
  – Appetite suppressants: 2%

Eating disorders began within the first 2 years after the diagnosis of PD in 65% of cases.

In this research—apart from AN, BN, and BED—the other frequencies suffer, of course, from the uncertainty related to the lack of shared diagnostic definitions.

However, more robust studies are lacking and this recent survey is useful because it indicates that disordered eating and weight control behaviors can occur in many patients with PD under dopaminergic treatment.

31.6 Diagnosis and Treatment

Diagnostic evaluation is based on anamnestic data, physical examination, and the possible use of instrumental and psychometric tests.

The doctor looks for prodromal symptoms (hyposmia, REM sleep behavior disorders, etc.), motor symptoms (stiffness, rest tremor, etc.), cognitive decline, and psychiatric symptoms.

In uncertain cases, magnetic resonance imaging can distinguish PD from other parkinsonisms, while dopamine transporter single-photon emission computed tomography permits to distinguish PD from essential tremor [40].

Some psychometric tools can help in the assessment of ICSDs and, in particular, of disordered eating behaviors:

- *Addiction-like Eating Behavior Scale*, AEBS [67]. AEBS investigates the presence of addictive-like eating behaviors (according to the food addiction behavioral approach).
- *Ardouin Scale of Behavior in Parkinson's Disease* [68]. The scale is designed for quantifying changes of mood and behavior related to PD and dopaminergic therapy.
- *Barratt Impulsiveness Scale*, BIS-11 [69], BIS-R-21 [70]. The questionnaire is the most used measure of self-reported impulsivity.
- *Questionnaire for Impulsive-Compulsive Disorders in Parkinson's Disease*, QUIP [38]. QUIP researches the presence of both overeating and binge eating episodes in PD patients.
- *Questionnaire on Eating and Weight Patterns-5, QEWP-5* [71, 72]. QEWP especially rates the symptoms of BED and night eating syndrome (NES).
- *Yale Food Addiction Scale, version 2.0, YFAS 2.0* [73]. YFAS evaluates eating behaviors related to the current construct of food addiction (according to the food addiction substance approach).

At present, there is no cure capable of resolving the disease or significantly halting its progression: the treatment is symptomatic [5, 40].

The improvement of motor symptoms is entrusted mainly to levodopa-carbidopa, monoamine oxidase-B inhibitors, and dopamine agonists. Typically, combinations of different drugs are used to achieve complementary benefits, reduce doses, and limit dose-dependent side effects. Over time, however, the effect of each dose lasts less and less, and when it runs out, symptoms reappear (*wearing off periods*). More and more frequent adjustments and administration are necessary, even every 2–3 h [40].

In more severe and advanced cases, surgical approaches can be used:

- Deep brain stimulation (DBS), with the surgical placement of unilateral or bilateral electrodes in the subthalamic nucleus or the globus pallidus
- Levodopa-carbidopa enteral suspension (CLES). CLES is delivered into the jejunum via a PEG-J (percutaneous endoscopic gastrostomy jejunal extension) tube implanted surgically.

These severe, advanced, or drug-resistant cases are usually characterized by wearing off (the effect of each dose fades faster and faster) and dyskinesias (involuntary dance-like choreoathetoid movements that generally coincide with the moment of maximum brain concentration of levodopa). In this regard, it should be remembered that, as the disease progresses, the therapeutic window within which dopaminergic drugs improve motor symptoms without causing dyskinesia becomes narrower and narrower.

Subthalamic nucleus DBS relieves motor symptoms but can cause neuropsychiatric disorders and, in particular, loss of motivation. Apathy is probably the most disabling side effect induced by DBS. Apathetic behaviors can be alleviated by D2 and D3 dopaminergic receptor agonists. However, apathy appears to be a direct effect of DBS, not due to post-surgical reduction of dopaminergic treatments [74].

The improvement of motor symptoms with dopaminergic therapy has made non-motor symptoms and their weight on patients' quality of life more evident: pain, autonomic nervous system disorders, psychiatric disorders including ICSDs, and decline in cognitive abilities.

There is still a lack of high-quality studies that provide robust evidence for the treatment of many non-motor symptoms of PD [40].

For psychotic symptoms—particularly hallucinatory ones—clozapine is helpful but requires careful attention to its side effects.

Cholinesterase inhibitors are used for cognitive deficits.

For anxious and depressive symptoms, mainly selective serotonin reuptake inhibitors are used as drugs along with therapeutic education, counseling, and psychotherapy.

Motor and cognitive rehabilitation programs are helpful.

Exercise and a well-balanced diet are beneficial [75]. Physical activity is considered useful both in the prevention and treatment of PD [20].

A randomized clinical trial recently compared outpatient palliative care with current care standards in patients with PD and related disorders [76]. A neurologist and a primary care practitioner provided standard care. A team composed of a neurologist, social worker, nurse, and chaplain administered integrated palliative care. A palliative medicine specialist offered guidance and selective involvement. Integrated palliative care was associated with greater improvements in patient and/or caregiver outcomes.

Perhaps the team should include a dietician, and the program should also address frequent eating and weight problems.

31.7 Concluding Remarks

Dopaminergic agonists directly activate post-synaptic receptors and resolve the deficit of functioning presynaptic terminals. Motor symptoms improve, but, in several cases, ICSDs occur that complicate and worsen patients' health and quality of life.

Among the non-motor symptoms and ICSDs are frequent disorders of feeding, eating, and body weight.

People with PD usually do not ask for help with their diet and weight problems, and neurologists, for their part, tend to underestimate them.

References

1. Parkinson J. An essay on the shaking palsy. London: printed by Whittingham and Rowland for Sherwood, Neely, and Jones; 1817.
2. Carlsson A. Thirty years of dopamine research. Adv Neurol. 1993;60:1–10.
3. Lees AJ, Tolosa E, Olanow CW. Four pioneers of L-dopa treatment: Arvid Carlsson, Oleh Hornykiewicz, George Cotzias, and Melvin Yahr. Mov Disord. 2015;30(1):19–36. https://doi.org/10.1002/mds.26120.
4. Spillantini MG, Crowther RA, Jakes R, Hasegawa M, Goedert M. alpha-Synuclein in filamentous inclusions of Lewy bodies from Parkinson's disease and dementia with Lewy bodies. Proc Natl Acad Sci U S A. 1998;95(11):6469–73. https://doi.org/10.1073/pnas.95.11.6469.
5. Braak H, Del Tredici-Braak K, Gasser T. Special issue "Parkinson's disease". Cell Tissue Res. 2018;373(1):1–7. https://doi.org/10.1007/s00441-018-2863-5.
6. Klein C, Westenberger A. Genetics of Parkinson's disease. Cold Spring Harb Perspect Med. 2012;2(1):1–15. https://doi.org/10.1101/cshperspect.a008888.
7. Cherian A, Divya KP. Genetics of Parkinson's disease. Acta Neurol Belg. 2020; https://doi.org/10.1007/s13760-020-01473-5.
8. Sito Italiano della malattia di Parkinson; 2020. Parkinson.it. https://www.parkinson.it/. Accessed 3 Oct 2020.
9. Melchionda N, Cuzzolaro M. Parkinson's disease, dopamine, and eating and weight disorders: an illness in the disease? Eat Weight Disord. 2019;24(3):383–4. https://doi.org/10.1007/s40519-019-00684-x.
10. GBD 2016 Parkinson's Disease Collaborators. Global, regional, and national burden of Parkinson's disease, 1990-2016: a systematic analysis for the Global Burden of Disease Study 2016. Lancet Neurol. 2018;17(11):939–53. https://doi.org/10.1016/S1474-4422(18)30295-3.
11. Hirsch L, Jette N, Frolkis A, Steeves T, Pringsheim T. The incidence of Parkinson's disease: a systematic review and meta-analysis. Neuroepidemiology. 2016;46(4):292–300. https://doi.org/10.1159/000445751.
12. Han C, Lu Y, Cheng H, Wang C, Chan P. The impact of long-term exposure to ambient air pollution and second-hand smoke on the onset of Parkinson disease: a review and meta-analysis. Public Health. 2020;179:100–10. https://doi.org/10.1016/j.puhe.2019.09.020.
13. Belvisi D, Pellicciari R, Fabbrini A, Costanzo M, Pietracupa S, De Lucia M, Modugno N, Magrinelli F, Dallocchio C, Ercoli T, Terravecchia C, Nicoletti A, Solla P, Fabbrini G, Tinazzi M, Berardelli A, Defazio G. Risk factors of Parkinson's disease: simultaneous assessment, interactions and etiological subtypes. Neurology. 2020; https://doi.org/10.1212/WNL.0000000000010813.
14. Erro R, Brigo F, Tamburin S, Zamboni M, Antonini A, Tinazzi M. Nutritional habits, risk, and progression of Parkinson disease. J Neurol. 2018;265(1):12–23. https://doi.org/10.1007/s00415-017-8639-0.
15. Gao X, Chen H, Fung TT, Logroscino G, Schwarzschild MA, Hu FB, Ascherio A. Prospective study of dietary pattern and risk of Parkinson disease. Am J Clin Nutr. 2007;86(5):1486–94. https://doi.org/10.1093/ajcn/86.5.1486.
16. Molsberry S, Bjornevik K, Hughes KC, Healy B, Schwarzschild M, Ascherio A. Diet pattern and prodromal features of Parkinson's disease. Neurology. 2020; https://doi.org/10.1212/WNL.0000000000010523.

17. Paknahad Z, Sheklabadi E, Moravejolahkami AR, Chitsaz A, Hassanzadeh A. The effects of Mediterranean diet on severity of disease and serum Total Antioxidant Capacity (TAC) in patients with Parkinson's disease: a single center, randomized controlled trial. Nutr Neurosci. 2020:1–8. https://doi.org/10.1080/1028415X.2020.1751509.
18. Boulos C, Yaghi N, El Hayeck R, Heraoui GN, Fakhoury-Sayegh N. Nutritional risk factors, microbiota and Parkinson's disease: what is the current evidence? Nutrients. 2019;11(8) https://doi.org/10.3390/nu11081896.
19. Barichella M, Severgnini M, Cilia R, Cassani E, Bolliri C, Caronni S, Ferri V, Cancello R, Ceccarani C, Faierman S, Pinelli G, De Bellis G, Zecca L, Cereda E, Consolandi C, Pezzoli G. Unraveling gut microbiota in Parkinson's disease and atypical parkinsonism. Mov Disord. 2019;34(3):396–405. https://doi.org/10.1002/mds.27581.
20. Fan B, Jabeen R, Bo B, Guo C, Han M, Zhang H, Cen J, Ji X, Wei J. What and how can physical activity prevention function on Parkinson's disease? Oxid Med Cell Longev. 2020;2020:4293071. https://doi.org/10.1155/2020/4293071.
21. Hong CT, Chan L, Bai CH. The effect of caffeine on the risk and progression of Parkinson's disease: a meta-analysis. Nutrients. 2020;12(6) https://doi.org/10.3390/nu12061860.
22. Crotty GF, Maciuca R, Macklin EA, Wang J, Montalban M, Davis SS, Alkabsh JI, Bakshi R, Chen X, Ascherio A, Astarita G, Huntwork-Rodriguez S, Schwarzschild MA. Association of caffeine and related analytes with resistance to Parkinson's disease among LRRK2 mutation carriers: a metabolomic study. Neurology. 2020; https://doi.org/10.1212/WNL.0000000000010863.
23. De Pablo-Fernandez E, Lees AJ, Holton JL, Warner TT. Prognosis and neuropathologic correlation of clinical subtypes of Parkinson disease. JAMA Neurol. 2019;76(4):470–9. https://doi.org/10.1001/jamaneurol.2018.4377.
24. Armstrong MJ, Okun MS. Time for a new image of parkinson disease. JAMA Neurol. 2020; https://doi.org/10.1001/jamaneurol.2020.2412.
25. Gowers WR. A Manual of Diseases of the Nervous System, vol. 1. London: J. & A. Churchill; 1886.
26. Suzuki K, Fujita H, Watanabe Y, Matsubara T, Kadowaki T, Sakuramoto H, Hamaguchi M, Nozawa N, Hirata K. Leg restlessness preceding the onset of motor symptoms of Parkinson disease: a case series of 5 patients. Medicine (Baltimore). 2019;98(33):e16892. https://doi.org/10.1097/MD.0000000000016892.
27. Marinus J, Zhu K, Marras C, Aarsland D, van Hilten JJ. Risk factors for non-motor symptoms in Parkinson's disease. Lancet Neurol. 2018;17(6):559–68. https://doi.org/10.1016/S1474-4422(18)30127-3.
28. Williams-Gray CH, Mason SL, Evans JR, Foltynie T, Brayne C, Robbins TW, Barker RA. The CamPaIGN study of Parkinson's disease: 10-year outlook in an incident population-based cohort. J Neurol Neurosurg Psychiatry. 2013;84(11):1258–64. https://doi.org/10.1136/jnnp-2013-305277.
29. Bove F, Fraix V, Cavallieri F, Schmitt E, Lhommée E, Bichon A, Meoni S, Pélissier P, Kistner A, Chevrier E, Ardouin C, Limousin P, Krack P, Benabid AL, Chabardès S, Seigneuret E, Castrioto A, Moro E. Dementia and subthalamic deep brain stimulation in Parkinson disease. A long-term overview. Neurology. 2020;95(4):e384–92. https://doi.org/10.1212/wnl.0000000000009822.
30. Chuquilin-Arista F, Alvarez-Avellon T, Menendez-Gonzalez M. Prevalence of depression and anxiety in Parkinson disease and impact on quality of life: a community-based study in Spain. J Geriatr Psychiatry Neurol. 2020;33(4):207–13. https://doi.org/10.1177/0891988719874130.
31. Lo Monaco MR, Di Stasio E, Zuccala G, Petracca M, Genovese D, Fusco D, Silveri MC, Liperoti R, Ricciardi D, Cipriani MC, Laudisio A, Bentivoglio AR. Prevalence of obsessive-compulsive symptoms in elderly Parkinson disease patients: a case-control study. Am J Geriatr Psychiatry. 2020;28(2):167–75. https://doi.org/10.1016/j.jagp.2019.08.022.
32. Piredda R, Desmarais P, Masellis M, Gasca-Salas C. Cognitive and psychiatric symptoms in genetically determined Parkinson's disease: a systematic review. Eur J Neurol. 2020;27(2):229–34. https://doi.org/10.1111/ene.14115.

33. Creese B, Albertyn CP, Dworkin S, Thomas RS, Wan YM, Ballard C. Executive function but not episodic memory decline associated with visual hallucinations in Parkinson's disease. J Neuropsychol. 2020;14(1):85–97. https://doi.org/10.1111/jnp.12169.
34. Dave S, Weintraub D, Aarsland D, Ffytche DH. Drug and disease effects in Parkinson's psychosis: revisiting the role of dopamine. Mov Disord Clin Pract. 2020;7(1):32–6. https://doi.org/10.1002/mdc3.12851.
35. Weintraub D, Mamikonyan E. Impulse control disorders in Parkinson's disease. Am J Psychiatry. 2019;176(1):5–11. https://doi.org/10.1176/appi.ajp.2018.18040465.
36. El Otmani H, Mouni FZ, Abdulhakeem Z, Attar Z, Rashad L, Saali I, El Moutawakil B, Rafai MA, Slassi I, Nadifi S. Impulse control disorders in Parkinson disease: a cross-sectional study in Morocco. Rev Neurol (Paris). 2019;175(4):233–7. https://doi.org/10.1016/j.neurol.2018.07.009.
37. de Chazeron I, Durif F, Chereau-Boudet I, Fantini ML, Marques A, Derost P, Debilly B, Brousse G, Boirie Y, Llorca PM. Compulsive eating behaviors in Parkinson's disease. Eat Weight Disord. 2019;24(3):421–9. https://doi.org/10.1007/s40519-019-00648-1.
38. Weintraub D, Hoops S, Shea JA, Lyons KE, Pahwa R, Driver-Dunckley ED, Adler CH, Potenza MN, Miyasaki J, Siderowf AD, Duda JE, Hurtig HI, Colcher A, Horn SS, Stern MB, Voon V. Validation of the questionnaire for impulsive-compulsive disorders in Parkinson's disease. Mov Disord. 2009;24(10):1461–7. https://doi.org/10.1002/mds.22571.
39. Gatto EM, Aldinio V. Impulse control disorders in Parkinson's disease. a brief and comprehensive review. Front Neurol. 2019;10:351. https://doi.org/10.3389/fneur.2019.00351.
40. Armstrong MJ, Okun MS. Diagnosis and treatment of parkinson disease: a review. JAMA. 2020;323(6):548–60. https://doi.org/10.1001/jama.2019.22360.
41. Castro-Martinez XH, Garcia-Ruiz PJ, Martinez-Garcia C, Martinez-Castrillo JC, Vela L, Mata M, Martinez-Torres I, Feliz-Feliz C, Palau F, Hoenicka J. Behavioral addictions in early-onset Parkinson disease are associated with DRD3 variants. Parkinsonism Relat Disord. 2018;49:100–3. https://doi.org/10.1016/j.parkreldis.2018.01.010.
42. Friedman JH. Punding on levodopa. Biol Psychiatry. 1994;36(5):350–1. https://doi.org/10.1016/0006-3223(94)90636-x.
43. Napier TC, Kirby A, Persons AL. The role of dopamine pharmacotherapy and addiction-like behaviors in Parkinson's disease. Prog Neuropsychopharmacol Biol Psychiatry. 2020;109942:102. https://doi.org/10.1016/j.pnpbp.2020.109942.
44. Weintraub D, Koester J, Potenza MN, Siderowf AD, Stacy M, Voon V, Whetteckey J, Wunderlich GR, Lang AE. Impulse control disorders in Parkinson disease: a cross-sectional study of 3090 patients. Arch Neurol. 2010;67(5):589–95. https://doi.org/10.1001/archneurol.2010.65.
45. Latella D, Maggio MG, Maresca G, Saporoso AF, Le Cause M, Manuli A, Milardi D, Bramanti P, De Luca R, Calabro RS. Impulse control disorders in Parkinson's disease: a systematic review on risk factors and pathophysiology. J Neurol Sci. 2019;398:101–6. https://doi.org/10.1016/j.jns.2019.01.034.
46. Farnikova K, Obereigneru R, Kanovsky P, Prasko J. Comparison of personality characteristics in Parkinson disease patients with and without impulse control disorders and in healthy volunteers. Cogn Behav Neurol. 2012;25(1):25–33. https://doi.org/10.1097/WNN.0b013e31824b4103.
47. Weintraub D, Papay K, Siderowf A, Parkinson's progression markers Initiative. Screening for impulse control symptoms in patients with de novo Parkinson disease: a case-control study. Neurology. 2013;80(2):176–80. https://doi.org/10.1212/WNL.0b013e31827b915c.
48. Joutsa J, Martikainen K, Kaasinen V. Parallel appearance of compulsive behaviors and artistic creativity in Parkinson's disease. Case Rep Neurol. 2012;4(1):77–83. https://doi.org/10.1159/000338759.
49. Inzelberg R. The awakening of artistic creativity and Parkinson's disease. Behav Neurosci. 2013;127(2):256–61. https://doi.org/10.1037/a0031052.
50. Walker RH, Warwick R, Cercy SP. Augmentation of artistic productivity in Parkinson's disease. Mov Disord. 2006;21(2):285–6. https://doi.org/10.1002/mds.20758.

51. Canesi M, Rusconi ML, Isaias IU, Pezzoli G. Artistic productivity and creative thinking in Parkinson's disease. Eur J Neurol. 2012;19(3):468–72. https://doi.org/10.1111/j.1468-1331.2011.03546.x.
52. Grall-Bronnec M, Victorri-Vigneau C, Donnio Y, Leboucher J, Rousselet M, Thiabaud E, Zreika N, Derkinderen P, Challet-Bouju G. Dopamine agonists and impulse control disorders: a complex association. Drug Saf. 2018;41(1):19–75. https://doi.org/10.1007/s40264-017-0590-6.
53. Hu G, Jousilahti P, Nissinen A, Antikainen R, Kivipelto M, Tuomilehto J. Body mass index and the risk of Parkinson disease. Neurology. 2006;67(11):1955–9. https://doi.org/10.1212/01.wnl.0000247052.18422.e5.
54. Roos E, Grotta A, Yang F, Bellocco R, Ye W, Adami HO, Wirdefeldt K, Trolle Lagerros Y. Body mass index, sitting time, and risk of Parkinson disease. Neurology. 2018;90(16):e1413–7. https://doi.org/10.1212/WNL.0000000000005328.
55. Nam GE, Kim SM, Han K, Kim NH, Chung HS, Kim JW, Han B, Cho SJ, Yu JH, Park YG, Choi KM. Metabolic syndrome and risk of Parkinson disease: a nationwide cohort study. PLoS Med. 2018;15(8):e1002640. https://doi.org/10.1371/journal.pmed.1002640.
56. Kim R, Jun JS. Impact of overweight and obesity on functional and clinical outcomes of early Parkinson's disease. J Am Med Dir Assoc. 2020;21(5):697–700. https://doi.org/10.1016/j.jamda.2019.11.019.
57. Goldman JG, Vernaleo BA, Camicioli R, Dahodwala N, Dobkin RD, Ellis T, Galvin JE, Marras C, Edwards J, Fields J, Golden R, Karlawish J, Levin B, Shulman L, Smith G, Tangney C, Thomas CA, Troster AI, Uc EY, Coyan N, Ellman C, Ellman M, Hoffman C, Hoffman S, Simmonds D. Cognitive impairment in Parkinson's disease: a report from a multidisciplinary symposium on unmet needs and future directions to maintain cognitive health. NPJ Parkinsons Dis. 2018;4(19) https://doi.org/10.1038/s41531-018-0055-3.
58. Miller N, Allcock L, Hildreth AJ, Jones D, Noble E, Burn DJ. Swallowing problems in Parkinson disease: frequency and clinical correlates. J Neurol Neurosurg Psychiatry. 2009;80(9):1047–9. https://doi.org/10.1136/jnnp.2008.157701.
59. Fagerberg P, Klingelhoefer L, Bottai M, Langlet B, Kyritsis K, Rotter E, Reichmann H, Falkenburger B, Delopoulos A, Ioakimidis I. Lower energy intake among advanced vs. early Parkinson's disease patients and healthy controls in a clinical lunch setting: a cross-sectional study. Nutrients. 2020;12(7) https://doi.org/10.3390/nu12072109.
60. Suzuki K, Okuma Y, Uchiyama T, Miyamoto M, Haruyama Y, Kobashi G, Sakakibara R, Shimo Y, Hatano T, Hattori N, Yamamoto T, Hirano S, Yamamoto T, Kuwabara S, Kaji Y, Fujita H, Kadowaki T, Hirata K. Determinants of low body mass index in patients with Parkinson's disease: a multicenter case-control study. J Park Dis. 2020;10(1):213–21. https://doi.org/10.3233/JPD-191741.
61. da Luz MCL, Bezerra GKA, Asano AGC, Chaves de Lemos MDC, Cabral PC. Determinant factors of sarcopenia in individuals with Parkinson's disease. Neurol Sci. 2020; https://doi.org/10.1007/s10072-020-04601-4.
62. Bannier S, Montaurier C, Derost PP, Ulla M, Lemaire JJ, Boirie Y, Morio B, Durif F. Overweight after deep brain stimulation of the subthalamic nucleus in Parkinson disease: long term follow-up. J Neurol Neurosurg Psychiatry. 2009;80(5):484–8. https://doi.org/10.1136/jnnp.2008.158576.
63. Locke MC, Wu SS, Foote KD, Sassi M, Jacobson CE, Rodriguez RL, Fernandez HH, Okun MS. Weight changes in subthalamic nucleus vs globus pallidus internus deep brain stimulation: results from the COMPARE Parkinson disease deep brain stimulation cohort. Neurosurgery. 2011;68(5):1233–7; discussion 1237-1238. https://doi.org/10.1227/NEU.0b013e31820b52c5.
64. Voon V, Fox SH. Medication-related impulse control and repetitive behaviors in Parkinson disease. Arch Neurol. 2007;64(8):1089–96. https://doi.org/10.1001/archneur.64.8.1089.
65. Lee JY, Kim JM, Kim JW, Cho J, Lee WY, Kim HJ, Jeon BS. Association between the dose of dopaminergic medication and the behavioral disturbances in Parkinson disease. Parkinsonism Relat Disord. 2010;16(3):202–7. https://doi.org/10.1016/j.parkreldis.2009.12.002.
66. Perez-Lloret S, Rey MV, Fabre N, Ory F, Spampinato U, Brefel-Courbon C, Montastruc JL, Rascol O. Prevalence and pharmacological factors associated with impulse-control disor-

der symptoms in patients with Parkinson disease. Clin Neuropharmacol. 2012;35(6):261–5. https://doi.org/10.1097/WNF.0b013e31826e6e6d.
67. Ruddock HK, Christiansen P, Halford JCG, Hardman CA. The development and validation of the Addiction-like Eating Behaviour Scale. Int J Obes (Lond). 2017;41(11):1710–7. https://doi.org/10.1038/ijo.2017.158.
68. Rieu I, Martinez-Martin P, Pereira B, De Chazeron I, Verhagen Metman L, Jahanshahi M, Ardouin C, Chereau I, Brefel-Courbon C, Ory-Magne F, Klinger H, Peyrol F, Schupbach M, Dujardin K, Tison F, Houeto JL, Krack P, Durif F. International validation of a behavioral scale in Parkinson's disease without dementia. Mov Disord. 2015;30(5):705–13. https://doi.org/10.1002/mds.26223.
69. Patton JH, Stanford MS, Barratt ES. Factor structure of the Barratt impulsiveness scale. J Clin Psychol. 1995;51(6):768–74. https://doi.org/10.1002/1097-4679(199511)51:6<768::aid-jclp2270510607>3.0.co;2-1.
70. Kapitany-Foveny M, Urban R, Varga G, Potenza MN, Griffiths MD, Szekely A, Paksi B, Kun B, Farkas J, Kokonyei G, Demetrovics Z. The 21-item Barratt Impulsiveness Scale Revised (BIS-R-21): an alternative three-factor model. J Behav Addict. 2020;9(2):225–46. https://doi.org/10.1556/2006.2020.00030.
71. Spitzer R, Yanovski S, Marcus M. Questionnaire on eating and weight patterns, revised. Pittsburgh, PA: Behavioral Measurement Database Services; 1994.
72. Yanovski SZ, Marcus MD, Wadden TA, Walsh BT. The Questionnaire on Eating and Weight Patterns-5: an updated screening instrument for binge eating disorder. Int J Eat Disord. 2015;48(3):259–61. https://doi.org/10.1002/eat.22372.
73. Gearhardt AN, Corbin WR, Brownell KD. Development of the Yale food addiction scale version 2.0. Psychol Addict Behav. 2016;30(1):113–21. https://doi.org/10.1037/adb0000136.
74. Vachez Y, Carcenac C, Magnard R, Kerkerian-Le Goff L, Salin P, Savasta M, Carnicella S, Boulet S. Subthalamic nucleus stimulation impairs motivation: implication for apathy in Parkinson's disease. Mov Disord. 2020;35(4):616–28. https://doi.org/10.1002/mds.27953.
75. Ray S, Agarwal P. Depression and anxiety in Parkinson disease. Clin Geriatr Med. 2020;36(1):93–104. https://doi.org/10.1016/j.cger.2019.09.012.
76. Kluger BM, Miyasaki J, Katz M, Galifianakis N, Hall K, Pantilat S, Khan R, Friedman C, Cernik W, Goto Y, Long J, Fairclough D, Sillau S, Kutner JS. Comparison of integrated outpatient palliative care with standard care in patients with Parkinson disease and related disorders: a randomized clinical trial. JAMA Neurol. 2020;77(5):551–60. https://doi.org/10.1001/jamaneurol.2019.4992.

Polycystic Ovary Syndrome and Eating and Weight Disorders

32

Francesco Pallotti and Francesco Lombardo

32.1 Introduction

Polycystic ovary syndrome (PCOS) is a complex and multifactorial condition that involves both metabolic and hormonal dysfunctions [1]. Historically, in the 1930s Stein and Leventhal were the first to describe a peculiar case series of amenorrhea associated with polycystic ovaries, grouping relatively frequent signs such as hirsutism and oligo-amenorrhea with ovary structural abnormalities under the banner of a new pathological entity [2]. Due to relevant social impact for both esthetic, metabolic, and reproductive issues associated with PCOS, research was particularly vivid since then, and several diagnostic criteria have been established. Clinicians investigating this condition should focus on anamnesis and physical examination, evaluating the presence of hirsutism (inappropriate presence of body and/or facial hair growth), alopecia, and acne as signs of androgen excess and menstruation abnormalities, and ultrasound examination of the ovaries looking for polycystic appearance. It is worth stressing that PCOS is a syndrome, and a single diagnostic sign has insufficient specificity; furthermore, several endocrinopathies and pathologies (Cushing syndrome, nonclassical congenital adrenal hyperplasia, adrenal/ovarian tumors, etc.) may have similar clinical manifestations and, thus, require to be excluded prior to establish a diagnosis. To this purpose, in 2003 the Rotterdam consensus provided a definition of PCOS as a syndrome with at least two among clinical/biochemical hyperandrogenism, oligo-anovulation, and specific ovary ultrasound polycystic appearance [1]. Although a unique PCOS definition is still a matter of debate, nowadays it is undoubtedly among the most common causes of female infertility, with a reported prevalence of at least 5–10% of women of

---

F. Pallotti (✉) · F. Lombardo
Department of Experimental Medicine, "Sapienza" University of Rome, Rome, Italy
e-mail: francesco.pallotti@uniroma1.it; francesco.lombardo@uniroma1.it

© Springer Nature Switzerland AG 2022
E. Manzato et al. (eds.), *Hidden and Lesser-known Disordered Eating Behaviors in Medical and Psychiatric Conditions*,
https://doi.org/10.1007/978-3-030-81174-7_32

reproductive age. Its pathogenesis has also some unclear aspects, but hyperandrogenism and hyperinsulinemia seem to drive the phenotypic aspects of PCOS: elevated circulating levels of testosterone (both total and free) and dehydroepiandrosterone sulfate (DHEAS) can be demonstrated up to 80–90% of women with PCOS, and insulin resistance with compensatory hyperinsulinemia can be detected in 50–70% of these subjects. Often, increased LH level and LH/FSH ratio, as well as impaired gonadotropin pulsatility, are present [3], but are not considered a diagnostic criteria. All these hormone abnormalities are able to disrupt paracrine follicle signaling and follicle growth: the aromatase activity is inhibited in antral follicle granulosa cells by the exceeding androgens causing a follicle maturation arrest, an effect which is further strengthened by a hyperinsulinism-induced androgen production in theca cells, a premature granulosa cell luteinization, and, possibly, AMH overproduction [1]. Genetic factors have also been investigated in PCOS pathogenesis: there is a higher prevalence of PCOS in familiar groups, with at least one third of female first-degree relatives sharing the presence of PCOS; also hyperandrogenism and hyperinsulinemia have shown to have an inheritable components in families with PCOS. However, even though several candidate genes have been identified, methodological issues and phenotypic heterogeneity lead to conflicting results in many association studies, currently allowing us to explain only a limited number of inheritable phenotypes [1, 4]. Treatment of PCOS can be a challenge as it may vary depending on the predominant clinical manifestation(s), and, often, combination therapy is necessary: anovulatory uterine bleeding may require the administration of either estrogen-progestin oral contraceptives or progestin alone treatment (oral or, in selected cases, as intrauterine device); hyperandrogenism dermatological manifestations may require peripheral androgen receptor blockade (preferably as a progestin with anti-androgenic activity associated in an oral contraceptive formulation); anovulatory infertility may need endogenous FSH secretion induction through clomiphene citrate or aromatase inhibitors (letrozole); hyperinsulinism with associated cardiometabolic dysfunctions (diabetes, cardiovascular disease, etc.) could benefit from metformin administration or other specific treatments (other antiglycemic drugs, anti-dyslipidemic drugs, etc.) [1, 5, 6]. However, it is widely accepted that lifestyle interventions, such as weight loss and physical exercise, should anticipate and accompany every pharmacological treatment [5, 7, 8]: in fact, even modest reduction in body weight in these women, in whom metabolic dysfunctions such as insulin resistance and obesity/overweight have higher prevalence than general population, should be able to improve insulin sensitivity and hyperandrogenism and restore regular menses and fertility [6, 9]. Though positive effects of lifestyle interventions are recognized, a recent meta-analysis suggest that good quality evidence is still required to clarify the effects on glucose tolerance [10].

32.2 PCOS and Eating Disorders

A less investigated and controversial aspect of PCOS is the association with eating disorders (EDs). It is unclear if EDs are causally linked to PCOS. PCOS women are reported to have a higher prevalence of several psychiatric comorbidities and, specifically, reduced mood/depression and anxiety [11], which in turn are known to be frequently associated with eating disorders [12]. Likewise, the ED prevalence increases with obesity, which is part of the PCOS spectrum of clinical manifestations [13]. It is hypothesized that EDs, intrinsically linked to increased body weight, may be secondary to a poor self-perceived body image in these women; in addition, completing a complex psychological background, a strong association has been reported between depression symptoms and unhappiness of personal physical appearance, as well as lower levels of self-esteem in PCOS women [14]. A distorted self-perception, with a certain level of disagreement between the perceived and expected body image, is the key in developing EDs in these women. Irrespective of their BMI, PCOS women experience greater concerns for their weight, for their physical appearance in relation to other hyperandrogenism signs (hirsutism, acne, and alopecia), and for the abnormal menses, with potential negative repercussions in their quality of life [15]. Depressed PCOS women have, thus, an increased risk of developing any eating disorder. Accordingly, when compared with unaffected controls, PCOS women show an increased tendency toward an abnormal eating behavior, which may develop into a specific ED diagnosis, ranging from anorexia to bulimia or may present as a binge eating disorder (BED) [16]. Reported prevalence of EDs in PCOS women may range from 10 to 25% but may vary in relation to the diagnostic methods (questionnaires, structured interviews, etc.) [17]. One of the largest population registry-based study available indicates that PCOS women have about 50% increased risk to have any ED, compared to controls [11, 17]. Taken together, these data suggest the need of exploring the presence of these comorbidities in PCOS women, but these aspects are sometimes overlooked in a clinical setting.

Anorexia nervosa (AN) and bulimia nervosa (BN) were episodically reported among psychiatric comorbidities in PCOS women. More recent papers, however, suggest that PCOS women show neither higher incidence of anorexia nervosa nor an increased risk to develop its symptoms, compared to the general population [11, 14, 16]. In regard to BN women, studies with relatively small caseloads found them to have a higher incidence of ultrasound-confirmed polycystic appearance of the ovaries than controls [18]. On the other hand, a large population study report that PCOS women have an increased risk (OR 1.3) to have bulimia nervosa, compared to the general population [11]. However, other recent studies do not confirm these findings [16, 17].

Binge eating episodes and BED are more frequently reported to be associated with PCOS [19]. In particular, diagnostic criteria for BED, a condition characterized by the uncontrolled eating of a large amount of food in a discrete amount of time, can be met in up to 25% of PCOS women [20], and it is linked to weight gain, obesity, and failure of weight loss treatments [16]. In the long term, BED is associated with cardiometabolic diseases such as diabetes and hypertension, thus requiring particular attention in the management and follow-up of PCOS women, who already present increased risk to develop these pathologies.

Night eating syndrome (NES), characterized by hyperphagia and binge eating episodes taking place specifically during the night, has also been recognized in women affected by PCOS. It shares the psychological comorbidities of the previously reported EDs and has a prevalence of 1.0–1.5% in the general population. There is paucity of data about NES in PCOS women, but a recent case-control study reported a nearly 13% prevalence in the PCOS cohort [16]. Other than being an obvious obstacle to weight loss treatment strategies, EDs represent possible factors in the exacerbation of PCOS clinical manifestations (Fig. 32.1). Binge eating has been associated with hyperandrogenism which may lead to menstrual abnormalities strengthening the pathological hormone pathways of PCOS. Furthermore, increased testosterone levels have been investigated as a possible etiological factor for EDs, as it may influence food cravings by reducing impulse control. This may be supported by the observation that antiandrogenic treatment may suppress the uncontrolled eating behavior. On the other hand, binge eating episodes may contribute to PCOS follicular arrest by influencing insulin levels which may act also by reducing circulating sex hormone binding globulin and, thus, further increasing free circulating androgens in the bloodstream [19]. Apart from hormonal dysregulation, cardiovascular and metabolic comorbidities of PCOS make it important to investigate and treat EDs, as they may lead to further weight increase and visceral adiposity, which in turn may exacerbate cardiometabolic diseases [21]. Weight loss strategies that consider a possible ED comorbidity are paramount to optimize PCOS non-pharmacological treatment, and overweight or obese patients (irrespective of PCOS) are recommended to be screened for BED and NES [22].

This, in association to other lifestyle changes (mainly physical activity) and possibly other psychological support (cognitive-behavioral therapy), can improve overall mental health and allow PCOS women to acquire coping strategies to oppose the depressive symptoms that provide the basis for the binge eating [23]. This is further strengthened by the evidence that overweight and/or obese PCOS women do not seem to have any biological hindrances in reducing weight compared to controls

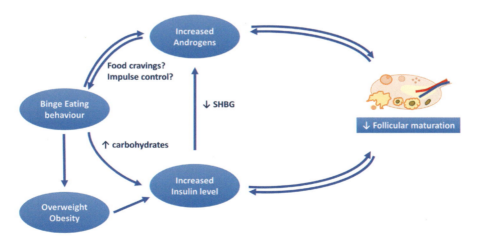

Fig. 32.1 Hypothetical interactions between binge eating behavior and PCOS hormonal imbalances

[15]. However, the relatively higher carbohydrate intake reported in PCOS women [15] may be target of dietary counselling, defining the amount of sugars and fiber-rich foods to control both weight and glucose tolerance.

In conclusion, the relation between EDs and PCOS poses an interesting conundrum as the weight loss suggested for PCOS may be in conflict with the ED treatment, which per se is not necessarily focused on weight loss, and may be also conflicting with the specific ED affecting the woman. In particular, women reporting binge eating episodes have difficulties in losing weight and are likely to be less compliant to weight loss treatments, thus hindering the treatment of PCOS.

References

1. Goodarzi MO, Dumesic DA, Chazenbalk G, Azziz R. Polycystic ovary syndrome: etiology, pathogenesis and diagnosis. Nat Rev Endocrinol. 2011;7:219–31.
2. Azziz R, Adashi EY. Stein and Leventhal: 80 years on. Am J Obstet Gynecol. 2016;214:247.e1–247.e11.
3. Taylor AE, McCourt B, Martin KA, Anderson EJ, Adams JM, Schoenfeld D, Hall JE. Determinants of abnormal gonadotropin secretion in clinically defined women with polycystic ovary syndrome. J Clin Endocrinol Metab. 1997;82:2248–56.
4. Crespo RP, Bachega TASS, Mendonca BB, Gomes LG. An update of genetic basis of PCOS pathogenesis. Arch Endocrinol Metab. 2018;62:352–61.
5. Teede HJ, Misso ML, Costello MF, Dokras A, Laven J, Moran L, Piltonen T, Norman RJ. Recommendations from the international evidence-based guideline for the assessment and management of polycystic ovary syndrome. Hum Reprod. 2018;33:1602–18.
6. Goodman NF, Cobin RH, Futterweit W, Glueck JS, Legro RS, Carmina E. American Association of Clinical Endocrinologists, American College of Endocrinology, and Androgen Excess and PCOS Society Disease state clinical review: guide to the best practices in the evaluation and treatment of polycystic ovary syndrome—part 2. Endocr Pract. 2015;21:1415–26.
7. Moran LJ, Ko H, Misso M, Marsh K, Noakes M, Talbot M, Frearson M, Thondan M, Stepto N, Teede HJ. Dietary composition in the treatment of polycystic ovary syndrome: a systematic review to inform evidence-based guidelines. J Acad Nutr Diet. 2013;113:520–45.
8. Marzouk TM, Sayed Ahmed WA. Effect of dietary weight loss on menstrual regularity in obese young adult women with polycystic ovary syndrome. J Pediatr Adolesc Gynecol. 2015;28:457–61.
9. Faghfoori Z, Fazelian S, Shadnoush M, Goodarzi R. Nutritional management in women with polycystic ovary syndrome: a review study. Diabetes Metab Syndr. 2017;11(Suppl 1):S429–32.
10. Lim SS, Hutchison SK, Van Ryswyk E, Norman RJ, Teede HJ, Moran LJ. Lifestyle changes in women with polycystic ovary syndrome. Cochrane Database Syst Rev. 2019;3:CD007506.
11. Cesta CE, Mansson M, Palm C, Lichtenstein P, Iliadou AN, Landen M. Polycystic ovary syndrome and psychiatric disorders: co-morbidity and heritability in a nationwide Swedish cohort. Psychoneuroendocrinology. 2016;73:196–203.
12. Hudson JI, Hiripi E, Pope HGJ, Kessler RC. The prevalence and correlates of eating disorders in the National Comorbidity Survey Replication. Biol Psychiatry. 2007;61:348–58.
13. Lee I, Cooney LG, Saini S, Sammel MD, Allison KC, Dokras A. Increased odds of disordered eating in polycystic ovary syndrome: a systematic review and meta-analysis. Eat Weight Disord. 2019;24:787–97.
14. Annagur BB, Kerimoglu OS, Tazegul A, Gunduz S, Gencoglu BB. Psychiatric comorbidity in women with polycystic ovary syndrome. J Obstet Gynaecol Res. 2015;41:1229–33.
15. Larsson I, Hulthen L, Landen M, Palsson E, Janson P, Stener-Victorin E. Dietary intake, resting energy expenditure, and eating behavior in women with and without polycystic ovary syndrome. Clin Nutr. 2016;35:213–8.

16. Lee I, Cooney LG, Saini S, Smith ME, Sammel MD, Allison KC, Dokras A. Increased risk of disordered eating in polycystic ovary syndrome. Fertil Steril. 2017;107:796–802.
17. Tay CT, Teede HJ, Hill B, Loxton D, Joham AE. Increased prevalence of eating disorders, low self-esteem, and psychological distress in women with polycystic ovary syndrome: a community-based cohort study. Fertil Steril. 2019;112:353–61.
18. Raphael FJ, Rodin DA, Peattie A, Bano G, Kent A, Nussey SS, Lacey JH. Ovarian morphology and insulin sensitivity in women with bulimia nervosa. Clin Endocrinol (Oxf). 1995;43:451–5.
19. Jeanes YM, Reeves S, Gibson EL, Piggott C, May VA, Hart KH. Binge eating behaviours and food cravings in women with Polycystic Ovary Syndrome. Appetite. 2017;109:24–32.
20. Algars M, Huang L, Von Holle AF, Peat CM, Thornton LM, Lichtenstein P, Bulik CM. Binge eating and menstrual dysfunction. J Psychosom Res. 2014;76:19–22.
21. Ehsani B, Moslehi N, Mirmiran P, Ramezani Tehrani F, Tahmasebinejad Z, Azizi F. A visceral adiposity index-related dietary pattern and the cardiometabolic profiles in women with polycystic ovary syndrome. Clin Nutr. 2016;35:1181–7.
22. Garvey WT, Mechanick JI, Brett EM, Garber AJ, Hurley DL, Jastreboff AM, Nadolsky K, Pessah-Pollack R, Plodkowski R. American Association of Clinical Endocrinologists and American College of Endocrinology comprehensive clinical practice guidelines for medical care of patients with obesity. Endocr Pract. 2016;22(Suppl 3):1–203.
23. Correa JB, Sperry SL, Darkes J. A case report demonstrating the efficacy of a comprehensive cognitive-behavioral therapy approach for treating anxiety, depression, and problematic eating in polycystic ovarian syndrome. Arch Womens Ment Health. 2015;18:649–54.

Prader-Willi Syndrome and Eating and Weight Disorders

Massimo Cuzzolaro

33.1 Historical Notes

The disease is called Prader-Willi syndrome (PWS), or Prader-Labhart-Willi syndrome, or also Prader, Labhart, Willi, and Fanconi syndrome.

The eponyms recall some facts. In 1956, Swiss endocrinologists Andrea Prader, Alexis Labhart, and Heinrich Willi published in German a description of a set of abnormalities they had observed in nine children: a syndrome of obesity, short growth, cryptorchidism, and mental retardation, with an amyotonia-like condition in the neonatal period [1]. In July of the same year, Prader, Labhart, Willi, and Fanconi presented the syndrome in Copenhagen, at the Eighth International Congress of Pediatrics. In 1961, Prader and Willi reviewed the disease and reported that diabetes mellitus can also occur during childhood [2].

Two decades later the genetic origin of the disease was discovered. The syndrome was associated with alterations of chromosome 15 [3, 4].

Lastly, in 1989 [5, 6], PWS was linked to a particular category of genes, the newly discovered imprinted genes [7, 8].

However, the British physician John Langdon Down (1828–1896)—famous for his description of Down's syndrome—was probably the first to write about this condition at the end of the nineteenth century [9].

In fact, those who leaf through the classic volume of Down [10], in the chapter dedicated to polysarcia (obesity), find the case E. C., a girl who at the age of 13 years was hospitalized in an Asylum for Idiots. At the time of admission, a mental retardation was noted along with excessive corpulence and a voracious appetite. E. C. was 141 cm. tall and weighed 51 kg.

M. Cuzzolaro (✉)
University of Roma Sapienza, Roma, Italy
e-mail: massimo.cuzzolaro@gmail.com

© Springer Nature Switzerland AG 2022
E. Manzato et al. (eds.), *Hidden and Lesser-known Disordered Eating Behaviors in Medical and Psychiatric Conditions*,
https://doi.org/10.1007/978-3-030-81174-7_33

At 20 years of age, the stature had remained the same, but the girl's weight had risen to 68 kg and a year later, when Down began to follow her, to 89 kg. She ate too much and moved very little. Down prescribed detailed dietary restrictions and exercise (walking). However, at 25 years of age, the weight had increased again (95.25 kg) with a waist circumference of 139.7 cm. Several observations by Down support the hypothesis that E. C. was affected by PWS.

> "My note-book states that in January, 1862, she remained the same height (four feet four inches), but had increased in weight. She was then 210 lbs. when weighed in her nightdress, and measured, round her waist, fifty-five inches. Her feet and hands remained small and contrasted remarkably with the appendages they terminated. She had no hair in the axillae and scarcely any on the pubis. Although twenty-five years of age she had never menstruated, nor did she exhibit the slightest sexual instinct … She suffered from dyspnœa, and her breathing at night was attended by so much noise that the occupants of the same room were much disturbed thereby." [10] (p. 172)

A data, reported and not observed, does not correspond to the most frequent forms of PWS in which hyperphagia and weight gain appear around 3 years of age. However, cases are also described in which these phenomena occur late, around 8 years, as perhaps happened to Down's patient.

> "From inquiries made of her friends, I found that … she had been delicate and thin up to seven years of age." [10] (p. 171)

33.2 Epidemiology and Genetics

PWS is the most common genetic cause of compulsive hyperphagia and severe early-onset obesity.

It is part of the rare secondary pediatric obesities, due to known genetic factors (such as Cohen syndrome, Klinefelter syndrome, Laurence-Moon syndrome, Turner syndrome) or endocrine diseases (such as adiposogenital dystrophy or Fröhlich's syndrome, pediatric Cushing disease, pediatric hypothyroidism).

The incidence is about 1 case per 10,000–30,000 live births [11, 12]. Males and, to a lesser extent, females of all ethnicities are affected. It mostly appears sporadically, but sometimes it affects several members of the same family.

PWS is a genetic disease. It is defined, in particular, as an *imprinting disease* or *genomic imprinting disorder* because genes called *imprinted genes* are at stake [12].

The most frequent genetic abnormality (about 70% of cases) is the de novo deletion of a region of the long arm of chromosome 15 of paternal origin (affected loci 15q11.2-q13). In other cases (about 25%, *nondeletion PWS*), the genetic abnormality is uniparental maternal disomy of chromosome 15 (both chromosomes 15 come from the mother). The remaining cases (about 5%) are due to other *imprinting defects* [13–15].

PWS and Angelman syndrome (AS) were the first *imprinting diseases* discovered in humans [5].

What are imprinting genes?

A brief recall to these concepts can be useful.

It is known that most autosomal genes are expressed from both alleles (paternal and maternal). For a small minority of genes (maybe around 1%), however, the expression is only from one of the two alleles. These genes are called *imprinted genes* [16].

Epigenetic marks are imprinted in the sperm or egg cells of the parents during gametogenesis; they are not lost at the time of fertilization and are maintained through mitotic cell divisions.

The genomic imprinting is an epigenetic process because it does not alter the sequence of DNA nucleotides but modulates gene expression. It involves DNA methylation and histone methylation. The different methylation of a particular gene locus is the imprinting that imposes the expression of only one of the two alleles of that locus, the paternal or maternal one.

Imprinted genes are few but play an essential role in normal embryogenesis, growth, and development, particularly in the formation of the nervous system. They have been found mainly in placental mammals. In the evolution of the species, they seem to represent a balancing mechanism in the transmission to the offspring of the characters of the two parents [16].

In the case of imprinting genes, since only one of the two allele genes, coming from the two parents, can be expressed, eventual anomalies are more often pathogenic.

The abnormalities of *imprinted genes* can be due to mutations that change DNA structure by altering the sequence of nucleotides or epigenetic modifications that affect the expression of genes without altering the DNA structure.

Genetic and epigenetic disruptions involving *imprinted genes* are responsible for phenomena studied in recent decades (*genomic imprinting disorders*) such as PWS and AS.

In PWS, the imprinting of the 15q11.2-q13 loci of the maternal allele prevents the expression of those genes. But the paternal allele is mutated, and the corresponding loci are missing by deletion, so the individual will develop a number of phenotypic anomalies. In a minority of cases, as already written, the phenomenon is due, instead, to other anomalies, for example, to a maternal uniparental dysomia of chromosome 15: in this case, in both the present alleles—both maternal—the imprinting imposes the non-expression of those genes.

Incidentally, even the manipulation of the cellular environment can interfere epigenetically with the proper functioning of *imprinted genes*.

It is believed, among other things, that conception by assisted reproductive technology (ART) may be a risk factor for *genomic imprinting disorders* [12, 17]. For PWS and AS, some studies report a positive association [18, 19]; others do not [20, 21], although there is a higher incidence of maternal disomy and 15/imprinting defects in cases of PWS born after ART [20].

33.3 Somatic Features and Medical Comorbidity

PWS is a multisystem genetic disorder. Genotype-phenotype correlations are still little known [22].

Common somatic features are short stature, already during the early years of life, light hair, fair skin, narrow forehead, almond-shaped eyes, epicanthus (vertical skin fold covering the inner corner of the eye), strabismus, hypertelorismus (eyes very far apart), thin lips, malformed ears with low implant, small hands and feet, and thick saliva.

Muscle hypotonia causes difficulty in sucking, delay in motor development, and difficulty in articulating words.

The threshold of reaction to pain is high. The ability to vomit is decreased. The regulation of body temperature is altered. Fatigue and drowsiness are common. Bone mineral density is low, and osteoporosis is frequent.

Many symptoms are related to a dysfunction of the hypothalamus that leads to endocrine disorders.

The main phenomena are growth hormone deficiency (GH), hypogonadism, hypothyroidism, and adrenal insufficiency.

Almost all men and most women with PWS suffer from hypogonadism. This affects the somatic aspect, physical and mental health, and quality of life. Hypogonadism has long been considered central of hypothalamic origin. However, a severe gonadotropin deficiency is rare, while primary gonadal dysfunction is frequent, especially in males [23, 24].

Already in the prepubertal period, signs of hypogenitalism and, in males, cryptorchidism and small penis are observed.

Insatiable hunger and severe and progressive obesity are characteristic of almost all patients.

Common obesity-related diseases are respiratory failure, obstructive sleep apnea (OSA), hypertension, cardiovascular disease, and reduced tolerance to carbohydrates that evolves over time into type 2 diabetes mellitus [11, 25–27].

Gastroenterological problems may be present: delayed gastric emptying, delayed colonic transit, constipation, dysphagia, decreased vomiting, and increased choking.

Compulsive hyperphagia, associated with decreased ability to vomit and to feel gastric filling, carries a high risk of gastric dilatation until rupture [28, 29].

Rare episodes of gastric dilatation, abdominal hypertension, and secondary shock not related to hyperphagic crisis but to gastroparesis have been described in some cases of PWS, in preschool age [30].

Individuals with PWS are at increased risk of prematurely developing age-related diseases [31], including demential symptoms [32].

33.4 Mortality

People with PWS have a shorter life expectancy than the general population.

A research by the PWS Association (USA) on 486 deaths (263 males) reported an average age of 29.5 ± 16 years (range, 2 months–67 years). In recent years life expectancy seems to have increased, probably due to earlier diagnosis and earlier interventions to prevent and limit obesity [33, 34].

Intellectual disability in general is associated with higher mortality. However, a longitudinal cohort study found that mortality rates of people with PWS were much higher than those of people with intellectual disabilities from other causes [35].

Hyperphagia and obesity are the main factors responsible for premature mortality [33, 35–37]. Respiratory failure, heart failure, and gastrointestinal disorders are the most common causes of death.

According to some studies [28], stomach rupture accounts for 3% of the causes of premature death in PWS. Suffocation from food is another not uncommon cause (8%) of death. It is related to hyperphagia, voracious eating behaviors with poor chewing, poor coordination of oral movements, and hypotonia.

33.5 Fertility

Sexual maturation and fertility are generally altered and compromised, but sexual and romantic interests and fantasies are often present.

Pregnancies have been reported in some women, but no cases of male fertility [23].

In men, PWS is a heterogeneous disease from the point of view of testicular histology, but spermatogenesis is mostly absent [38].

In women, follicle maturation and complete pubertal development are usually impaired. But, in some cases, ovulation and conception are possible [39].

It has been published the case of a woman with PWS (deletion of 15q11-q13 of the paternal chromosome) who generated a daughter with Angelman syndrome (inherited deletion of the same region but in the maternal chromosome 15) [40].

33.6 Neurocognitive Development, Psychosocial Adaptation, and Psychiatric Comorbidity

PWS is a neurodevelopmental genetic disease.

Children with PWS have a mild to moderate cognitive disability with an IQ that in most cases falls between 70 and 35. Sometimes the deficit is severe with IQ < 35. Language understanding is better than production [41, 42].

Sleep disorders are generally present. There are difficulties in starting and maintaining sleep, sleep breathing disorders, and obstructive sleep apnea (OSA) [43].

The facial and bodily expression of one's emotions are poor and equivocal [44].

The incidence of emotional instability, tantrums, disturbed behavior, and other psychopathological symptoms is high.

The most frequent challenging behaviors are food seeking and other food-related problems, skin picking, repetitive questioning, obsessive speech, difficulty transitioning, and non-compliance [45, 46].

Skin picking is a very frequent symptom in PWS. It mainly affects skin imperfections with a tendency to pinch and scratch [47]. Cases of rectal picking with rectal bleeding and ulceration are described [29].

In the first years of life, individuals with Prader-Willi syndrome are usually sociable and communicative. But then appear obsessive symptoms, impulsive behaviors, low tolerance of frustrations, and explosions of anger up to frankly aggressive and antisocial behaviors, often related to compulsive food seeking.

There are frequent outbursts of anger and stubborn and repetitive behaviors that increase over the years. The ability to take part in group activities and share food and objects is lacking. In general, social adaptation is full of difficulties.

Sometimes there are frank psychotic manifestations (auditory and visual hallucinations, depressive states, mystical exaltations) and states of agitation. In other cases, rejection and lethargy prevail: the patient avoids all contact, confines himself in bed, and even rejects food and drink.

An Irish study [45] found that at least one other psychiatric diagnosis was reported in more than half of the cases of PWS. The most common was anxiety disorder, but also rates of psychosis, autism spectrum disorders, obsessive-compulsive disorder, and self-harm had increased [15].

Immune-inflammatory alterations have been observed in association with various mental disorders. A case-control study showed in children with PWS the presence of elevated levels of interleukin, related to the presence of psychopathological symptoms [48].

Individuals with PWS are therefore at high risk of psychiatric disorders. But is it correct to apply DSM-5 and ICD-11 categories and talk about comorbidity [49–51]?

For example, should skin picking in patients with PWS receive a second diagnosis of associated obsessive-compulsive disorder? The specific genetic abnormality of PWS should be considered directly or indirectly responsible for this challenging behavior. However, skin picking does not occur only in this syndrome, and the compromised genetic loci in PWS are not involved in the etiology of similar symptoms in non-PWS subjects.

Likewise, what is the relationship between PWS compulsive hyperphagia and the feeding and eating disorders described by DSM-5 and ICD-11?

Questions like these have inspired the Research Domain Criteria (RDoC, National Institute of Mental Health) [52]. The project was launched in 2009 to offer psychiatric research a new conceptual grid beyond categorical diagnoses. It aims to identify constructs relevant to psychopathology, to be explored in terms of biological substrates and observable behaviors, but in a transdiagnostic and dimensional perspective [53].

33.7 Feeding, Eating, and Weight Disorders

Children with PWS, at birth and in the first 2 years of life, have hypotonia, weak sucking capacity, difficulty in nutrition, developmental delays, and often poor weight growth (*failure-to-thrive*).

Then, the feeding behavior takes the characters of hyperphagia with rapid weight gain and early obesity, usually evident at 2–4 years of age.

Table 33.1 Nutritional phases in PWS [55]

Median age of onset	Features
In utero	– Decreased fetal movements, growth restriction
9 months	– Hypotonia, difficulty feeding with or without failure to thrive – Then, the weight increases at a normal rate
2 years	– Weight gain without significant change in appetite – Then, weight gain and increased interest in food
8 years	– Weight gain, lack of satiety, compulsive hyperphagia
Adulthood	– Some adults with PWS no longer have an insatiable hunger

Obesity is severe and progressive and is associated with compulsive hyperphagia, i.e., the tendency to eat, in an ungovernable and repetitive way, enormous amounts of food, up to 5000 calories per day [54]. Hyperphagia can be associated with the tendency to steal food, money, and rummage through garbage.

There are usually two nutritional stages in PWS:

– Poor feeding and, in many cases, *failure to thrive* in infancy
– Hyperphagia and obesity in later childhood

A longitudinal study of the eating behavior of people with PWS showed a more gradual and complex pattern [55]. Table 33.1 summarizes the results of that work.

Hyperphagia is not directly related to intellectual disorders as in other conditions with tendency to obesity (e.g., Down's syndrome) [56]. Food preferences go toward sweet tastes and calorie-dense foods [57].

In PWS there is rather a specific disorder of the sense of satiation (that marks the end of the meal) and satiety (that determines the interval between meals) [57, 58]:

– Satiation occurs later than that in normal subjects during meals.
– Satiety lasts less between meals with a frequent urge to eat.

This hypothesis is reinforced by brain imaging studies [59, 60].

Rumination behaviors have been described in 10% of cases. Their frequency seems to increase when the control of diet and weight is very tight [61] and involves the risk of aspiration of gastric contents [62].

33.8 Differential Diagnosis

The diagnosis of PWS is based on clinical criteria and must be confirmed by genetic analysis. It is usually formulated before puberty, but rare diseases such as PWS are often undiagnosed or misdiagnosed [15].

With regard to obesity and metabolic syndrome indices, body mass index (BMI) values, with appropriate thresholds for sex and age, are still the best and simplest choice [63].

Some symptoms may be evident already at birth (e.g., muscle hypotonia) or even in utero (e.g., reduced fetal movements).

It may be useful to note that Angelman syndrome (AS) is a sister of PWS, because it affects the same region but in chromosome 15 of maternal origin.

AS affects both sexes and is characterized by short stature, morphological abnormalities, severe mental retardation, epilepsy, hypotonia, and unnatural joy.

In early childhood there are difficulties in nutrition, then obesity, but not compulsive hyperphagia [64–66]. Problematic behavior related to food (such as impaired satiety, preoccupation with food, taking and storing food) have been described in over 50% of persons with AS [67].

The fragile X syndrome (FXS) is another genetic disorder characterized by intellectual disability, hypotonia, deficit in motor activities, and behavioral disorders. It is associated with an abnormality in the FMR1 gene, which is found on the X chromosome, and plays an essential role in the development of the brain. The incidence is double in males.

A subgroup (10%) of individuals with FXS shows hyperphagia, lack of satiation/satiety, and severe obesity. They are described as the PWS phenotype of FXS [68, 69].

33.9 Treatment

The genetic defects underlying PWS would be the primary goal of the therapy [70]. PWS is due to an absence of expression of some genes of paternal origin located in the central part of chromosome 15. The same genes are present in chromosome 15 of maternal origin but are repressed at the transcriptional level. The epigenetic therapy aims to activate the expression of those genes but has not yet made sufficient progress.

PWS patients must be followed throughout their lifespan.

Recent guidelines recommend a multidisciplinary approach to the clinical management of PWS patients, patient- and family-centered [71]. It is crucial that parents are informed about the disease early and helped over time because long-term caring for offspring with PWS is stressful. Practical and emotional supports are necessary [72].

The high frequency of psychiatric disorders and problematic behaviors requires the regular availability of psychological and psychiatric care [73], still inadequate [45]. Psychiatric drugs are used on the basis of clinical judgment, but there are no randomized controlled trials that demonstrate their effectiveness [71]. For skin picking, interventions aimed at improving the modulation of emotions and control of compulsive behaviors can be helpful [47].

Cyclical rehabilitation programs (behavior rehabilitation, speech-language therapy, physiotherapy, physical exercise training, nutritional management) may be beneficial [74].

The treatment of endocrine problems is essential for the health of people with PWS [27]. In particular, growth hormone (GH) therapy improves stature, body composition, and BMI. Early and prolonged treatment with GH can also have some beneficial effects on motor and cognitive abilities [41, 75].

PWS patients have a lower salivary flow with a more acidic pH. They very often suffer from caries and gingivitis, and dental care is a necessary component of treatment [76].

Controlling nutrition is essential to prevent serious weight gain.

During childhood, feeding control is sometimes possible because it is largely entrusted to parents. But in adolescence, dietary transgressions become increasingly frequent, and attempts to regulate nutrition often lead to violent reactions.

Various dietary strategies have been used in the treatment of obesity of people with PWS, including the Modified Atkins Diet (high fat and low carbohydrate) [77], with modest and uncertain results. The abovementioned guidelines recommend [71]:

- Caloric restriction depending on physical activity
- Vegetables and grains
- No sugars and artificial sweeteners
- Protein at every meal
- Water consumption (that PWS patients tend to reject)

A study of gut microbiota components in a cohort of children and adolescents with PWS suggested that increasing fruit intake and limiting meat could be helpful in managing body weight [78].

In the treatment of an 18-year-old girl with PWS and a body weight of 161 kg, it was found useful in the short term to associate liraglutide with an aggressive restriction of calories (200 kcal/day). After discharge, she maintained a weight of just over 100 kg with 1000 kcal/day for 1 year [79].

PWS patients, compared to people with non-PWS obesity, show less spontaneous physical activity and more sedentary time. Supervised home-based exercise sessions are recommended [80].

Bariatric surgery is used in PWS [81], even in children and adolescents [82, 83], with severe obesity and after the failure of noninvasive treatments.

Intellectual disabilities and young age pose important ethical problems, even in case of serious life-threatening conditions [84]. A multidisciplinary team should evaluate the surgical indication and follow the patient and her/his family for a long time after the operation.

A study analyzed the results of laparoscopic sleeve gastrectomy (LSG) in 24 pediatric patients (mean age 10.7, range 4.9–18) with PWS. Follow-up data for up to 5 years showed significant weight loss without mortality or slowing of growth. Many medical comorbidities improved [83].

However, there is still a lack of convincing data and long-term follow-up on the efficacy and safety of bariatric surgery in PWS patients. Some studies are not encouraging.

A prospective multidisciplinary survey evaluated five patients with PWS (two males, mean age 19.2 ± 3.0 years) 10 years after surgery (two sleeve gastrectomy, two one-anastomosis-gastric-bypass, and one Roux-en-Y gastric bypass). The average percentage of total weight loss was highest after 2 years (24.7%). It dropped to 11.9% after 5 years and to 0% after 10 years. None of the comorbidities present at the beginning had disappeared [85].

In four patients (two men) with PWS and severe obesity, bilateral electrode implantation in the lateral hypothalamic area was used. Deep brain stimulation was ineffective: body weight increased, and two patients developed manic symptoms [86].

33.10 Concluding Remarks

At present, it is not possible to achieve a stable recovery of many medical problems, challenging behaviors, and psychiatric symptoms of PWS, including eating and weight disorders. The disease creates a troublesome burden for patients and their caregivers.

The family should be helped from the first detection of the disease with information and psycho-educational interventions directed to behavioral problems as well as diet and physical activity management.

In the future, while waiting for epigenetic therapies, new drugs in the study might enrich the therapeutic resources [87].

Despite its current limitations, the treatment of PWS is expensive. A study found that the total annual direct medical costs of patients with PWS were 8.8 times higher than those of a control group [88].

References

1. Prader A, Labhart A, Willi H. Ein Syndrom von Adipositas, Kleinwuchs, Kryptorchismus und Oligophrenie nach myatonieartigem Zustand im neugeborenenalter. Schweiz Med Wochenschr. 1956;86:1260–1.
2. Prader A, Willi H, editors. Das Syndrom von Imbezilität, Adipositas, Muskelhypotonie, Hypogenitalismus, Hypogonadismus und Diabetes mellitus mit "Anamnese". Vienna, 2nd International Congress of Mental Retardation Part 1, 353. Basel & New York: Basel, Karger; 1961.
3. Hawkey CJ, Smithies A. The Prader-Willi syndrome with a 15/15 translocation. Case report and review of the literature. J Med Genet. 1976;13(2):152–7.
4. Ledbetter DH, Riccardi VM, Airhart SD, Strobel RJ, Keenan BS, Crawford JD. Deletions of chromosome 15 as a cause of the Prader-Willi syndrome. N Engl J Med. 1981;304(6):325–9.
5. Knoll JH, Nicholls RD, Magenis RE, Graham JM Jr, Lalande M, Latt SA. Angelman and Prader-Willi syndromes share a common chromosome 15 deletion but differ in parental origin of the deletion. Am J Med Genet. 1989;32(2):285–90.
6. Nicholls RD, Knoll JH, Butler MG, Karam S, Lalande M. Genetic imprinting suggested by maternal heterodisomy in nondeletion Prader-Willi syndrome. Nature. 1989;342(6247):281–5.
7. Surani MA, Barton SC, Norris ML. Development of reconstituted mouse eggs suggests imprinting of the genome during gametogenesis. Nature. 1984;308(5959):548–50.
8. McGrath J, Solter D. Completion of mouse embryogenesis requires both the maternal and paternal genomes. Cell. 1984;37(1):179–83.

9. Brain R. Chairman's opening remarks: historical introduction. In: Wolstenholme G, Porter R, editors. Mongolism, Ciba Foundation Study Group Number 25. Boston: Little Brown & Co; 1967. p. 1–5.
10. Down JLH. On some of the mental affections of childhood and youth: being the Lettsomian lectures delivered before the Medical society of London in 1887, together with other papers. London: J. & A. Churchill; 1887.
11. Crino A, Fintini D, Bocchini S, Grugni G. Obesity management in Prader-Willi syndrome: current perspectives. Diabetes Metab Syndr Obes. 2018;11:579–93.
12. Butler MG. Genomic imprinting disorders in humans: a mini-review. J Assist Reprod Genet. 2009;26(9-10):477–86.
13. Cassidy SB, Driscoll DJ. Prader-Willi syndrome. Eur J Hum Genet. 2009;17(1):3–13.
14. Butler MG. Prader-Willi syndrome: obesity due to genomic imprinting. Curr Genomics. 2011;12(3):204–15.
15. Butler MG, Kimonis V, Dykens E, Gold JA, Miller J, Tamura R, et al. Prader-Willi syndrome and early-onset morbid obesity NIH rare disease consortium: a review of natural history study. Am J Med Genet A. 2018;176(2):368–75.
16. Ishida M, Moore GE. The role of imprinted genes in humans. Mol Aspects Med. 2013;34(4):826–40.
17. Hara-Isono K, Matsubara K, Mikami M, Arima T, Ogata T, Fukami M, et al. Assisted reproductive technology represents a possible risk factor for development of epimutation-mediated imprinting disorders for mothers aged >/= 30 years. Clin Epigenetics. 2020;12(1):111.
18. Cortessis VK, Azadian M, Buxbaum J, Sanogo F, Song AY, Sriprasert I, et al. Comprehensive meta-analysis reveals association between multiple imprinting disorders and conception by assisted reproductive technology. J Assist Reprod Genet. 2018;35(6):943–52.
19. Han JY, Park J, Jang W, Chae H, Kim M, Kim Y. A twin sibling with Prader-Willi syndrome caused by type 2 microdeletion following assisted reproductive technology: a case report. Biomed Rep. 2016;5(1):18–22.
20. Gold JA, Ruth C, Osann K, Flodman P, McManus B, Lee HS, et al. Frequency of Prader-Willi syndrome in births conceived via assisted reproductive technology. Genet Med. 2014;16(2):164–9.
21. Henningsen AA, Gissler M, Rasmussen S, Opdahl S, Wennerholm UB, Spangsmose AL, et al. Imprinting disorders in children born after ART: a Nordic study from the CoNARTaS group. Hum Reprod. 2020;35(5):1178–84.
22. Ehrhart F, Janssen KJM, Coort SL, Evelo CT, Curfs LMG. Prader-Willi syndrome and Angelman syndrome: visualisation of the molecular pathways for two chromosomal disorders. World J Biol Psychiatry. 2019;20(9):670–82.
23. Eldar-Geva T, Hirsch HJ, Gross-Tsur V. The reproductive system in Prader-Willi syndrome. Harefuah. 2015;154(3):178–82, 211.
24. Hirsch HJ, Eldar-Geva T, Bennaroch F, Pollak Y, Gross-Tsur V. Sexual dichotomy of gonadal function in Prader-Willi syndrome from early infancy through the fourth decade. Hum Reprod. 2015;30(11):2587–96.
25. Vogels A, Fryns JP. Age at diagnosis, body mass index and physical morbidity in children and adults with the Prader-Willi syndrome. Genet Couns. 2004;15(4):397–404.
26. Krochik AG, Ozuna B, Torrado M, Chertkoff L, Mazza C. Characterization of alterations in carbohydrate metabolism in children with Prader-Willi syndrome. J Pediatr Endocrinol Metab. 2006;19(7):911–8.
27. Alves C, Franco RR. Prader-Willi syndrome: endocrine manifestations and management. Arch Endocrinol Metab. 2020;64(3):223–34.
28. Stevenson DA, Heinemann J, Angulo M, Butler MG, Loker J, Rupe N, et al. Gastric rupture and necrosis in Prader-Willi syndrome. J Pediatr Gastroenterol Nutr. 2007;45(2):272–4.
29. Salehi P, Lee D, Ambartsumyan L, Sikka N, Scheimann AO. Rectal picking masquerading as inflammatory bowel disease in Prader-Willi syndrome. J Pediatr Gastroenterol Nutr. 2018;67(1):59–63.

30. Blat C, Busquets E, Gili T, Caixas A, Gabau E, Corripio R. Gastric dilatation and abdominal compartment syndrome in a child with Prader-Willi syndrome. Am J Case Rep. 2017;18:637–40.
31. Donze SH, Codd V, Damen L, Goedegebuure WJ, Denniff M, Samani NJ, et al. Evidence for accelerated biological aging in young adults with Prader-Willi syndrome. J Clin Endocrinol Metab. 2020;105(6)
32. Whittington JE, Holland AJ, Webb T. Ageing in people with Prader-Willi syndrome: mortality in the UK population cohort and morbidity in an older sample of adults. Psychol Med. 2015;45(3):615–21.
33. Butler MG, Manzardo AM, Heinemann J, Loker C, Loker J. Causes of death in Prader-Willi syndrome: Prader-Willi Syndrome Association (USA) 40-year mortality survey. Genet Med. 2017;19(6):635–42.
34. Manzardo AM, Loker J, Heinemann J, Loker C, Butler MG. Survival trends from the Prader-Willi Syndrome Association (USA) 40-year mortality survey. Genet Med. 2018;20(1):24–30.
35. Einfeld SL, Kavanagh SJ, Smith A, Evans EJ, Tonge BJ, Taffe J. Mortality in Prader-Willi syndrome. Am J Ment Retard. 2006;111(3):193–8.
36. Lionti T, Reid SM, Rowell MM. Prader-Willi syndrome in Victoria: mortality and causes of death. J Paediatr Child Health. 2012;48(6):506–11.
37. Proffitt J, Osann K, McManus B, Kimonis VE, Heinemann J, Butler MG, et al. Contributing factors of mortality in Prader-Willi syndrome. Am J Med Genet A. 2019;179(2):196–205.
38. Vogels A, Moerman P, Frijns JP, Bogaert GA. Testicular histology in boys with Prader-Willi syndrome: fertile or infertile? J Urol. 2008;180(4 Suppl):1800–4.
39. Siemensma EP, van Alfen-van der Velden AA, Otten BJ, Laven JS, Hokken-Koelega AC. Ovarian function and reproductive hormone levels in girls with Prader-Willi syndrome: a longitudinal study. J Clin Endocrinol Metab. 2012;97(9):E1766–73.
40. Schulze A, Mogensen H, Hamborg-Petersen B, Graem N, Ostergaard JR, Brondum-Nielsen K. Fertility in Prader-Willi syndrome: a case report with Angelman syndrome in the offspring. Acta Paediatr. 2001;90(4):455–9.
41. Donze SH, Damen L, Mahabier EF, Hokken-Koelega ACS. Cognitive functioning in children with Prader-Willi syndrome during 8 years of growth hormone treatment. Eur J Endocrinol. 2020;182(4):405–11.
42. Curfs LM, Fryns JP. Prader-Willi syndrome: a review with special attention to the cognitive and behavioral profile. Birth Defects Orig Artic Ser. 1992;28(1):99–104.
43. Queiroga TLO, Damiani D, Lopes MC, Franco R, Bueno C, Soster L. A questionnaire study on sleep disturbances associated with Prader-Willi syndrome. J Pediatr Endocrinol Metab. 2020;33(3):397–401.
44. Famelart N, Diene G, Cabal-Berthoumieu S, Glattard M, Molinas C, Guidetti M, et al. Equivocal expression of emotions in children with Prader-Willi syndrome: what are the consequences for emotional abilities and social adjustment? Orphanet J Rare Dis. 2020;15(1):55.
45. Feighan SM, Hughes M, Maunder K, Roche E, Gallagher L. A profile of mental health and behaviour in Prader-Willi syndrome. J Intellect Disabil Res. 2020;64(2):158–69.
46. Gantz MG, Andrews SM, Wheeler AC. Food and non-food-related behavior across settings in children with Prader-Willi Syndrome. Genes (Basel). 2020;11(2)
47. Bull LE, Oliver C, Woodcock KA. Skin picking in people with Prader-Willi syndrome: phenomenology and management J Autism Dev Disord. 2020.
48. Krefft M, Frydecka D, Zalsman G, Krzystek-Korpacka M, Smigiel R, Gebura K, et al. A proinflammatory phenotype is associated with behavioural traits in children with Prader-Willi syndrome. Eur Child Adolesc Psychiatry. 2020;
49. Whittington J, Holland A. A review of psychiatric conceptions of mental and behavioural disorders in Prader-Willi syndrome. Neurosci Biobehav Rev. 2019;95:396–405.
50. Whittington J, Holland A. Developing an understanding of skin picking in people with Prader-Willi syndrome: a structured literature review and re-analysis of existing data. Neurosci Biobehav Rev. 2020;112:48–61.

51. Holland AJ, Aman LCS, Whittington JE. Defining mental and behavioural disorders in genetically determined neurodevelopmental syndromes with particular reference to Prader-Willi syndrome. Genes (Basel). 2019;10(12)
52. Salles J, Lacassagne E, Benvegnu G, Berthoumieu SC, Franchitto N, Tauber M. The RDoC approach for translational psychiatry: could a genetic disorder with psychiatric symptoms help fill the matrix? the example of Prader-Willi syndrome. Transl Psychiatry. 2020;10(1):274.
53. Cuthbert BN. The role of RDoC in future classification of mental disorders. Dialogues Clin Neurosci. 2020;22(1):81–5.
54. Bray G, Dahms W, Swerdloff RS, Fiser RH, Atkinson RL, Carrel RE. The Prader-Willi syndrome: a study of 40 patients and a review of the literature. Medicine (Baltimore). 1983;62(2):59–80.
55. Miller JL, Lynn CH, Driscoll DC, Goldstone AP, Gold J-A, Kimonis V, et al. Nutritional phases in Prader-Willi syndrome. Am J Med Genet A. 2011;155A(5):1040–9.
56. Holland AJ, Treasure J, Coskeran P, Dallow J, Milton N, Hillhouse E. Measurement of excessive appetite and metabolic changes in Prader-Willi syndrome. Int J Obes Relat Metab Disord. 1993;17(9):527–32.
57. Martinez Michel L, Haqq AM, Wismer WV. A review of chemosensory perceptions, food preferences and food-related behaviours in subjects with Prader-Willi Syndrome. Appetite. 2016;99:17–24.
58. Lindgren AC, Barkeling B, Hagg A, Ritzen EM, Marcus C, Rossner S. Eating behavior in Prader-Willi syndrome, normal weight, and obese control groups. J Pediatr. 2000;137(1):50–5.
59. Hinton EC, Holland AJ, Gellatly MS, Soni S, Patterson M, Ghatei MA, et al. Neural representations of hunger and satiety in Prader-Willi syndrome. Int J Obes (Lond). 2006;30(2):313–21.
60. Reinhardt M, Parigi AD, Chen K, Reiman EM, Thiyyagura P, Krakoff J, et al. Deactivation of the left dorsolateral prefrontal cortex in Prader-Willi syndrome after meal consumption. Int J Obes (Lond). 2016;40(9):1360–8.
61. Alexander RC, Greenswag LR, Nowak AJ. Rumination and vomiting in Prader-Willi syndrome. Am J Med Genet. 1987;28(4):889–95.
62. Sloan TB, Kaye CI. Rumination risk of aspiration of gastric contents in the Prader-Willi syndrome. Anesth Analg. 1991;73(4):492–5.
63. Radetti G, Fanolla A, Lupi F, Sartorio A, Grugni G. Accuracy of different indexes of body composition and adiposity in identifying metabolic syndrome in adult subjects with Prader-Willi syndrome. J Clin Med. 2020;9(6)
64. Dagli AI, Mueller J, Williams CA. Angelman syndrome. In: Adam MP, Ardinger HH, Pagon RA, Wallace SE, Bean LJH, Stephens K, et al., editors. GeneReviews((R)). Seattle (WA); 1993.
65. Brennan ML, Adam MP, Seaver LH, Myers A, Schelley S, Zadeh N, et al. Increased body mass in infancy and early toddlerhood in Angelman syndrome patients with uniparental disomy and imprinting center defects. Am J Med Genet A. 2015;167A(1):142–6.
66. Gillessen-Kaesbach G, Demuth S, Thiele H, Theile U, Lich C, Horsthemke B. A previously unrecognised phenotype characterised by obesity, muscular hypotonia, and ability to speak in patients with Angelman syndrome caused by an imprinting defect. Eur J Hum Genet. 1999;7(6):638–44.
67. Welham A, Lau J, Moss J, Cullen J, Higgs S, Warren G, et al. Are Angelman and Prader-Willi syndromes more similar than we thought? Food-related behavior problems in Angelman, Cornelia de Lange, fragile X, Prader-Willi and 1p36 deletion syndromes. Am J Med Genet A. 2015;167A(3):572–8.
68. Muzar Z, Lozano R, Kolevzon A, Hagerman RJ. The neurobiology of the Prader-Willi phenotype of fragile X syndrome. Intractable Rare Dis Res. 2016;5(4):255–61.
69. Dy ABC, Tassone F, Eldeeb M, Salcedo-Arellano MJ, Tartaglia N, Hagerman R. Metformin as targeted treatment in fragile X syndrome. Clin Genet. 2018;93(2):216–22.
70. Mian-Ling Z, Yun-Qi C, Chao-Chun Z. Prader-Willi syndrome: molecular mechanism and epigenetic therapy. Curr Gene Ther. 2020;

71. Duis J, van Wattum PJ, Scheimann A, Salehi P, Brokamp E, Fairbrother L, et al. A multidisciplinary approach to the clinical management of Prader-Willi syndrome. Mol Genet Genomic Med. 2019;7(3):e514.
72. Thomson A, Glasson E, Roberts P, Bittles A. "Over time it just becomes easier…": parents of people with Angelman syndrome and Prader-Willi syndrome speak about their carer role. Disabil Rehabil. 2017;39(8):763–70.
73. Benchikhi L, Nafiaa H, Zaroual A, Ouanass A. Psychological management of a patient with Prader Willi syndrome: case study of a young Moroccan girl. Pan Afr Med J. 2019;33:115.
74. Grolla E, Andrighetto G, Parmigiani P, Hladnik U, Ferrari G, Bernardelle R, et al. Specific treatment of Prader-Willi syndrome through cyclical rehabilitation programmes. Disabil Rehabil. 2011;33(19-20):1837–47.
75. Passone CGB, Franco RR, Ito SS, Trindade E, Polak M, Damiani D, et al. Growth hormone treatment in Prader-Willi syndrome patients: systematic review and meta-analysis. BMJ Paediatr Open. 2020;4(1):e000630.
76. Munne-Miralves C, Brunet-Llobet L, Cahuana-Cardenas A, Torne-Duran S, Miranda-Rius J, Rivera-Baro A. Oral disorders in children with Prader-Willi syndrome: a case control study. Orphanet J Rare Dis. 2020;15(1):43.
77. Felix G, Kossoff E, Barron B, Krekel C, Testa EG, Scheimann A. The modified Atkins diet in children with Prader-Willi syndrome. Orphanet J Rare Dis. 2020;15(1):135.
78. Garcia-Ribera S, Amat-Bou M, Climent E, Llobet M, Chenoll E, Corripio R, et al. Specific dietary components and gut microbiota composition are associated with obesity in children and adolescents with Prader-Willi syndrome. Nutrients. 2020;12(4)
79. Kim YM, Lee YJ, Kim SY, Cheon CK, Lim HH. Successful rapid weight reduction and the use of liraglutide for morbid obesity in adolescent Prader-Willi syndrome. Ann Pediatr Endocrinol Metab. 2020;25(1):52–6.
80. Bellicha A, Coupaye M, Hocquaux L, Speter F, Oppert JM, Poitou C. Increasing physical activity in adult women with Prader-Willi syndrome: a transferability study. J Appl Res Intellect Disabil. 2020;33(2):258–67.
81. Kobayashi J, Kodama M, Yamazaki K, Morikawa O, Murano S, Kawamata N, et al. Gastric bypass in a Japanese man with Prader-Willi syndrome and morbid obesity. Obes Surg. 2003;13(5):803–5.
82. Tripodi M, Casertano A, Peluso M, Musella M, Berardi G, Mozzillo E, et al. Prader-Willi syndrome: role of bariatric surgery in two adolescents with obesity. Obes Surg. 2020; (Epub date 2020/05/27).
83. Alqahtani AR, Elahmedi MO, Al Qahtani AR, Lee J, Butler MG. Laparoscopic sleeve gastrectomy in children and adolescents with Prader-Willi syndrome: a matched-control study. Surg Obes Relat Dis. 2016;12(1):100–10.
84. Di Pietro ML, Zace D. Three scenarios illustrating ethical concerns when considering bariatric surgery in obese adolescents with Prader-Willi syndrome. J Med Ethics. 2020;
85. Liu SY, Wong SK, Lam CC, Ng EK. Bariatric surgery for Prader-Willi syndrome was ineffective in producing sustainable weight loss: long term results for up to 10 years. Pediatr Obes. 2020;15(1):e12575.
86. Franco RR, Fonoff ET, Alvarenga PG, Alho EJL, Lopes AC, Hoexter MQ, et al. Assessment of safety and outcome of lateral hypothalamic deep brain stimulation for obesity in a small series of patients with Prader-Willi syndrome. JAMA Netw Open. 2018;1(7):e185275.
87. Tan Q, Orsso CE, Deehan EC, Triador L, Field CJ, Tun HM, et al. Current and emerging therapies for managing hyperphagia and obesity in Prader-Willi syndrome: a narrative review. Obes Rev. 2020;21(5):e12992.
88. Shoffstall AJ, Gaebler JA, Kreher NC, Niecko T, Douglas D, Strong TV, et al. The high direct medical costs of Prader-Willi syndrome. J Pediatr. 2016;175:137–43.

Turner's Syndrome and Eating and Weight Disorders

34

Massimo Cuzzolaro

34.1 Turner's Syndrome or Ullrich-Turner's Syndrome: Some Historical Steps

In 1930 Otto Ullrich (1894–1957), a German pediatrician, described the case of an 8-year-old girl with low-set auricles, webbed neck, short stature, and lymphedema of the hands and feet [1].

Eight years later, the American endocrinologist Henry H. Turner (1892–1970) published an article [2] about the syndrome that now bears his name: *Turner's syndrome* (TS).

Turner described seven women, between the ages of 15 and 23, with the following features: webbed neck, low posterior hairline, cubitus valgus, short stature, and lack of sexual development. Symptoms and signs were very similar to those of Ullrich's case. Turner tried to treat his patients with pituitary extracts, but without any result.

In the 1940s, endocrinological studies revealed primary ovarian failure associated with elevated levels of gonadotropins in TS, and Turner himself observed that his patients responded to estrogen therapy with an increase in uterine and breast volume [3, 4].

In the following decade, TS was linked to a genetic anomaly.

In 1954 a brief article was published on three cases of TS with aortic coarctation and sex chromosome abnormality [5]. Then, in 1959, Charles Ford and colleagues published a case report about a 14-year-old girl with gonadal dysgenesis, TS symptoms and signs, and a 45,X karyotype [6].

M. Cuzzolaro (✉)
University of Roma Sapienza, Roma, Italy
e-mail: massimo.cuzzolaro@gmail.com

© Springer Nature Switzerland AG 2022
E. Manzato et al. (eds.), *Hidden and Lesser-known Disordered Eating Behaviors in Medical and Psychiatric Conditions*,
https://doi.org/10.1007/978-3-030-81174-7_34

A few years later, in 1963, Ferris Pitts and Samuel Guze published the first known case report of an association of TS with anorexia nervosa (AN) [7].

Lastly, Ullrich's patient was studied again in 1987, and a cytogenetic analysis found a 45,X chromosomal constitution [8].

The eponym *Ullrich-Turner's syndrome*, sometimes used in Europe, is due to Ullrich's first description of this clinical picture.

34.2 Definition and Epidemiology

TS is a sex chromosome disorder with a complete or partial absence of the second X chromosome. In about 60% of TS cases, the karyotype is a pure X monosomy (45,X). 20% of women with TS have two X chromosomes (46,XX), but one is incomplete or has a different structure, e.g., a ring or two long arms instead of one long and the other short. It is also possible that, in the same individual, there are cell lines with different karyotypes (mosaicism). Different types of mosaicism are described, such as 45X/46XX, 45X/46XXX, and 45X/46XY [4, 9].

TS has often been defined as agenesis or gonadal dysgenesis to indicate total or partial gonadal developmental defects [10, 11]. In TS, gonadal degeneration is mostly late fetal/neonatal. The ovarian lesion ("streak gonads") leads to hypergonadotropic hypogonadism, amenorrhea, sexual infantilism, and metabolic and endocrine disorders.

In a fair percentage of cases, up to 40%, spontaneous pubertal development occurs before premature gonadal failure [12].

The presence of cells with Y chromosome material (45X/46XY mosaicism), a rare occurrence, generally does not determine male characteristics, nor does it absolutely exclude the possibility of spontaneous pubertal development and spontaneous menarche, but there is a risk of malignancy (gonadoblastoma) [13].

Persons with TS are short in stature. Mosaicism is generally associated with taller stature and less marked phenotypic alterations. However, the correlations between genotypic and phenotypic characters are still little known [4, 14, 15].

TS is one of the most frequent chromosome abnormalities and is the most common sex chromosome anomaly in women.

TS affects about 1 in 2500 female live births [9]. The number of women with TS in the world would be around 1.5–2 million.

It is much more common in stillbirths and spontaneous abortions. It is believed to be present in about 3% of all female fetuses and is responsible for 7–10% of all miscarriages [12].

34.3 Turner's Syndrome, Medical Comorbidity, and Mortality

Throughout life, TS is associated with increased medical morbidity and premature mortality. Diseases, of course, contribute to worsening the quality of life, in particular the health-related quality of life (HR-QoL) [16].

Hypogonadism with estrogen deficiency and infertility are characteristic clinical data of TS. Hypogonadism is hypergonadotropic, but a rare case of TS with hypogonadotropic hypogonadism and hyperthyroidism (Graves' disease) has been described [17].

Congenital cardiovascular, kidney, and skeleton malformations (e.g., micrognathia, ogival palate, short fourth metacarpal, scoliosis), aortic diseases (dilation, coarctation, dissection), hypertension, lymphedema of hands and feet, and hypoacusis are frequent. There is an increased risk of diabetes (both type 1 and 2), autoimmune disorders, coeliac disease, hypothyroidism and other endocrinological diseases, inflammatory bowel disease, intestinal angiodysplasia, obesity, and osteoporosis.

A retrospective study of 317 patients with TS followed from 1950 to 2017 [18] found the following results:

- Average age at the beginning of the study 22 ± 18 years old
- Average age at diagnosis 9 years (range 2–12)
- Pure X monosomy 37%
- Weight kg 57 ± 11
- Height cm 143 ± 16
- Body mass index kg/m^2 26 ± 8
- Hypertension 31%
- Hyperlipidemia 25%
- Diabetes mellitus types 1 and 2 12%
- Hypothyroidism 33%
- 46 patients died (mean age at the time of death, 53 ± 17 years)
- Major causes of death: cardiovascular disease, liver disease, and malignancy.

34.4 Fertility

In TS, there is a very high risk of premature ovarian failure (POF), mostly occurring before puberty.

However, 5%–20% of women with TS have spontaneous pubertal development with menarche [19, 20].

2%–8% of women with TS have spontaneous pregnancies, mostly reported in TS with mosaicism. Frequent outcomes of pregnancies in TS are miscarriages, perinatal deaths, and malformations (TS, Down's syndrome), while only in 38% of cases, infants are healthy [12, 21, 22].

In addition to adoption, for about 30 years, women with TS who want to have a child and have not yet lost their ovarian reserve may be offered in vitro fertilization of their oocytes with subsequent intrauterine embryo transfer. Embryonic biopsy with preimplantation genetic diagnosis is recommended [23, 24].

In cases of TS with spontaneous menarche, fertility preservation strategies have also been available for use before ovarian failure occurs. The method is controlled ovarian stimulation with cryopreservation of oocytes [25, 26]. An international panel of experts (gynecologists, endocrinologists, medical ethicists, and 20 women with TS) concluded that ovarian tissue cryopreservation (OTC) should be offered to young women with TS and spontaneous menarche [27].

A recent study described its application in three women with spontaneous menarche and no spontaneous pregnancy [28]. The intervention took place when they were 17, 26, and 27 years old, respectively. BMI values were normal. There was a success in all three cases, including the pure monosomy case (45,X), without negative side effects. At the time the work was published, oocytes had not yet been used for in vitro fertilization.

Other possibilities offered to meet the maternity demand of women with TS are currently the donation of oocytes or embryos and gestational surrogacy [26, 29, 30].

It is argued that infertility severely damages the quality of life of women with TS [26]. But what psychic effects does a spontaneous pregnancy have on a woman with TS? And how can be experienced motherhood achieved with the new technical devices, more or less authorized by the various legislations?

New possibilities raise further and challenging questions.

34.5 Turner's Syndrome, Neurocognitive Development, Psychosocial Adjustment, and Psychiatric Comorbidity

Neuroimaging studies have reported several anatomical and functional differences in the brain of women with TS, at various levels, compared to age-matched controls. Decreased gray matter volumes appear in the premotor, somatosensory, and parieto-occipital cortex. The neuroanatomical profile observed in adulthood is already present at the age of 1 year [31, 32].

A study of temperamental characteristics and cognitive and adaptive functioning in 1-year-old girls with TS found no major differences from controls and normative values. The early neuroevolutionary profile (1–2 years) appeared overall positive except for some deficits in fine movements and visual-perceptual abilities [33].

In school age and adolescence, from the neurocognitive point of view, verbal skills and language are generally normal; on the contrary, TS girls may perform more poorly than control girls on mathematical and non-verbal abilities (visual-motor skills, attention, etc.) [34, 35].

The ability to read facial expressions and recognize emotions, especially fear, seems, in some cases, diminished as in autism spectrum disorders [36, 37].

With regard to psychosocial adaptation, Ullrich's first patient was studied again in 1987 at the age of 66. In all cells examined, she showed a karyotype 45,X which confirmed the diagnosis of TS and excluded that of Noonan syndrome. She was 144.5 cm tall and had primary amenorrhea and a lack of maturation of secondary sexual characteristics. Nevertheless, according to the authors, she had adapted quite well to her condition both personally and at work [8].

However, in TS, various factors may favor psychic suffering and the development of psychopathological symptoms, including negative body image and disturbed eating behavior, already in adolescence:

- Physical abnormalities
- Tendency to obesity
- Pharmacological induction of puberty
- Need for regular medical check-ups and ongoing care

TS almost always results in short stature with short legs and a short neck. Cubitus valgus (the forearm is angled out of the body when the arm is fully extended) and Madelung deformity (bayonet deformity of the wrist) are frequent, due to defects in the development of the ulna and radius.

Various other anomalies of physical appearance may be more or less evident such as low posterior hairline, low-set ears, micrognathia, high arched palate, and pterigium colli (webbed neck).

These characteristics are the same in different ethnic groups [38] and influence, obviously, the discomfort and dissatisfaction of the body and the difficulties in social relations.

On the psychological level, in many cases of TS immaturity, low self-esteem, social insecurity, and excessive shyness were found [39–41].

Young women with TS explicitly report anxiety and difficulties in social relationships that tend to intensify in adolescence, when they feel "out of sync" in the peer group [42].

Even in adulthood, the quality of psychological and social as well as physical life is significantly lower than in controls [16, 40].

Skuse and colleagues have found poorer social skills and greater difficulty of adaptation in women with TS whose X chromosome derives from the mother than those in which it derives from the father [43].

Regarding the association with mental disorders, Cardoso and colleagues examined 100 women with TS with structured clinical interview for DSM-IV after suspending hormone replacement treatment for 2 weeks. The average age was 34.7 years (range 16–61). The criteria for the diagnosis of an anxiety or depression disorder, current or past, were met in 52 cases and those for an eating disorder in the past in 6 cases [44].

The research is among the few to have used a structured clinical interview on a large sample. It has the limit of having used a sample of volunteers, presumably healthier and more willing to social contact than the average of people with TS.

Moreover, a recent systematic review of the literature [45] found that, in controlled studies, women with TS suffer from more frequent and more severe depressive symptoms than controls, already in adolescence and even more so in adulthood.

34.6 Turner's Syndrome, Feeding, Eating, and Weight Disorders

In life, a woman with TS can present feeding and eating disorders and body weight abnormalities by default or excess.

A case-control study [46] of ten infants with TS observed during meals found, in addition to other well-known abnormalities:

- Marked hypotonia of lips and cheeks
- Ogival palate, high narrow, hyper-convex (high-arched)
- Dysfunctional tongue movements
- Less developed chewing skills
- Shorter mealtimes
- Lower body weight than controls at 6, 12, and 15 months of age
- Parents reported that difficulties in feeding girls with TS were present from birth.

Other works have confirmed that in most cases of TS, from birth to 3 years of age, there is poor appetite, difficulty in chewing solid food, and frequent vomiting [47, 48].

Since 1963 [7], several cases of association of TS with AN and one with bulimia nervosa (BN) [44] have been reported. These are mostly case reports. In 1973 there were at least seven published cases of association of TS with AN [49], in 1975 nine [50], and 1983 twelve [51].

A question immediately arose: should TS be considered a risk factor for the development of AN?

In 1981 Darby and collaborators described the eleventh documented co-occurrence of TS with AN [52]. They reported that for some authors the association was not accidental [53] but added that subsequent evidence depicted that the frequency of the association between the two clinical pictures was no higher than that expected by chance.

Larocca, discussing a clinical case, advanced the hypothesis that the TS-AN relationship was mediated by a mood disorder and that anorexic symptoms were secondary to depression [54].

As already mentioned, in a sample of 100 TS patients examined with SCID-DSM-IV, six had previously suffered from eating disorders (five AN and one BN) [44].

Darby's question—cause or coincidence—has come back systematically and has entered into the framework of a multifactorial, multidimensional vision of the AN etiology. Cognitive deficits that invest the social relationship skills associated with low levels of self-esteem and body dissatisfaction are common in TS [39, 55] and represent possible premises for the development of anorexic symptoms.

In commenting on the onset of AN in a girl with Turner's mosaic (X0/XX), Fieldsend has opportunely recalled that the eating disorder has a multifactorial etiology and the chromosomal anomaly with its consequences can be a not determining but concurrent factor [56].

Thirty years later, this position is still to be shared. The frequency of the association between TS and AN does not seem significantly higher than a random coincidence. But this does not take away the fact that, in every single life story, the connections between being affected by TS and developing psychopathological symptoms must be sought.

The case of a woman, described with care and acumen in 1975 by a psychiatrist and a gynecologist, is still instructive [50]. The diagnosis of TS had already been suspected on a clinical basis (growth retardation, primary amenorrhea) but was confirmed, by chromosomal analysis (45,X), only at the age of 37 years when she was admitted for the third time for AN.

The girl was treated from the age of 15 with Physex (human chorionic gonadotropin, hCG) and then, from the age of 27, with Anovlar, an oral estroprogestin contraceptive.

She was married at 21 years. At the time of the wedding, she weighed 60 kg and kept that weight for a long time. At 29, with her husband, she adopted a child.

After a short time, this woman began to feel too fat, started a diet, and dropped to 29 kg (height 152 cm) with various hospitalizations. She seemed depressed and non-committed, manifested thoughts and behaviors typical of AN, was physically overactive, and pushed her son to overeat. The personality was very immature. She used to dress "in a very feminine way … to underline her gender role, as several Turner patients do [57]" [50] (p. 32).

About the relationship between adoption of a child and onset of AN symptoms, the authors wrote: "(…) she in the past had tried to reestablish a small girl status in her own home, which resulted in rivalry with her adopted 7-year-old son for her husband's attention. She often by slip of the tongue referred to her husband as 'father'" [50] (p. 33). The fear of growing up—"flight from growth"—is a feature of the AN [58].

This medical history suggests ancient and still open questions:

- Is TS' association with AN meaningful?
- What weight can TS be given as a risk factor for the development of AN?
- Can hormone treatments be precipitating factors?
- What is the role of biological factors related to the chromosomal anomaly?
- What is the role of psychological factors and life events?

In 1993, Muhs and Lieberz published a literature review of 21 cases of association between AN and TS reviewed from a psychodynamic point of view [59].

Some observations continue to be valid and useful for medical and psychological interventions that should always take individual differences into account. It's worth remembering three notes:

- The childhood and adolescence of a girl with TS are marked by somatic deformities, starting with her short stature, and other deficits that lead to painful narcissistic wounds
- In this season of life, the quality of family relationships plays an essential part.
- It should be remembered that AN mostly occurs after puberty. Drives, emotions, and conflicts related to sexuality and gender role can intervene in the connection between the onset of hormonal treatment and the development of anorexic symptoms in a girl with TS.

Already in 1989, the authors of a case study wondered whether the hormonal treatment needed for TS could contribute to the pathogenesis of AN: in a

14-year-old girl with TS, anorexic symptoms appeared shortly after the start of treatment with estrogen [60]. This relationship is frequent in cases of AN in TS.

It's not just estrogen that's at stake. Nicholls and Stanhope, in 1998, published a letter in which they described two cases of TS with AN, arising from a weight slightly above normal (109% and 107%) [61]. One girl's AN started at 16, and the other at 15.5. For both the treatment protocol included in addition to ethinylestradiol an anabolic steroid, oxandrolone. Oxandrolone stimulates appetite and promotes weight gain through lean mass gain. In these two cases, it was interrupted after the appearance of AN, but its possible pathogenetic contribution remains uncertain.

In TS eating symptoms can be associated or alternate with other psychopathological symptoms. In a young girl with TS, depressive symptoms appeared at the age of 11; at 17 years of age, those of AN were added; and, when eating habits normalized, the depression continued [54]. A young woman with TS at 19 years of age met diagnostic criteria for AN, attention-deficit/hyperactivity disorder (ADHD), bipolar disorder type 1, and obsessive-compulsive disorder (OCD) [62].

The co-occurrence with AN is the one that has attracted the most attention. However, the association of TS with overweight and obesity is much more frequent.

Turner's seminal article [2] included a picture of six women observed in the 1930s. The women were photographed naked. A height marker demonstrates short stature, but in none is an obesity condition recognizable [4].

On the other hand, case reports from the 1960s and 1970s [63, 64] already spoke of obesity, and it has long been known that overweight/obesity and obesity-related diseases are frequently observed in TS. They contribute to worsening morbidity, mortality, and quality of life and may be associated with disturbed and unhealthy eating behaviors.

In a large long-term outcome study of 317 patients [18], body mass index (BMI) was 26 ± 8. BMI was >25 in 50% of patients, and many cases showed signs of metabolic syndrome.

A Japanese study found that in a sample of 426 patients with TS aged 15–39 years, 106 had a BMI ≥ 25 kgm^2: the prevalence (24.7%) was significantly higher than that of the general female population (9.4%). Many women had obesity-related diseases [65].

One of the rare longitudinal cohort studies followed 98 TS patients (30 with monosomy 45,X) from childhood to early adulthood. BMI percentiles and metabolic comorbidities significantly increased over time, and group 45.X was at greater risk [66].

Hormone replacement therapy and, in particular, progestins contribute to body weight gain from adolescence onward [67].

34.7 Differential Diagnosis

The diagnosis of TS is based on the karyotype analysis.

It can also be performed in prenatal age when the fetal ultrasound shows elements of suspicion (e.g., cystic hygroma, kidney, or heart abnormalities) or at birth, but mostly the condition is recognized during childhood.

In several cases, especially in girls who have spontaneous puberty, the diagnosis is made only in adulthood.

TS must not be confused with Noonan syndrome.

Some symptoms are similar, such as short stature, webbed neck, facial dysmorphism, developmental retardation, and congenital heart defects. Relatively frequent are psychopathological symptoms [68] and childhood feeding disorders [69]. A case of association with AN has also been described [70], while obesity rates seem lower than that in the control population [71].

However, Noonan syndrome is a genetic disease, but there are no chromosomal abnormalities. It is more prevalent than TS and affects both men and women [72].

34.8 Treatment

TS is a lifelong diagnosis. Therapeutic interventions and their frequency must be cut on an individual basis. The rate of follow-ups depends on the morbidity burden.

A recent case study may be educational because it reports some particular consequences of non-treatment [73].

In a 64-year-old woman treated for microcytic anemia, the diagnosis of TS was suspected based on two characteristic signs: the fourth finger of her left hand (ring finger) was very short, and her left wrist had a Madelung's deformity. The X-ray showed abnormal shortness of the left fourth metacarpal and subluxation of the distal part of the ulna. The patient reported untreated primary amenorrhea, and the karyogram showed total monosomy X confirming the diagnosis of TS.

Why did anemia occur? The cause was blood loss due to an ulcer in the gastric cavity, secondary to prolonged use of non-steroidal anti-inflammatory drugs. The low level of estrogen had always caused severe osteoporosis with vertebral fractures, chronic osteoarticular pain, and continued use of painkillers without gastroprotection.

In fact, in TS female hormone replacement therapy (HRT) is necessary. After puberty induction, women with TS generally continue to receive cyclic estro-progestin therapy.

But what are its long-term effects?

A Danish study compared women treated with women never treated: HRT did not reduce mortality but showed beneficial effects on comorbidity with less drug use and less hospitalization [74].

Therapies affect appetite and eating behavior of girls with TS and parents' attitudes.

Oxandrolone has already been mentioned [61] and is used to promote growth, even stature [75]. Furthermore, TS is a registered indication for treatment with growth hormone (GH). It has been found that girls with TS treated with growth hormone (GH) eat more, have less fat mass, and have less conflict with their parents over food [76].

The risk of developing an excess of adiposity, a metabolic syndrome, and a non-alcoholic fatty liver disease (NAFLD) is rather high in TS, and cardiovascular disease and NAFLD disease are two leading causes of premature mortality.

Treatment suggests:

- Avoiding excessive increases in body weight
- Paying attention to lifestyle
- Promoting a healthy diet and an adequate level of physical activity
- Controlling liver function once a year

Women with TS, both teenagers and adults, tend to engage little in physical activity and to overestimate it [77]. This attitude is consequent to the physical and psychological problems associated with TS but tends, on the other hand, to accentuate them, including overweight and associated pathologies [78].

Pterigium colli, when accentuated, can contribute to aesthetic discomfort and require surgical correction.

Puberty is, in general, a time of risk for the development of psychopathological symptoms. This remark also applies when puberty is artificially induced.

Recent guidelines recommend the development of social skill training interventions [42], but in several cases, this kind of psycho-educational help may not be sufficient.

As already mentioned, women with TS have long been reported to have psychosocial problems and psychiatric comorbidities, including eating and weight disorders [40]. And it is likely that many psychopathological symptoms escape observation by doctors or are underestimated in the face of physical problems [62].

Periodic checks and treatment plans should also take these aspects into account, but the attention is still inadequate [79].

34.9 Conclusive Remarks

No psychiatric component is a regular part of TS. However, depressive disorders, anxiety disorders, and anorexia nervosa have been documented in several cases of TS.

Although there is no evidence in the literature that women with TS have a higher risk of developing AN or other eating disorders, treatment must be adequate in cases where comorbidity occurs.

Especially the most recent studies show that the prevalence of overweight, obesity, and obesity-related diseases in TS is high. This fact suggests that attention should be paid to eating patterns and physical activity.

References

1. Ullrich O. Über typische Kombinationsbilder multipler Abartungen. Z Kinderheilkd. 1930;49(3):271–6.
2. Turner HH. A syndrome of infantilism, congenital webbed neck, and cubitus valgus. Endocrinology. 1938;23(5):566–74.
3. Schaefer GB, Riley HDJA. Tribute to Henry H. Turner, MD (1892–1970): a pioneer endocrinologist. Endocrinologist. 2004;14(4):179–84.

4. Saenger P, Bondy CA. Turner syndrome. In: Sperling MA, editor. Pediatric endocrinology. 4th ed. Philadelphia: Elsevier; 2014. p. 664–96.
5. Polani PE, Hunter WF, Lennox B. Chromosomal sex in Turner's syndrome with coarctation of the aorta. Lancet. 1954;267(6829):120–1.
6. Ford CE, Jones KW, Polani PE, De Almeida JC, Briggs JH. A sex-chromosome anomaly in a case of gonadal dysgenesis (Turner's syndrome). Lancet. 1959;1(7075):711–3.
7. Pitts FN Jr, Guze SB. Anorexia nervosa and gonadal dysgenesis (Turner's syndrome). Am J Psychiatry. 1963;119(11):1100.
8. Wiedemann HR, Glatzl J. Follow-up of Ullrich's original patient with "Ullrich-Turner" syndrome. Am J Med Genet. 1991;41(1):134–6.
9. Gravholt CH, Viuff M, Stochholm K, Andersen NH. Adult care of Turner syndrome. In: Huhtaniemi H, Martini L, editors. Encyclopedia of endocrine diseases, vol. 2. 2nd ed. San Diego: Elsevier Academic Press; 2019. p. 482–9.
10. Russell A, Levin B, Wilmers M. The webbing syndrome (Ullrich-Turner) with and without gonadal agenesis: chromosomal sex typing by skin cell or leucocyte examination in diagnosis. Proc R Soc Med. 1955;48(4):318–20.
11. Bush RT. Turner's syndrome and gonadal dysgenesis. N Z Med J. 1960;59:45–9.
12. Elsheikh M, Dunger DB, Conway GS, Wass JA. Turner's syndrome in adulthood. Endocr Rev. 2002;23(1):120–40.
13. Dabrowski E, Johnson EK, Patel V, Hsu Y, Davis S, Goetsch AL, et al. Turner syndrome with Y chromosome: spontaneous thelarche, menarche, and risk of malignancy. J Pediatr Adolesc Gynecol. 2020;33(1):10–4.
14. Gravholt CH, Andersen NH, Conway GS, Dekkers OM, Geffner ME, Klein KO, et al. Clinical practice guidelines for the care of girls and women with Turner syndrome: proceedings from the 2016 Cincinnati International Turner Syndrome Meeting. Eur J Endocrinol. 2017;177(3):G1–G70.
15. Turner syndrome society of the United States. https://www.turnersyndrome.org/ [cited 2020 19 June].
16. van den Hoven AT, Bons LR, Dykgraaf RHM, Dessens AB, Pastoor H, de Graaff LCG, et al. A value-based healthcare approach: health-related quality of life and psychosocial functioning in women with Turner syndrome. Clin Endocrinol (Oxf). 2020;92(5):434–42.
17. Zhang H, Zhang X, Yang M. Clinical case report: a case of Turner syndrome with Graves' disease. Medicine (Baltimore). 2020;99(11):e19518.
18. Fuchs MM, Attenhofer Jost C, Babovic-Vuksanovic D, Connolly HM, Egbe A. Long-term outcomes in patients with Turner syndrome: a 68-year follow-up. J Am Heart Assoc. 2019;8(11):e011501.
19. Pasquino AM, Passeri F, Pucarelli I, Segni M, Municchi G. Spontaneous pubertal development in Turner's syndrome. Italian Study Group for Turner's Syndrome. J Clin Endocrinol Metab. 1997;82(6):1810–3.
20. Kim MJ, Jeong HR. Spontaneous sexual development and heavy menstrual bleeding in 45,X monosomy and 45,X/47,XXX mosaic Turner syndrome and a review of the literature. J Pediatr Adolesc Gynecol. 2020;33(5):602–6.
21. Tarani L, Lampariello S, Raguso G, Colloridi F, Pucarelli I, Pasquino AM, et al. Pregnancy in patients with Turner's syndrome: six new cases and review of literature. Gynecol Endocrinol. 1998;12(2):83–7.
22. Ramage K, Grabowska K, Silversides C, Quan H, Metcalfe A. Maternal, pregnancy, and neonatal outcomes for women with Turner syndrome. Birth Defects Res. 2020;112(14):1067–73.
23. Ditkoff EC, Vidali A, Sauer MV. Pregnancy in a woman with Turner mosaicism following ovarian stimulation and in vitro fertilization. J Assist Reprod Genet. 1996;13(5):447–8.
24. Osorio-Ramirez W, Giraldo-Moreno J, Gomez-Cortes D, Olive D, Cano-Franco J, Tamayo-Hussein S. Birth of healthy neonate following preimplantation genetic diagnosis in a mother with mosaic Turner syndrome. Case report and review of the literature. Rev Colomb Obstet Ginecol. 2020;71(1):56–62.

25. Kavoussi SK, Fisseha S, Smith YR, Smith GD, Christman GM, Gago LA. Oocyte cryopreservation in a woman with mosaic Turner syndrome: a case report. J Reprod Med. 2008;53(3):223–6.
26. Ye M, Yeh J, Kosteria I, Li L. Progress in fertility preservation strategies in Turner syndrome. Front Med (Lausanne). 2020;7:3.
27. Schleedoorn MJ, Mulder BH, Braat DDM, Beerendonk CCM, Peek R, Nelen W, et al. International consensus: ovarian tissue cryopreservation in young Turner syndrome patients: outcomes of an ethical Delphi study including 55 experts from 16 different countries. Hum Reprod. 2020;35(5):1061–72.
28. Vergier J, Bottin P, Saias J, Reynaud R, Guillemain C, Courbiere B. Fertility preservation in Turner syndrome: karyotype does not predict ovarian response to stimulation. Clin Endocrinol (Oxf). 2019;91(5):646–51.
29. Gutierrez Gutierrez AM, Grimalt L, Remohi J, Pellicer A. Twin pregnancy after oocyte donation in a woman with Turner syndrome. Ginecol Obstet Mex. 1994;62:182–4.
30. Obata S, Tsuburai T, Shindo R, Aoki S, Miyagi E, Sakakibara H. Current situation and outcomes of pregnancy in women with Turner syndrome in Japan. J Obstet Gynaecol Res. 2020;46:1728–34.
31. O'Donoghue S, Green T, Ross JL, Hallmayer J, Lin X, Jo B, et al. Brain development in school-age and adolescent girls: effects of Turner syndrome, estrogen therapy, and genomic imprinting. Biol Psychiatry. 2020;87(2):113–22.
32. Davenport ML, Cornea E, Xia K, Crowley JJ, Halvorsen MW, Goldman BD, et al. Altered brain structure in infants with Turner syndrome. Cereb Cortex. 2020;30(2):587–96.
33. Pretzel RE, Knickmeyer RC, DeRamus M, Duquette P, Okoniewski KC, Reinhartsen DB, et al. Early development of infants with Turner syndrome. J Dev Behav Pediatr. 2020;41:470–9.
34. Ross JL, Stefanatos G, Roeltgen D, Kushner H, Cutler GB Jr. Ullrich-Turner syndrome: neurodevelopmental changes from childhood through adolescence. Am J Med Genet. 1995;58(1):74–82.
35. Baker JM, Klabunde M, Jo B, Green T, Reiss AL. On the relationship between mathematics and visuospatial processing in Turner syndrome. J Psychiatr Res. 2020;121:135–42.
36. Lawrence K, Kuntsi J, Coleman M, Campbell R, Skuse D. Face and emotion recognition deficits in Turner syndrome: a possible role for X-linked genes in amygdala development. Neuropsychology. 2003;17(1):39–49.
37. Mazzola F, Seigal A, MacAskill A, Corden B, Lawrence K, Skuse DH. Eye tracking and fear recognition deficits in Turner syndrome. Soc Neurosci. 2006;1(3–4):259–69.
38. Kruszka P, Addissie YA, Tekendo-Ngongang C, Jones KL, Savage SK, Gupta N, et al. Turner syndrome in diverse populations. Am J Med Genet A. 2020;182(2):303–13.
39. Delooz J, Van den Berghe H, Swillen A, Kleczkowska A, Fryns JP. Turner syndrome patients as adults: a study of their cognitive profile, psychosocial functioning and psychopathological findings. Genet Couns. 1993;4(3):169–79.
40. Liedmeier A, Jendryczko D, van der Grinten HC, Rapp M, Thyen U, Pienkowski C, et al. Psychosocial well-being and quality of life in women with Turner syndrome. Psychoneuroendocrinology. 2020;104548:113.
41. Schmidt PJ, Cardoso GM, Ross JL, Haq N, Rubinow DR, Bondy CA. Shyness, social anxiety, and impaired self-esteem in Turner syndrome and premature ovarian failure. JAMA. 2006;295(12):1374–6.
42. Wolstencroft J, Mandy W, Skuse D. Experiences of social interaction in young women with Turner syndrome: a qualitative study. Child Care Health Dev. 2020;46(1):46–55.
43. Skuse DH, James RS, Bishop DV, Coppin B, Dalton P, Aamodt-Leeper G, et al. Evidence from Turner's syndrome of an imprinted X-linked locus affecting cognitive function. Nature. 1997;387(6634):705–8.
44. Cardoso G, Daly R, Haq NA, Hanton L, Rubinow DR, Bondy CA, et al. Current and lifetime psychiatric illness in women with Turner syndrome. Gynecol Endocrinol. 2004;19(6):313–9.
45. Morris LA, Tishelman AC, Kremen J, Ross RA. Depression in Turner syndrome: a systematic review. Arch Sex Behav. 2020;49(2):769–86.

46. Mathisen B, Reilly S, Skuse D. Oral-motor dysfunction and feeding disorders of infants with Turner syndrome. Dev Med Child Neurol. 1992;34(2):141–9.
47. Frias JL, Davenport ML, Committee on Genetics, Section on Endocrinology. Health supervision for children with Turner syndrome. Pediatrics. 2003;111(3):692–702.
48. Hjerrild BE, Mortensen KH, Gravholt CH. Turner syndrome and clinical treatment. Br Med Bull. 2008;86:77–93.
49. Liston EH, Shershow LW. Concurrence of anorexia nervosa and gonadal dysgenesis. A critical review with practical considerations. Arch Gen Psychiatry. 1973;29(6):834–6.
50. Theilgaard A, Philip J. Concurrence of Turner's syndrome and anorexia nervosa. Acta Psychiatr Scand. 1975;52(1):31–5.
51. Dougherty GG Jr, Rockwell WJ, Sutton G, Ellinwood EH Jr. Anorexia nervosa in treated gonadal dysgenesis: case report and review. J Clin Psychiatry. 1983;44(6):219–21.
52. Darby PL, Garfinkel PE, Vale JM, Kirwan PJ, Brown GM. Anorexia nervosa and 'Turner syndrome': cause or coincidence? Psychol Med. 1981;11(1):141–5.
53. Kron L, Katz JL, Gorzynski G, Weiner H. Anorexia nervosa and gonadal dysgenesis. Further evidence of a relationship. Arch Gen Psychiatry. 1977;34(3):332–5.
54. Larocca FE. Concurrence of Turner's syndrome, anorexia nervosa, and mood disorders: case report. J Clin Psychiatry. 1985;46(7):296–7.
55. Wolstencroft J, Skuse D. Social skills and relationships in Turner syndrome. Curr Opin Psychiatry. 2019;32(2):85–91.
56. Fieldsend B. Anorexia nervosa and Turner's syndrome. Br J Psychiatry. 1988;152:270–1.
57. Theilgaard A. Cognitive style and gender role in persons with sex chromosome aberrations. Dan Med Bull. 1972;19(8):276–86.
58. Crisp AH. Anorexia nervosa as flight from growth: assessment and treatment based on the model. In: Garner DM, Garfinkel PE, editors. Handbook of treatment for eating disorders. New York: Guilford Press; 1997. p. 248–77.
59. Muhs A, Lieberz K. Anorexia nervosa and Turner's syndrome. Psychopathology. 1993;26(1):29–40.
60. Ohzeki T, Hayashi K, Higurashi M, Hanaki K, Ishitani N, Shiraki K. Ullrich-Turner syndrome and anorexia nervosa. Am J Med Genet. 1989;32(1):87–9.
61. Nicholls D, Stanhope R. Turner's syndrome, anorexia nervosa, and anabolic steroids. Arch Dis Child. 1998;79(1):94.
62. Moonga SS, Pinkhasov A, Singh D. Obsessive-compulsive disorder in a 19-year-old female adolescent with Turner syndrome. J Clin Med Res. 2017;9(12):1026–8.
63. Mellinger RC. Turner's syndrome with X0-XX mosaicism. A case presentation. Henry Ford Hosp Med Bull. 1964;12:181–6.
64. Givens JR, Wilroy RS, Summitt RL, Andersen RN, Wiser WL, Fish SA. Features of Turner's syndrome in women with polycystic ovaries. Obstet Gynecol. 1975;45(6):619–24.
65. Hanew K, Tanaka T, Horikawa R, Hasegawa T, Fujita K, Yokoya S. Women with Turner syndrome are at high risk of lifestyle-related disease. From questionnaire surveys by the Foundation for Growth Science in Japan. Endocr J. 2016;63(5):449–56.
66. Lebenthal Y, Levy S, Sofrin-Drucker E, Nagelberg N, Weintrob N, Shalitin S, et al. The natural history of metabolic comorbidities in Turner syndrome from childhood to early adulthood: comparison between 45,X monosomy and other karyotypes. Front Endocrinol. 2018;9:27.
67. Mathez ALG, Monteagudo PT, do Nascimento Verreschi IT, Dias-da-Silva MR. Levonorgestrel correlates with less weight gain than other progestins during hormonal replacement therapy in Turner syndrome patients. Sci Rep. 2020;10(1):8298.
68. Roelofs RL, Wingbermuhle E, van der Heijden PT, Jonkers R, de Haan M, Kessels RPC, et al. Personality and psychopathology in adults with Noonan syndrome. J Clin Psychol Med Settings. 2020;27(2):256–67.
69. Geelan-Hansen K, Anne S. Otolaryngologic manifestations of Noonan syndrome. Ear Nose Throat J. 2015;94(9):E4–6.
70. Arvaniti A, Samakouri M, Keskeridou F, Veletza S. Concurrence of anorexia nervosa and Noonan syndrome. Eur Eat Disord Rev. 2014;22(1):83–5.

71. da Silva FM, Jorge AA, Malaquias A, da Costa Pereira A, Yamamoto GL, Kim CA, et al. Nutritional aspects of Noonan syndrome and Noonan-related disorders. Am J Med Genet A. 2016;170(6):1525–31.
72. Bhangoo A, editor. Noonan syndrome. Characteristics and interventions. London: Academic Press—Elsevier; 2019.
73. Major J, Pusztai P, Igaz P. A short ring finger points to a diagnosis of Turner syndrome again. Lancet. 2020;395(10227):e51.
74. Viuff MH, Berglund A, Juul S, Andersen NH, Stochholm K, Gravholt CH. Sex hormone replacement therapy in Turner syndrome: impact on morbidity and mortality. J Clin Endocrinol Metab. 2020;105(2):dgz039.
75. Gault EJ, Cole TJ, Casey S, Hindmarsh PC, Betts P, Dunger DB, et al. Effect of oxandrolone and timing of pubertal induction on final height in Turner syndrome: final analysis of the UK randomised placebo-controlled trial. Arch Dis Child. 2021;104:74–6.
76. Blissett J, Harris G, Kirk J. Effect of growth hormone therapy on feeding problems and food intake in children with growth disorders. Acta Paediatr. 2000;89(6):644–9.
77. Sienkiewicz-Dianzenza E, Milde K, Tomaszewski P, Frac M. Physical activity of girls with Turner's syndrome. Pediatr Endocrinol Diabetes Metab. 2011;17(3):134–7.
78. Thompson T, Zieba B, Howell S, Karakash W, Davis S. A mixed methods study of physical activity and quality of life in adolescents with Turner syndrome. Am J Med Genet A. 2020;182(2):386–96.
79. Kruszka P, Silberbach M. The state of Turner syndrome science: are we on the threshold of discovery? Am J Med Genet C Semin Med Genet. 2019;181(1):4–6.

Eating Behavior and Psychopathology in Non-HIV Lipodystrophic Patients

35

Federica Ferrari, Pasquale Fabio Calabrò, Giovanni Ceccarini, and Ferruccio Santini

35.1 Background

Lipodystrophic disorders are a heterogeneous group of rare syndromes characterized by an abnormal physical appearance, due to a generalized or partial loss of subcutaneous adipose tissue [1]. The worldwide prevalence of non-HIV-related lipodystrophy is estimated to be 3.07 cases per million [2]; however, since the disease is unknown to most clinicians, the true prevalence is thought to be higher. Lipodystrophic patients are mainly females [3, 4], possibly because adipose tissue abnormalities and the related metabolic alterations become more evident than in males.

Due to the reduction of physiological sites of energy stores, triglycerides of exogenous and endogenous origin are accumulated in places such as the liver, skeletal muscle, heart, kidneys, and pancreas, predisposing to the development of insulin resistance and its complications: diabetes mellitus, dyslipidemia, hepatosteatosis, acanthosis nigricans, and polycystic ovary syndrome [1, 5, 6]. Loss of adipose tissue leads also to a proportional reduction of serum leptin levels, an adipokine produced exclusively by adipocytes. Leptin acts as a modulator of appetite (reducing caloric intake acting on both homeostatic and hedonic components of eating regulation), prevents lipotoxicity, increases glucose uptake in skeletal muscle, reduces hepatic gluconeogenesis, modulates immune responses, and influences bone remodelling and gonadotropins release. This state of leptin deficiency triggers hyperphagia and a vicious circle supporting the ectopic accumulation of lipids [1, 5–10].

F. Ferrari (✉) · P. F. Calabrò · G. Ceccarini · F. Santini (✉)
Obesity and Lipodystrophy Center, Endocrinology Unit, University Hospital of Pisa, Pisa, Italy
e-mail: giovanni.ceccarini@unipi.it; ferruccio.santini@med.unipi.it

Lipodystrophic syndromes are characterized by a very heterogenous phenotype and are usually classified as acquired or inherited (Fig. 35.1). There are partial forms, characterized by a regional fat loss, and generalized forms where subcutaneous adipose tissue is completely absent [1, 5, 7, 9]. Besides the metabolic complications, changes of the body shape and the related psychological distress are a major concern for patients suffering from this disease. Loss or abnormal distribution of adipose tissue produces different phenotypes that characterize the various types of lipodystrophies [5]. Patients with familial partial lipodystrophy of Dunnigan type, one of the most common subtypes, are characterized by a Cushingoid appearance with thin limbs, hump, moon face, and marked fat accumulation at the level of the neck [1, 5, 11]. Another partial familial form, known as Kobberling syndrome, is characterized by a marked loss of adipose tissue in the limbs (mainly lower) and in the buttocks, associated with abdominal obesity [12]. In patients with Barraquer-Simons syndrome, an acquired partial lipodystrophy, the loss of fatty tissue follows a craniocaudal progression pattern: there is an initial loss of fat in the face, followed by the shoulders, the upper limbs, and the abdomen, while fat is preserved in the lower limbs [5]. There are many other forms of lipodystrophy with peculiar phenotypes, which impact body shape: in some congenital lipodystrophies, the loss of adipose tissue is associated with an accelerated aging causing severe aesthetic impairment [9]. Prominent musculature and subcutaneous veins; buffalo hump; small size breast; acromegaloid features such as enlarged feet, hands, and jaw; mandibular and clavicular hypoplasia; elfic/triangular face; beak/pointed nose or wide nasal bridge; and various progeroid features may characterize specific lipodystrophy subtypes. In some partial forms, the normal body shape is preserved with a minimal loss of fat in very localized areas. Some syndromes may be associated with

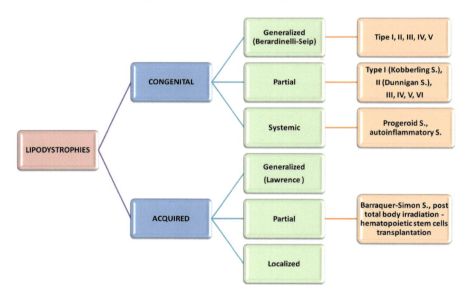

Fig. 35.1 Classification of lipodystrophies, from (Ref. [9]), modified

peculiar comorbidities such as deafness, immune defects, bone cysts, cardiomyopathies, or heart conduction defects [1, 5, 4, 11].

Fat loss is permanent, and treatment aims at improving the associated complications, first of all the metabolic abnormalities, by dietary intervention (hypolipidic, hypoglucidic, and normal or low-calorie diet), physical activity, and, when indicated, conventional drugs [4, 9]. Unfortunately, the compliance to dietary and lifestyle modifications is not always optimal, mainly because of the voracity driven by hypoleptinemia. In the most severe forms, hormonal replacement therapy by recombinant human leptin, named metreleptin, is an option. Approved by the Food and Drug Administration (FDA) in the USA since 2012 and by the European Medicines Agency (EMA) in Europe since July 2018, metreleptin induces satiety allowing easier adherence to dietary indications [4, 13]. Moreover, it has been recently shown that metreleptin therapy is capable of producing metabolic improvement, independently of the reduction of caloric intake [14].

35.2 Historical Perspectives

Case reports describing an association between the onset of lipodystrophy and mental illness have been published since the 1920s. Initially, a possible involvement of the central nervous system in the etiology of the syndrome was postulated. The onset of lipodystrophy was described after organic brain diseases: traumatisms (cerebral concussion), infections (encephalitis, meningitis), and neuroendocrine disorders (anterior hypothalamus lesions and pituitary diseases). Lipodystrophy was also described in patients affected by epilepsy or chorea, and the etiology of the disease was initially attributed to a primary neural alteration [15, 16]. Fascinated by the hypothesis of a connection between brain diseases and lipodystrophy, in the 1950s, R. Gibson, the director of an institution for the treatment of mental disorders, conducted a survey among 400 patients of his institute and found three patients with a lipodystrophic phenotype: a high prevalence for such a rare disease [17].

In the same years, some cases of psychological flare-up associated with lipodystrophy were reported; in particular, the onset of lipodystrophy was described in conjunction with personality changes (e.g., mental instability, aggressiveness and suicide attempts, psychosis), supporting the idea that lipodystrophy can predispose to psychological and psychiatric disorders [16].

The efforts of those authors to identify an etiological association between brain diseases and lipodystrophies were subsequently proven to be unsupported; indeed, only in very rare cases a connection between lipodystrophy and neurological diseases does actually exist. This is the case of the Berardinelli-Seip type II congenital lipodystrophy (BSCL-2), one of the most severe types of lipodystrophy, characterized by a generalized lack of adipose tissue, which in 80% of subjects is associated with a mild/severe mental retardation. BSCL-2 is transmitted as an autosomal recessive trait, and the disease-determining gene (BSCL-2), identified in 2001, encodes for an integral membrane protein of the endoplasmic reticulum, named Seipin, with an established role in the adipogenesis (it is involved in the formation of lipid droplets, lipolysis, metabolism of phospholipids, and calcium homeostasis in the endoplasmic reticulum); even if its function in the brain is not fully known, it is highly expressed in this site, and it is supposed to be responsible of the intellectual impairment associated with lipodystrophy, probably by a dysregulation of synaptic function [18–23]. A role for Seipin in neurological diseases is proved also by its involvement in some types of neuropathies, such as Celia's encephalopathy, a severe progressive neurodegenerative disease that can be associated with lipodystrophy. It has been postulated that the peculiar mutation of BSCL-2 leads to the accumulation of an aberrant protein (Celia seipin) in the neurons, responsible for cellular apoptosis [23].

Recently, different authors described four cases of children affected by acquired lipodystrophy associated with brain tumors (one craniopharyngioma and three astrocytomas). In these cases there was a temporal connection between removal of the tumor and an improvement of the lipodystrophy. The involvement of paraneoplastic autoantibodies in the etiology of lipodystrophy has been hypothesized, and an imaging study of brain in all children affected by acquired lipodystrophy is advised to exclude the coexistence of a cerebral neoplasia [24, 25].

35.3 Psychopathological Comorbidities

After the cases described in the 1950s, research has focused primarily on the metabolic complications related to lipodystrophies, and only recently there has been a renewed interest in the study of psychiatric comorbidities in affected patients. Indeed, both the European and American guidelines recommend the assessment of the psychopathological profile of lipodystrophic patients, to refer them to mental health professional for psychiatric and psychological support, if needed [4, 9, 16].

Scientific evidence indicates how lipodystrophic patients experience more psychological distress (Fig. 35.2) compared to the normal population or to patients affected by diabetes or morbid obesity [26, 27]. In two studies, comprising a total sample of 39 lipodystrophic subjects, 54% were affected by mood disorders [28, 29]. In the study conducted on 23 subjects with partial lipodystrophy (18 women and 5 men), the predominant mood disorder was depression, which affected 43% of the subjects, a higher proportion than that reported in diabetic patients (32%) [26, 29]. At variance, in the study conducted on a heterogeneous population of 16 lipodystrophic patients affected by partial or generalized forms, anxiety disorders were predominant (50%) [28]. There are many potential causes for the psychological distress observed in these patients. They report a sense of frustration due to the diagnostic delay. Achievement of a proper diagnosis may represent a positive, albeit transient, aid, and new frustration arises from the awareness that lipodystrophy is a chronic condition. A partial relief can be obtained by treatment of metabolic comorbidities, but aesthetic affliction has little chance to benefit from various therapies. Another frequent complaint of patients with lipodystrophy regards the need to provide to other people frequent explanations for their condition, denying, for example, of being anorectic and often not being taken seriously [30].

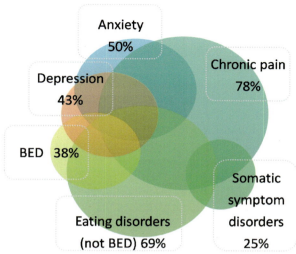

Fig. 35.2 Psychopathological and psychiatric disorders associated with lipodystrophy (*BED* Binge eating disorder). Data obtained from (Refs. [28, 29])

Lipodystrophic patients may exhibit body image disorders and develop chronic distress similarly to obese patients [28]. An altered distribution of adipose tissue modifies the body shape, and the risk of developing anxiety, depression, and low self-esteem is higher in lipodystrophic patients, especially women, in analogy with what occur to people suffering from other dysmorphisms [30]. In a study that evaluated the impact of lipodystrophy on body image, the sample of patients who consented to participate to the study consisted mainly of women, and only one man out of the five selected agreed to be enrolled [30]. The authors hypothesized that lipodystrophic men may be less influenced by changes of their body appearance and therefore would not be interested or not feel comfortable talking about this issue. At variance, women would be more frustrated by the dysmorphic features that characterize the disease and negatively affect their canons of femininity. Indeed, the lipodystrophic phenotype may be associated with muscular hypertrophy; hirsutism; masculinization; loss of female shapes caused by lack of adipose tissue from cheeks, buttocks, legs, and breasts; and adipose accumulation in abnormal sites such as neck, hump, and pubis [30]. Patients report that a critical time for the appearance of psychological distress is during adolescence, when the differences between male and female become more pronounced. It is common in clinical practice to find lipodystrophic women who complain having been bullied for their physical appearance and ask to undergo surgical procedures for aesthetic purposes (such as breast enlargement, liposuction of fat accumulated in ectopic sites) [30]. The chronic discomfort that patients affected by lipodystrophy experience in their daily lives, feeling observed and judged, could lead them to paranoid ideation [28].

Not all subjects are equally affected by the distressing effect of physical defects. The environment, e.g., the familiar support, could be crucial in this regard. Different authors report that lipodystrophic patients do not feel sufficiently understood by family members; it is possible that an effective support may derive from getting to know other people affected by a similar condition through patient associations or social networks, since it is easier to interact with people who have a direct experience of the disease, without having to give them discomforting explanations [28, 30].

A relevant proportion of patients (78.3%) suffer from chronic pain of different origins: neuropathic, arthritic, fibromyalgic, and myopathic [28, 29]. The prevalence of a somatic symptom disorder with predominant pain has been found in up to 25% of lipodystrophic patients; the origin of pain could depend on the ectopic accumulation of lipids in the muscles or the nerves. Chronic pain interferes with daily life by multiple means, and the consequent reduction of physical activity contributes to worsening of metabolic complications. Chronic pain, anxiety, and depression are overlapping disorders, and each one concurs to the development or the worsening of the others [31]. By assessing pain on WHYMPI (West Haven-Yale Multidimensional Pain Inventory) scale, it has been shown that pain negatively affects social and personal life, similarly to what occurs to oncologic patients [28]. Another psychopathological feature of lipodystrophic patients is represented by eating behavior disorders: a binge eating disorder (BED) has been reported in almost 40% of patients and an eating disorder not otherwise specified in an even greater percentage (69%); this second group of disorders includes emotional eating, night eating syndrome, bulimia nervosa, dysfunctional eating, atypical anorexia nervosa, and sub-threshold binge eating disorders [28]. BED is considerably more prevalent than in severe obese individuals, among whom it is estimated to be around 17%; moreover, at variance with obese subjects, food craving is influenced mainly by internal cues rather than by external stimuli (such as the environment, conviviality, the appearance of food). Furthermore, evidence has been provided that the food-related reward in lipodystrophic patients is reduced as compared with obese or normal subjects [27, 28, 32, 33]. We can speculate that hypoleptinemia is the most important internal cue, responsible for food craving in lipodystrophic patients [28]. Indeed, leptin is a fundamental hormone in the regulation of hunger, by acting as an indicator of body energy reserves; an increase in leptin levels stimulates the hypothalamic neurons to release satiety signals. Since leptin is produced only in the adipose tissue, in lipodystrophic patients there is a characteristic state of hypoleptinemia, which can be mild (as in some partial forms) or complete (as in generalized forms) [6]. Lack of leptin action is therefore responsible for hyperphagia that characterizes the more severe forms of lipodystrophy.

Obese subjects affected by congenital leptin deficiency, due to missense mutations of the leptin gene, undergo normalization of body weight, hunger, and caloric intake when treated with the lacking hormone. Metreleptin administration leads to an activation of the brain regions that exert an inhibitory control of appetite, while reducing the activity of areas that stimulate hunger, as assessed in functional imaging studies [33–37]. In two studies comprising a sample of 19 lipodystrophic patients (10 affected by generalized forms and 9 by partial lipodystrophies), a functional brain MRI was performed in different conditions: before and after meal and before and after metreleptin treatment (up to 52 weeks of therapy) [10, 38]. The results of these studies show that the satiety after a meal (as evaluated by questionnaires and behavioral tests) is reduced in lipodystrophic patients compared to the healthy controls and that the feeling of fullness after a meal is implemented by metreleptin therapy. Consistent with these findings, functional imaging showed increased brain activity after metreleptin therapy in different areas such as the hypothalamus, insula/superior temporal gyrus, medial prefrontal cortex, and amygdala (areas involved in the homeostatic and hedonic control of food behavior). These results support the pathophysiological role of leptin deficiency in driving eating behavior disorders in lipodystrophic patients [10, 38].

Leptin is also considered a player involved in mood regulation. Experiments on adult mice, made leptin-resistant by the deletion of leptin receptor in the hippocampus, show behaviors compatible with a depressive attitude, as assessed by multiple tests (tail suspension test, preference test for sucrose, and learned helplessness test). Therefore, in animal models it is possible to induce a "depressive state" only by altering the leptin signaling pathway at the hippocampal level. In line with these findings, systemic leptin administration or direct injection in the hippocampus reverses the depression-like behavior of mice, with an effect similar to that of antidepressant drugs [39, 40].

A role for leptin in the pathogenesis of depression is also supported by the finding that the leptin receptor gene is expressed in serotonergic, gabaergic, and dopaminergic neurons, neurotransmitters that are all involved in mood control. Additional studies have shown a role for leptin in inducing the expression of the brain-derived neurotrophic factor (BDNF) mRNA, whose deficit, according to current neurotrophic theory, would be responsible for the development of depression [41, 42].

Based on these observations, we may hypothesize that therapy with recombinant human leptin, which in the context of lipodystrophy is primarily employed to treat metabolic comorbidities, might also be effective to improve the associated psychopathological symptoms. This view can be hardly reconciled with results of studies conducted in obese patients, which correlate increased leptin serum values with depression phenotypes [39, 41, 43, 44]. This controversy can be explained by the state of leptin resistance that characterizes obesity: obese patients have high serum leptin levels, but the efficacy of the hormone is reduced in the central nervous system, mimicking a leptin deficiency state [39, 41, 43, 44]. In these conditions, the absolute value of leptinemia can be misleading, and indicators better than leptin alone have been studied, for example, IGFBP-2 (insulin growth factor binding protein type 2), a leptin-regulated serum protein, as possible markers of leptin action [45]. Likewise, the BDNF/leptin ratio has been proposed as a prognostic index for the response to antidepressant therapy [46].

35.4 Conclusions

Lipodystrophy is frequently associated to psychopathological and psychiatric disorders that must be effectively researched and treated; too often, at least in the past, clinicians have focused on treating the metabolic aspects of the disease, with limited attention to the psychological well-being. Lipodystrophic patients themselves report to perceive lack of psychological support and ask for it. Evaluating psychological distress, even when mild, appears to be very important, and improving it can indeed impact positively on the other comorbidities. Since the cornerstone of the treatment of metabolic complications of lipodystrophy is a constant (long-life) adherence to diet and physical activity, any form of psychophysical distress (such as anxiety, depression, pain) could worsen the compliance to the dietary-behavioral advices. Nevertheless, scientific evidence available to date is scarce and derives from heterogeneous casistics. Studies on larger and more homogeneous samples, which take into account the genetic background and use modified scales for the assessment of psychopathological features, first of all food behavior disorders, are the next steps to be taken for a better understanding of these aspects and to guide the treatment of lipodystrophic patients.

References

1. Garg A. Acquired and Inherited Lipodystrophies. N Engl J Med. 2004;350:1220–34.
2. Chiquette E, Oral EA, Garg A, Araujo-Vilar D, Dhankhar P. Estimating the prevalence of generalized and partial lipodystrophy: findings and challenges. Diabetes Metab Syndr Obes. 2017;10:375–83.
3. Garg A. Gender differences in the prevalence of metabolic complications in familial partial lipodystrophy (Dunnigan variety). J Clin Endocrinol Metab. 2000;85:1776–82.
4. Brown RJ, Cheung PT, Dunger D, Garg A, Jack M, Mungai L, Oral EA, Patni N, Rother KI, von Schnurbein J, Sorkina E, Stanley T, Vigouroux C, Wabitsch M, Williams R, Yorifuji T. The diagnosis and management of lipodystrophy syndromes: a multi-society practice guideline. J Clin Endocrinol Metab. 2016;101:4500–11.
5. Hussain I, Garg A. Lipodystrophy Syndromes. Endocrinol Metab Clin North Am. 2016;45:783–97.
6. Florenza C, Chou S, Mantzoros S. Lipodystrophy: pathophysiology and advances in treatment. Nat Rev Endocrinol. 2011;7:137–50.
7. Patni N, Garg A. Congenital generalized lipodystrophies-new insights into metabolic dysfunction. Nat Rev Endocrinol. 2015;11:522–34.
8. Berger S, Ceccarini G, Scabia G, Barone I, Pelosini C, Ferrari F, Magno S, Dattilo A, Chiovato L, Vitti P, Santini F, Maffei M. Lipodystrophy and obesity are associated with decreased number of T cells with regulatory function and pro-inflammatory macrophage phenotype. Int J Obes (Lond). 2017;11:1676–84.
9. Araùjo-Vilar D, Santini F. Diagnosis and treatment of lipodystrophy: a step-by-step approach. J Endocrinol Invest. 2018;1:61–73.
10. Schlögl H, Müller K, Horstmann A, Miehle K, Püschel J, Villringer A, Pleger B, Stumvoll M, Fasshauer M. Leptin substitution in patients with lipodystrophy: neural correlates for long-term success in the normalization of eating behavior. Diabetes. 2016;65:2179–86.
11. Lightbourne M, Brown RJ. Genetics of lipodystrophy. Endocrinol Metab Clin North Am. 2017;2:539–54.
12. Guillín-Amarelle C, Sánchez-Iglesias S, Castro-Pais A, Rodríguez-Cañete L, Ordóñez-Mayán L, Pazos M, González-Méndez B, Rodríguez-García S, Casanueva F, Fernández-Marmiesse A, Araújo-Vilar D. Type 1 familial partial lipodystrophy: understanding the Köbberling syndrome. Endocrine. 2016;2:411–21.
13. https://www.ema.europa.eu/en/medicines/human/EPAR/myalepta
14. Brown RJ, Valencia A, Startzell M. Metreleptin-mediated improvements in insulin sensitivity are independent of food intake in humans with lipodystrophy. J Clin Invest. 2018;8:3504–16.
15. Warin RP, Ingram JT. Progressive lipodystrophy report of two cases. Lancet. 1950;6619:55–7.
16. Fowler PBS. Lipodystrophia progressiva and temporary hydronephrosis. Br Med J. 1955;4924:1249–51.

17. Gibson R. The occurrence of progressive lipodystrophy in mental defectives. Can Med Assoc J. 1957;3:217–9.
18. Shawky RM, Gamal R, Seifeldin NS. Berardinelli–Seip syndrome type 2—an Egyptian child. Egypt J Med Human Genet. 2015;16:189–93.
19. Van Maldergem L. Berardinelli-Seip congenital lipodystrophy. In: Adam MP, Ardinger HH, Pagon RA, Wallace SE, LJH B, Stephens K, Amemiya A, editors. GeneReviews. Seattle: University of Washington; 2003. p. 1993–2020.
20. Ding L, Yang X, Tian H, Liang J, Zhang F, Wang G, Wang Y, Ding M, Shui G, Huang X. Seipin regulates lipid homeostasis by ensuring calcium-dependent mitochondrial metabolism. EMBO J. 2018;37:1–17.
21. Van Maldergem L, Magré J, Khallouf TE, Gedde-Dahl T Jr, Delépine M, Trygstad O, Seemanova E, Stephenson T, Albott CS, Bonnici F, Panz VR, Medina JL, Bogalho P, Huet F, Savasta S, Verloes A, Robert JJ, Loret H, De Kerdanet M, Tubiana-Rufi N, Mégarbané A, Maassen J, Polak M, Lacombe D, Kahn CR, Silveira EL, D'Abronzo FH, Grigorescu F, Lathrop M, Capeau J, O'Rahilly S. Genotype-phenotype relationships in Berardinelli-Seip congenital lipodystrophy. PLoS One. 2016;7:e0158874.
22. Wei S, Soh SL, Qiu W, Yang W, Seah CJ, Guo J, Ong WY, Pang ZP, Han W. Seipin regulates excitatory synaptic transmission in cortical neurons. J Neurochem. 2013;4:478–89.
23. Sánchez-Iglesias S, Unruh-Pinheiro A, Guillín-Amarelle C, González-Méndez B, Ruiz-Riquelme A, Rodríguez-Cañete BL, Rodríguez-García S, Guillén-Navarro E, Domingo-Jiménez R, Araújo-Vilar D. Skipped BSCL2 transcript in Celia's encephalopathy (PELD): new insights on fatty acids involvement, senescence and adipogenesis. J Med Genet. 2002;10:722–33.
24. Patni N, Alves C, von Schnurbein J, Wabitsch M, Tannin G, Rakheja D, Garg A. A novel syndrome of generalized lipodystrophy associated with pilocytic astrocytoma. J Clin Endocrinol Metab. 2015;10:3603–6.
25. Lockemer HE, Sumpter KM, Cope-Yokoyama S, Garg A. A novel paraneoplastic syndrome with acquired lipodystrophy and chronic inflammatory demyelinating polyneuropathy in an adolescent male with craniopharyngioma. J Pediatr Endocrinol Metab. 2017;4:479–83.
26. Anderson RJ, Clouse RE, Freedland KE, Lustman PJ. The prevalence of comorbid depression in adults with diabetes: a meta-analysis. Diabetes Care. 2011;6:1069–78.
27. Dawes AJ, Maggard-Gibbons M, Maher AR, Booth MJ, Miake-Lye I, Beroes JM, Shekelle PG. Mental health conditions among patients seeking and undergoing bariatric surgery: a meta-analysis. JAMA. 2016;2:150–63.
28. Calabrò PF, Ceccarini G, Calderone A, Lippi C, Piaggi P, Ferrari F, Magno S, Pedrinelli R, Santini F. Psychopathological and psychiatric evaluation of patients affected by lipodystrophy. Eat Weight Disord. 2019; https://doi.org/10.1007/s40519-019-00716-6.
29. Ajluni N, Meral R, Neidert AH, Brady GF, Buras E, McKenna B, DiPaola F, Chenevert TL, Horowitz JF, Buggs-Saxton C, Rupani AR, Thomas PE, Tayeh MK, Innis JW, Omary MB, Conjeevaram H, Oral EA. Spectrum of disease associated with partial lipodystrophy (PL): lessons from a trial cohort. Clin Endocrinol (Oxf). 2017;5:698–707.
30. Adams C, Stears A, Savage D, Deaton C. "We're stuck with what we've got": the impact of lipodystrophy on body image. J Clin Nurs. 2018;9–10:1958–68.
31. Katz J, Rosenbloom BN, Fascler S. Chronic pain, psychopathology, and DSM-5 somatic symptom disorder. Can J Psychiatry. 2015;4:160–7.
32. Innamorati M, Imperatori C, Balsamo M. Food craving questionnaire-trait (FCQ-T) discriminates between obese and overweight patients with and without binge eating tendencies: the italian version of the FCQ-T. J Pers Assess. 2014;6:632–9.
33. Farooqi IS, Bullmore E, Keogh J, Gillard J, O'Rahilly S, Fletcher PC. Leptin regulates striatal regions and human eating behavior. Science. 2007;5843:1–3.
34. Baicy K, London ED, Monterosso J, Wong ML, Delibasi T, Sharma A, Licinio J. Leptin replacement alters brain response to food cues in genetically leptin-deficient adults. Proc Natl Acad Sci U S A. 2007;46:18,276–9.
35. Frank S, Heni M, Moss A, von Schnurbein J, Fritsche A, Häring HU, Farooqi S, Preissl H, Wabitsch M. Leptin therapy in a congenital leptin-deficient patient leads to acute and long-

term changes in homeostatic, reward, and food-related brain areas. J Clin Endocrinol Metab. 2011;8:E1283–7.
36. Frank S, Heni M, Moss A, von Schnurbein J, Farooqi S, Häring H-U, Fritsche A, Preissl H, Wabitsch M. Long-term stabilization effects of leptin on brain functions in a leptin-deficient patient. PLoS One. 2013;6:e65893.
37. Farr OM, Florenza C, Papageorgiou P. Leptin therapy alters appetite and neural responses to food stimuli in brain areas of leptin-sensitive subjects without altering brain structure. J Clin Endocrinol Metab. 2014;12:E2529–38.
38. Aotani D, Ebihara K, Sawamoto N, Kusakabe T, Aizawa-Abe M, Kataoka S, Sakai T, Iogawa H, Ebihara C, Fujikura J, Hosoda K, Fukuyama H, Nakao K. Functional magnetic resonance imaging analysis of food-related brain activity in patients with lipodystrophy undergoing leptin replacement therapy. J Clin Endocrinol Metab. 2012;10:3663–71.
39. Zaraouna S, Wozniak G, Papachristou AI. Mood disorders: a potential link between ghrelin and leptin on human body? World J Exp Med. 2015;2:103–9.
40. Lu XY. The leptin hypothesis of depression: a potential link between mood disorders and obesity? Curr Opin Pharmacol. 2007;6:648–52.
41. Yildiz G, Senturk MB, Yildiz P, Cakmak Y, Budak MS, Cakar E. Serum serotonin, leptin and adiponectin changes in women with postpartum depression: controlled study. Arch Gynecol Obstet. 2017;4:853–8.
42. Zou X, Zhong L, Zhu C, Zhao H, Zhao F, Cui R, Gao S, Li B. Role of leptin in mood disorder and neurodegenerative disease. Front Neurosci. 2019;378:1–8.
43. Cernea S, Both E, Huțanu A, Șular FL, Roiban AL. Correlation of serum leptin and leptin resistance with depression and anxiety in patient with type 2 diabetes. Psychiatry Clin Neurosci. 2019;12:745–53.
44. Syk M, Ellström S, Mwinyi J, Schiöth HB, Ekselius L, Ramklint M, Cunningham JL. Plasma levels of leptin and adiponectin and depressive symptoms in young adults. Psychiatry Res. 2018;272:1–7.
45. Ceccarini G, Pelosini C, Ferrari F, Magno S, Vitti J, Salvetti G, Moretto C, Marioni A, Buccianti P, Piaggi P, Maffei M, Santini F. Serum IGF-binding protein 2 (IGFBP-2) concentrations change early after gastric bypass bariatric surgery revealing a possible marker of leptin sensitivity in obese subjects. Endocrine. 2019;65:86–93.
46. An JH, Jang EH, Kim AY, Fava M, Mischoulon D, Papakostas GI, Na EJ, Jang J, Yu HY, Hong JP, Jeon HJ. Ratio of plasma BDNF to leptin levels are associated with treatment response in major depressive disorder but not in panic disorder: a 12-week follow-up study. J Affect Disord. 2019;259:349–54.

36

Adipositas Athletica, Anorexia Athletica, Chewing and Spitting, Eating Disorders by Proxy, Emetophobia, Picky Eating ... Symptoms, Syndromes, or What?

Massimo Cuzzolaro

36.1 Introduction

In the field of feeding and eating disorders, DSM-5 [1] and ICD-11 [2] list six major diagnostic categories: pica, rumination-regurgitation disorder, avoidant-restrictive food intake disorder (ARFID), anorexia nervosa (AN), bulimia nervosa (BN), and binge eating disorder (BED). In addition to these six full syndromes, subliminal clinical pictures are collected in the seventh category, other specified feeding and eating disorders: e.g., purging disorder [3] and atypical anorexia nervosa not underweight [4, 5]. Finally, feeding or eating disorder, unspecified, is the eighth residual category.

Some behavioral frameworks such as *night eating syndrome* and *orthorexia nervosa* are the subject of increasing studies and could become autonomous categories in future taxonomies.

Furthermore, new expressions used to describe other phenomena related to food and eating are continually appearing in the scientific literature.

Feederism, gourmand syndrome, mukbang, pregorexia, and wannarexia are terms to which it may be useful to devote a brief citation.

Feederism appears in some articles [6–8] to indicate a connection between feeding and eroticism: feeders are sexually aroused by feeding their partners and encouraging them to gain weight, while feedees are individuals sexually aroused by being fed and the idea of gaining weight.

The expression *gourmand syndrome* is sometimes used to refer to an abnormal preoccupation with preparing and eating fine-quality food, associated with a neurological disease. Gourmand syndrome involves lesions of anterior portions of the

M. Cuzzolaro (✉)
University of Roma Sapienza, Roma, Italy
e-mail: massimo.cuzzolaro@gmail.com

© Springer Nature Switzerland AG 2022
E. Manzato et al. (eds.), *Hidden and Lesser-known Disordered Eating Behaviors in Medical and Psychiatric Conditions*,
https://doi.org/10.1007/978-3-030-81174-7_36

right cerebral hemisphere involving cortical areas, basal ganglia, amygdala, and other limbic structures [9, 10]. It has been described in both adults and children [11].

The Korean word *mukbang* (eating broadcast) indicates an increasingly widespread Internet phenomenon. It started in South Korea around 2014 and has become a global phenomenon. It consists of video recordings spread online in which a person is seen eating. The most popular mukbang YouTube videos are those with provocative content, such as eating large amounts of food [12]. Some studies suggest that individuals who frequently watch mukbang are at higher risk of disordered eating behaviors [13, 14].

Only one article available in PubMed is dedicated to the term *pregorexia* [15]. The word refers to cases in which a woman adopts or resumes unhealthy behaviors (such as extreme dieting, excessive exercise, self-induced vomiting) to avoid pregnancy weight gain. The phenomenon is notable and harmful, but the neologism has not had any luck.

Wannarexia is a derogatory term. It is used mainly by teenagers to indicate those who claim to be part of the diagnosis of anorexia nervosa without having the characteristics of that disease [16]. The word has had some use, particularly in pro-ana and pro-mia groups but no scientific literature.

This chapter will focus at greater length on six terms that have appeared in recent decades and have received significant attention in the scientific literature: *adipositas athletica*, *anorexia athletica*, *chewing and spitting*, *eating disorders by proxy*, *emetophobia*, and *picky eating*.

36.2 Adipositas Athletica

Some athletes seek a large body with excess body fat because they benefit from it in competitions. The reasons may be various:

- Fat increases energy reserves.
- Fat increases the thermal insulation of the body.
- A heavier body allows a sailor to better resist the wind and balance a racing boat.
- A larger and heavier body makes one more competitive in physical confrontations or explosive muscular efforts.

Some sports especially favor this condition:

- American football
- Hammer throw
- Open-water long-distance swimming
- Sailing (crewmembers)
- Shot put
- Sumo wrestling [17].

Berglund and collaborators introduced the expression adipositas athletica in 2011 and proposed two criteria [18]:

- Being an elite athlete
- Having a higher than athletic normal (Greek Olympic ideals) fat mass. It is essential to refer to the body composition and not to the body mass index (BMI): an athlete can have a high body weight due to lean body mass [19].

However, this definition includes both elite athletes who become obese intentionally and those to whom this happens without the intention of gaining weight.

Second, the term elite athlete is not well defined and is used in scientific literature in different ways based on professionalism, years of experience, or achievements [20].

Finally, a higher fat mass than athletic normal is a vague criterion.

The concept of adipositas athletica has not had much luck so far and does not appear in research papers in recent years.

However, overweight and obese athletes do exist, and their condition has not been adequately studied. Little is known about their diet, morbidity, mortality, and short- and long-term quality of life, apart from a few old studies devoted to sumo wrestlers [21, 22]. Adequate studies on prevention and treatment interventions for these particular clinical pictures and motivational processes are lacking.

As a side note, regarding the relationship between sport and obesity, it is known that several retired athletes develop overweight/obesity. This phenomenon also deserves prevention and treatment interventions [23].

36.3 Anorexia Athletica

Few studies have been devoted to anorexia athletica (AA), using this term, and even fewer to male cases [24].

The expression—*Sportanorexie* in German [25]—was coined to denote a sport-related eating disorder. The term refers to unhealthy eating and weight control behaviors of athletes engaged in sports in which achieving and maintaining low body weight are required or are an advantage in competitions.

In 1980, an article published in *Pediatrics* reported excessive weight loss and food aversion in athletes [26]. According to the author, this condition closely resembled anorexia nervosa but occurred more often in men than in women, was not underlain by severe emotional problems, and had a good prognosis if appropriately treated medically and nutritionally.

Despite the statement just above, AA studies have involved female athletes more often than men [27].

In a pioneering and still interesting Norwegian research of 1994, Jorunn Sundgot-Borgen examined 603 elite female athletes (ages 12–35 years) who practiced different sports [28]:

- Aesthetic or appearance-oriented sports (e.g., gymnastics)
- Ball games (e.g., tennis)
- Endurance sports (e.g., biathlon)
- Power sports (e.g., shot put)
- Technical sports (e.g., alpine skiing)
- Weight-dependent sports (e.g., judo).

In this study, "an elite athlete was defined as one who qualified for the national team at junior or senior levels or was a member of a recruiting squad for those teams" (p. 414).

Based on a self-administered questionnaire—Eating Disorder Inventory [29]—the authors identified 117 women at risk for eating disorders. Ninety-two of them, examined with a clinical interview, met the criteria for eating disorders:

- 7 anorexia nervosa (AN)
- 42 bulimia nervosa (BN)
- 43 anorexia athletica (AA).

The prevalence of eating disorders was higher among those who practiced sports that require leanness (aesthetic sports) or a specific weight (weight-dependent sports).

The DSM-III-R was used as diagnostic criteria for AN and BN [30]. For AA diagnosis, the authors used six criteria. It may be useful to summarize them (Table 36.1).

Davison et al. observed that weight concerns begin early, as early as 5–7 years of age, in girls engaged in aesthetic sports [31].

Matejek et al. compared a group of elite gymnasts with AA with a sample of girls with AN: girls with AA had percentages of fat mass and blood levels of leptin even more decreased and had delays in bone maturation and menarche [32].

Significant quantitative and qualitative nutritional deficiencies were found in female elite athletes: low mean intake of energy, carbohydrates, calcium, iron, and vitamin D [33].

Table 36.1 Anorexia athletica. Diagnostic criteria used by Sundgot-Borgen [28]

• Weight loss >5% of expected body weight
• Absence of medical illness or affective disorder explaining the weight reduction
• Excessive fear of becoming obese
• Restriction of caloric intake
• Gastrointestinal complaints

• One or more of the following features:
  – Binge eating
  – Body image disturbance
  – Compulsive exercising
  – Delayed puberty
  – Menstrual dysfunction
  – Purging

Female athlete triad (FAT) is the expression used to indicate the pathological interaction in female athletes between three components: energy availability, menstrual function, and bone mineral density.

The three components should be considered along with a continuum model, from health to disease. At the pathological end of the spectrum (FAT), they combine together:

- Low energy availability, with or without a recognizable clinical eating disorder
- Functional hypothalamic amenorrhea or menstrual disorder
- Osteopenia/osteoporosis.

The prevalence of FAT is highest among aesthetic athletes, including dancers. In these populations, educational interventions that increase knowledge of the triad [34] may be useful to prevent serious consequences, particularly bone stress injuries and spontaneous fractures [35].

Assessment tools have been developed to identify athletes at increased risk for low energy availability. Concordance in recognition of risk is quite good but is lower in the assignment of risk levels (high, moderate, or low) [36]:

- Female Athlete Triad Coalition cumulative risk assessment (Triad CRA) [37]
- Relative energy deficiency in sport clinical assessment tool (RED-S CAT) [38].

Male athlete triad (MAT) is the expression used to indicate that similar processes can also occur in male athletes: low energy availability (with or without disordered eating), hypogonadotropic hypogonadism, and low bone mineral density. They require attention for the consequences on bone health and reproductive function [39, 40].

In a sample of male distance runners, higher scores in a modified Triad CRA were associated with higher rates of bone stress injuries [41].

Coaches and athletic trainers have essential responsibilities.

In 2008, the American Athletic Trainers' Association published a position statement with recommendations for preventing, detecting, and comprehensively managing disordered eating behaviors in athletes [42].

The paper emphasized the high frequency of eating disorders in these populations, with prevalence estimates ranging up to 33% among male athletes and 62% among female athletes. However, in the text, the expression anorexia athletica never appears, and the pathologies reported were only those of the DSM-IV [43]: AN, BN, and eating disorders not otherwise specified (EDNOS) with particular attention to the female athlete triad. The term AA does not appear even in the same association's subsequent position statement dedicated to safe weight loss and maintenance practices in sport and exercise [44].

It is not easy to think that AA deserves diagnostic autonomy.

In several female athletes [27] and some male athletes—e.g., low weight category rowers and wrestlers [45]—the pressure to improve performance and physical appearance and maintain a low body weight may be added to other predisposing and precipitating factors, both personal and familial [46]. This concurrence of elements that induce the pursuit of unrealistic body weight goals precipitates persistent and dangerous pathology.

Eating disorder prevention programs specific to athletes involved in weight-sensitive sports are desirable [47]. A randomized controlled trial showed that a brief (4 h) intervention produces some small benefits through 18-month follow-up: reduced dietary restraint, lower thin-ideal internalization, and increased BMI [48].

The intersection of physical activity and sports and disturbed eating behaviors needs to be looked at from several perspectives. The relationships that link them are multiple and contradictory.

First, regular exercise improves health and well-being and is a protective, preventive, and curative factor for many long-term illnesses, including eating and weight disorders [49]. For example, dance movement therapy is part of such complementary treatment options, particularly for AN [50].

However, as we have seen, physical activity and sports can promote the development of eating-related pathology. Competitive and aesthetic sports, including dance [51], are considered for a long time among the risk factors for developing sport-related eating disorders because they emphasize thinness and physical appearance [52].

Lastly, compulsive exercise is a symptom of many patients diagnosed with AN and BN [49].

More than a century ago, Max Wallet already reported the need to move continuously to counteract the effects of food on body weight. Mademoiselle B (kg 27, m. 1.60, BMI 10.5), forced to stay in bed, "jumped on the bed, moved her arms and legs, did somersaults, and gesticulations of all sorts" [53] (p. 276).

In this regard, it should be noted that sometimes the expression AA is also used for non-athletes, in cases of eating disorders in which excessive/compulsive exercise is one of the main symptoms directed to weight control [54]. *Hypergymnasia* and *exercise bulimia* are other terms used for this symptom.

The boundaries of the concept of AA become, thus, even broader and more uncertain.

36.4 Chewing and Spitting

Chewing and spitting out food without swallowing (CHSP) is a behavior described as early as the end of the nineteenth century in a girl with anorexia nervosa. She was another patient of Max Wallet—Mademoiselle V (kg 35.4, m. 1.57, BMI 14.4)—who, obsessed with the fear of gaining weight, "put food in her mouth to taste it, but then spit it out" [53] (p. 276).

CHSP is a disordered eating behavior defined in 1995 as a neglected symptom [55] and, according to a 2016 systematic review, still poorly studied [56].

It has the character of a weight management technique or compensatory behavior to lose weight or not gain it while still enjoying the taste of food. It is mostly associated with other AN and BN symptoms, full syndrome or subliminal.

The amount of food chewed and spat out is sometimes very large [57]. However, Guarda et al. found that CHSP is more closely associated with restrictive behaviors than binge eating [58]. This finding suggests that most chewers/spitters use small amounts of food. The presence of a sense of loss of control is not clear.

In the DSM-IV, CHSP was among the examples of eating disorders not otherwise specified (EDNOS) and associated with large amounts of food: "Repeatedly chewing and spitting out, but not swallowing, large amounts of food" [59] (p. 550). This feature was disproved by the survey already mentioned [58].

CHSP does not appear among the diagnostic categories of the DSM-5 and ICD-11, nor among the symptoms required for the diagnosis of feeding and eating disorders, and not even among the examples of other specified feeding and eating disorders (OSFED) [1, 2]. This absence probably depends on an underestimation of the prevalence of the phenomenon.

In treatment-seeking individuals with eating disorders (ED), CHSP lifetime prevalences range from 22% [60] to 64.5% [61].

In a sample of 972 outpatients with ED, Durkin et al. found a lifetime prevalence of 30.4% and a current prevalence of 20.7%. CHSP was more frequent among younger patients, with lower BMI and more severe symptoms (restriction, compensatory behaviors). CHSP was more common among patients with AN and BN than among those with subthreshold disorders [62].

A further study of 359 patients with ED found a similar lifetime prevalence of CHSP (24.5%) and, again, an association with more pathologic eating behaviors [63].

Makhzoumi et al. studied 324 inpatients with ED. Approximately one in five reported CHSP at least once a week in the 2 months before admission. CHSP appeared again as a marker of increased severity for eating behaviors, body dissatisfaction, depression, and neuroticism [64].

Surveys such as the above were conducted in clinical samples with eating disorders. Little was known about the prevalence of CHSP in general population samples until two recent Australian papers.

The first study examined a sample of 3047 persons aged 15 years and older. CHSP point prevalence was 0.4%. This behavior was associated with other compensatory disordered eating behaviors and reduced physical and mental health-related quality of life. The median age of participants with CHSP was 39 years [65].

The second study examined 5111 adolescents (11–19 years of age) and found a 12.2% point prevalence rate for CHSP. Adolescents reporting CHSP also reported higher levels of psychological distress and lower levels of health-related quality of life [66].

A qualitative study of 18 cases with CHSP—conducted using the methodology of interpretative phenomenological analysis—found that CHSP can be [67]:

- Associated with negative emotions, particularly shame
- Accentuated by stressful situations
- A way of giving oneself pleasure, relief, and distraction
- Addictive
- Ritualistic
- Harmful to physical, psychological, and social health.

There is no evidence for specific treatments. As for medications, an article reported benefits with selective serotonin reuptake inhibitors (SSRIs) in one case of AN with CHSP and severe weight loss [68].

36.5 Eating Disorders by Proxy

Some historical references can be useful to frame the phenomenon.

In 1951, Asher proposed the expression Münchausen's syndrome to indicate the condition of a patient who invents and produces signs and symptoms, physical and/or psychological, to assume the role of sick and get attention, diagnostic investigations, hospitalization, and treatment [69]. He was inspired by Baron Münchausen, the protagonist of a book by Rudolf Erich Raspe (1736–1794), whose characteristic was to tell grandiose and false stories.

In 1977, Meadow published a paper on a form of child abuse that he called Münchausen's syndrome by proxy [70]. He applied it to the case where an adult—mostly a parent, more often the mother—invents or produces symptoms in a child. In DSM-5 [1] and ICD-11 [2], the formula "by proxy" has been replaced by "Factitious disorder imposed on another." The core feature is intentionally feigning, falsifying, inducing, or aggravating physical and psychological signs, symptoms, and injuries in another person (in most cases, a small and dependent child, sometimes an adult, and even an animal).

In all of these cases—as opposed to malingering—there is no discernible practical advantage (such as obtaining compensation, escaping prosecution). The motivation is linked to personal problems, conscious and, above all, unconscious.

36.5.1 Anorexia Nervosa by Proxy

The expression was used in 1985 by Katz et al. [71] and again in 1996 by the Japanese physician Honjo [72].

Honjo described a mother who brought her daughter to the hospital reporting that the child had been overeating for over a year. The child was 25 months old, underfed, and of low weight. The mother, who had suffered from AN, subjected her daughter to severe dietary restrictions. The author suggested that the mother projected her body weight and shape concerns onto her daughter [72].

Since then, the expression "AN by proxy" has rarely reappeared in the scientific literature [73], although several papers have been published on the impact of maternal eating disorders on child nutrition.

In the late 1980s, van Wezel-Meijler and Wit studied seven children with low weight-for-height and stunting. They were underfed and were children of three mothers with a history of AN. The authors advanced the hypothesis that children of mothers with a history of AN constitute a high-risk group for malnutrition and stunted growth [74].

Gerald Russell et al. studied the children of eight mothers who had suffered from AN [75]. Nine children (one girl and eight boys) had suffered from food deprivation, but the authors did not use the term AN by proxy. In one of these cases, lengthy treatment of the mother with various hospitalizations and family therapy produced benefits.

A recent systematic review found that mothers with a history of eating disorders often manifest problems in feeding their children, starting from breastfeeding, but the term "by proxy" was never used in this article [76].

36.5.2 Orthorexia Nervosa by Proxy

Although orthorexia nervosa is not yet a recognized diagnostic category, it seems possible to attribute the expression "orthorexia nervosa by proxy" to some recent cases [77].

In July 2016, a 13-month-old child was admitted to a Milan hospital against parental advice. He weighed 5.2 kilos, and his growth was below the third percentile. Doctors were faced with an emaciated body, muscular hypotonia, and severe motor and cognitive skills impairment. The results of laboratory and instrumental tests were very alarming and consistent with a state of extreme malnutrition. An inflexible vegan diet, imposed by the parents, was at the origin of the problem. It is known that veganism, even in adults, requires a well-balanced diet that includes adequate nutritional supplements. In infants, uncontrolled vegan diets are dangerous.

36.5.3 Treatment

In all cases of Factitious disorder imposed on another, the first goal must be protecting the child. The team that handles these cases should usually include a social worker. Judicial measures may be necessary. Effective interventions on perpetrators are problematic because they tend to deny the problem, lie, and evade treatment.

When possible, therapy is psychological, directed at helping the person discover the secret motivations for their behavior, the thoughts, desires, and emotions at play.

36.6 Emetophobia

The word is derived from ancient Greek: ἔμεσις (vomiting) + φόβος (fear). The term indicates an intense and irrational fear of vomiting and avoidance behaviors of situations associated with nausea and vomiting.

The DSM-5 [1] classifies emetophobia among anxiety disorders as a specific phobia, other type, of vomiting (SPOV). The diagnosis requires that the symptoms last for at least 6 months and create significant distress or impairment. Unlike DSM-IV [43], DSM-5 does not require the patient to acknowledge the irrationality of her/his behavior.

Epidemiological studies suffer from many uncertainties.

In Florida, about 5% of a sample of undergraduate students reported significant emetophobia symptoms [78] and, in El Salvador, about 7.5% [79]. A community-based study on the epidemiology of specific phobia subtypes found lower values: in a sample of young German women, the lifetime prevalence of emetophobia was 0.2% [80].

It is seen in adults as well as in children and adolescents [81, 82].

In 2001, Lipsitz et al. studied 56 participants (50 women, 6 men, mean age 31) in an Internet support group for emetophobia [83]. They found that the symptom generally had an early onset and a chronic course, damaging personal, social, and work life. Depression, panic attacks, eating rituals, and notable limitations in food choices to eat were common.

Emetophobia is related to the experience of disgust [84, 85]. In this regard, two distinct constructs have been proposed:

- Disgust propensity (how quickly the individual experiences disgust)
- Disgust sensitivity (how negatively the individual evaluates disgust).

An Internet-based survey found that disgust sensitivity is a good predictor of emetophobic symptoms [84].

Two psychometric instruments are designed to assess cognitive processes and behaviors that characterize emetophobia:

- The Specific Phobia of Vomiting Inventory (SPOVI), a 14-item self-report measure. It has a two-factor structure: avoidance symptoms and threat monitoring [86].
- The Emetophobia Questionnaire (EmetQ-13), a 13-item self-report scale. It has a three-factor structure: avoidance symptoms, dangerousness of exposure to vomit stimuli, and avoidance of others who may vomit [87].

36.6.1 Emetophobia and Eating Disorders

Fear of vomiting is considered an anxiety disorder (a specific phobia) that can occur alone or associated with other syndromes: avoidant restrictive food intake disorder, anorexia nervosa, other specified feeding and eating disorders, depression, obsessive-compulsive disorder, social anxiety disorder, panic disorder, generalized anxiety disorder, hypochondriasis, and somatization disorder [82, 87–89].

Uncertainties in the use of current diagnostic categories and recourse to multiple diagnoses are inevitable. In particular, people with emetophobia often report abnormal eating behaviors and are underweight in several cases [90].

Garfinkel et al. observed that emetophobia is a symptom that can result in food restriction and weight loss, but the absence of drive for thinness distinguishes this condition from AN [91].

In 1990, Manassis and Kalman described four girls, ranging in age from 9.5 to 15 years, hospitalized for suspected AN [92]. All had lost at least 15% of their body weight, had refused to eat for several weeks, and were severely dehydrated. Nevertheless, AN was ruled out because body image distortion was absent: they denied wanting to lose weight and recognized that they were too thin. In all four patients, an extreme fear of vomiting prevented them from eating regularly. The very sight of food caused intense anxiety. Both the thought of vomiting in solitude and the shame-filled thought of vomiting in public were unbearable. The onset of emetophobia had coincided with a viral disease (in three cases, gastrointestinal). Two girls were diagnosed with over-anxious disorder in childhood. Another was diagnosed with panic disorder with agoraphobia. The last patient "was more difficult to diagnose and was labeled as having query conversion disorder" [92] (p. 549).

Sometimes, after treatment of emetophobia, weight regain unmasks a desire for thinness and fitness and body image concerns [82].

36.6.2 Treatment

Emetophobia is considered challenging-to-treat disorder [93–95].

There is a lack of randomized controlled trials with adequate samples apart from a pilot study with a small sample [96]. This study found that 6 of 12 patients treated with CBT showed improvement compared to only 2 of 12 patients allocated to a waitlist.

Most of the information comes from case reports.

Cases of vomiting phobia treated with hypnosis and brief interventions were reported in the 1970s [97, 98].

In the four cases described by Manassis and Kalman, the fear of vomiting resolved within about 3 months with individual psychotherapy, family counseling, and, in one case, psychotropic medication (imipramine) [92].

The cognitive-behavioral approach (CBT) has treated emetophobia as an anxiety disorder, resulting from a combination of factors [89]:

– General anxiety vulnerability factor
– Tendency to somatize anxiety at the gastrointestinal level
– Exaggerated attention to gastrointestinal symptoms
– Tendency to evaluate nausea in a catastrophic way
– Belief that vomiting is an unacceptable phenomenon
– Avoidance behaviors.

Maak et al. described the case of a girl with emetophobia treated with exposure-based behavioral therapy. The good results were maintained during a 3-year follow-up [99].

Exposure therapy combined with parental education was also used to reintroduce avoided foods in an 8-year-old child with emetophobia and secondary food restriction [81].

Metacognitive therapy—an approach focused on the patient's meta-beliefs about how she/he thinks—gave benefits to three adolescents with emetophobia [100].

Vomiting-related traumatizing experiences are considered crucial. Intrusive imagery—a typical post-traumatic disorder phenomenon—is frequent in the specific phobia of vomiting and significantly related to the phobia severity [93].

In a 46-year-old woman, emetophobia improved durably (3-year follow-up) after a brief trauma-focused treatment (eye movement desensitization and reprocessing, EMDR) [94].

Imagery rescripting (ImRs) is an experiential technique that aims to change intrusive imagery's content and meaning by imagining alternative outcomes for traumatic events. ImRs is used in post-traumatic stress disorder with results comparable to EMDR [101]. ImRs was a component of the intervention in eight patients with emetophobia treated with cognitive-behavior therapy: SPOVI scores improved significantly [95].

In Japan, a traditional treatment, Morita therapy, is also used for emetophobia [102]. This therapeutic and spiritual approach developed by psychiatrist Shoma Morita (1874–1938) has received international interest [103].

As for medications, antianxiety drugs are used in conjunction with psychological interventions [104]. In an adolescent girl with severe emetophobia and dehydration, the slow introduction of foods with high water content and two medications (a selective serotonin reuptake inhibitor and hydroxyzine, a sedating antihistamine) promoted an improvement [105].

36.7 Picky Eating

Selective eating, food neophobia, picky eating, fussy eating, faddy eating, choosy eating, fussy/picky eating, and picky/fussy eating are eight different expressions used, often as synonyms, to describe the habitual tendency to limit the variety and, sometimes, even the quantity of foods eaten.

Food neophobia and picky eating are distinct but intertwined constructs that relate to feeding difficulties and represent child development aspects.

Personality factors, family system dysfunctions, feeding styles, and social and cultural influences play an important role, through caregivers, in the genesis and evolution of these eating patterns [106–108]. For example, exclusive breastfeeding for 6 months seems to reduce the odds of picky eating in early childhood [109].

Clear and shared definitions are missing [110, 111].

Food neophobia is generally used to refer to avoidance of and reluctance to eat new foods. Picky/fussy eating, on the other hand, refers to individuals who reject many foods, both familiar and unfamiliar; eat a very narrow variety of foods; avoid, in particular, vegetables, fruits, and fish; and frequently change food preferences [111]. Food neophobia and picky eating can result in qualitative and quantitative dietary deficiencies [112, 113].

The attempt to design a distinct behavior profile for picky eating in toddlers and children has suggested some characteristics [112, 114]:

- High food fussiness
- Slowness in eating
- Higher satiety responsiveness
- Low enjoyment of food
- Lower intake of vegetables and fish.

A recent systematic review of ten qualitative studies on childhood fussy/picky eating behaviors [111] added knowledge on child characteristics, parent feeding beliefs and practices, and emotional climate at mealtimes.

Adults can also be picky eaters [115, 116].

The study of an adult population found that, compared to non-picky eaters, picky eaters presented [117]:

- Low enjoyment of food
- Disgust sensitivity
- Food neophobia
- Higher obsessive-compulsive disorder symptoms
- Higher depression symptoms.

Psychometric tools can be helpful in the study of picky eating in pediatric age:

- The Child Eating Behaviour Questionnaire [118]
- The Child Feeding Questionnaire [119]
- The Infant and Child Feeding Questionnaire [120].

The Adult Picky Eating Questionnaire was designed for adulthood [121].

As to epidemiology, a meta-analysis calculated that, in children aged ≤30 months, the prevalence of picky eating was 22% [122].

The highest prevalence of picky eating is observed in preschool children. It then appears to decrease. A population-based study of 4018 participants [114] found that the prevalence of picky eating was:

- 26.5% at 18 months of age
- 27.6% at 3 years of age
- 13.2% at 6 years of age.

However, two Chinese studies of healthy preschool (3–7 years) and school-aged (7–12 years) children found that the prevalence of picky eating was, respectively, 54% and 59% [123, 124].

A survey found that in 40% of cases, picky eating lasted more than 2 years [125]. Another cohort study found that male sex, lower birth weight, low parental income, and non-Western maternal ethnicity predicted persistent picky eating [126].

Some studies found that picky eaters under 3–4 years of age are at increased risk of being underweight [127, 112]. Kwon et al. also found that picky eating behaviors are associated with children's negative growth patterns [128]. In the two Chinese surveys already mentioned, picky eating was significantly associated with lower weight and height [123, 124].

In contrast, in one study, picky eating at 5 years was associated with normal weight status at 15 years [129], and another prospective study of 120 children, followed from 2 to 11 years of age, found no significant effect on growth [125].

Several studies mitigate parents' and physicians' concerns because they show that picky eating can be a normal developmental stage without substantial consequences on nutrient intakes [130].

Mak rightly pointed out the risk of turning even non-harmful variants of childhood eating behavior into "picky eating syndrome" and the influence of the market and the medical system in this process [131].

In most children, picky eating is a transient phase, and parents should relax their feeding efforts [132]. Not picky eating but parental pressure to eat during childhood seems to be predictive of disordered eating symptoms in adulthood [133].

It is always necessary to evaluate, together with the feeding behavior, the growth curve, the body composition, the nutritional status, and, above all, the psychic conditions of the child and her/his family.

Epidemiological and clinical discrepancies are mainly related to the lack of a reliable and shared definition of the phenomenon [134].

The new diagnostic category "avoidant/restrictive food intake disorder" (ARFID), introduced in DSM-5 and ICD-11, did not solve diagnostic and clinical problems. ARFID refers to unhealthy eating behaviors that are typically restrictive, but not controlling weight, and not associated with body image issues [135]. Picky eating can be one of ARFID symptoms, but only a subset of picky eaters meet all the criteria for this diagnostic category [136].

36.8 Conclusive Remarks

In the field of human eating behaviors, more or less disturbed, the scientific language uses some diagnostic categories defined quite clearly in the DSM-5 [1] and ICD-11 [2] and, then, a set of expressions and definitions still confused, inconsistent, or not widely accepted.

Such terms refer to feeding or eating behaviors that can have (but do not always have) a significant negative impact on people's physical or psychological well-being.

To speak is to classify. However, definitions need to be clear and shared so that the words used to describe phenomena are useful and allow for comparative research.

The medicalization of life, including the so-called nosologomania [137], is a critical psychiatry problem. Media hype and diagnostic fad are different from genuine disorders [138]. Adding a name is not enough to add knowledge, and coining a neologism is not the same as discovering a new disease.

References

1. American Psychiatric Association DSM-5 Task Force. Diagnostic and statistical manual of mental disorders, DSM-5™. 5th ed. Arlington, VA: American Psychiatric Publishing, Inc.; 2013.
2. World Health Organization. ICD-11, International classification of diseases for mortality and morbidity statistics. Geneva: World Health Organization; 2019. https://icd.who.int/browse11/l-m/en. Accessed 11 Dec 2020.
3. Forney KJ, Crosby RD, Brown TA, Klein KM, Keel PK. A naturalistic, long-term follow-up of purging disorder. Psychol Med. 2020:1–8. https://doi.org/10.1017/S0033291719003982.
4. Sawyer S, Whitelaw M, Le Grange D, et al. Physical and psychological morbidity in adolescents with atypical anorexia nervosa. Pediatrics. 2016;137(4):e20154080. https://doi.org/10.1542/peds.2015-4080.
5. Strand M, Zvrskovec J, Hubel C, Peat CM, Bulik CM, Birgegard A. Identifying research priorities for the study of atypical anorexia nervosa: a Delphi study. Int J Eat Disord. 2020;53(10):1729–38. https://doi.org/10.1002/eat.23358.
6. Terry LL, Vasey PL. Feederism in a woman. Arch Sex Behav. 2011;40(3):639–45. https://doi.org/10.1007/s10508-009-9580-9.
7. Terry LL, Suschinsky KD, Lalumiere ML, Vasey PL. Feederism: an exaggeration of a normative mate selection preference? Arch Sex Behav. 2012;41(1):249–60. https://doi.org/10.1007/s10508-012-9925-7.
8. Obreja LD. Feederism as coercive control: connecting the dots between sexuality and law. Cult Health Sex. 2020;22(11):1207–21. https://doi.org/10.1080/13691058.2019.1668058.
9. Regard M, Landis T. "Gourmand syndrome": eating passion associated with right anterior lesions. Neurology. 1997;48(5):1185–90. https://doi.org/10.1212/wnl.48.5.1185.
10. Gallo M, Gamiz F, Perez-Garcia M, Del Moral RG, Rolls ET. Taste and olfactory status in a gourmand with a right amygdala lesion. Neurocase. 2014;20(4):421–33. https://doi.org/10.1080/13554794.2013.791862.
11. Kurian M, Schmitt-Mechelke T, Korff C, Delavelle J, Landis T, Seeck M. "Gourmand syndrome" in a child with pharmacoresistant epilepsy. Epilepsy Behav. 2008;13(2):413–5. https://doi.org/10.1016/j.yebeh.2008.04.004.
12. Kang E, Lee J, Kim KH, Yun YH. The popularity of eating broadcast: Content analysis of "mukbang" YouTube videos, media coverage, and the health impact of "mukbang" on public. Health Informatics J. 2020;26(3):2237–48. https://doi.org/10.1177/1460458220901360.
13. Strand M, Gustafsson SA. Mukbang and disordered eating: an ethnographic analysis of online eating broadcasts. Cult Med Psychiatry. 2020;44(4):586–609. https://doi.org/10.1007/s11013-020-09674-6.
14. Yun S, Kang H, Lee H. Mukbang- and Cookbang-watching status and dietary life of university students who are not food and nutrition majors. Nutr Res Pract. 2020;14(3):276–85. https://doi.org/10.4162/nrp.2020.14.3.276.
15. Mathieu J. What is pregorexia? J Am Diet Assoc. 2009;109(6):976–9. https://doi.org/10.1016/j.jada.2009.04.021.
16. Cohen D. The worrying world of eating disorder wannabes. BMJ. 2007;335(7618):516. https://doi.org/10.1136/bmj.39328.510880.59.
17. Kenji Tierney R. Bodies steeped in stew: sport, tradition and the bodies of the sumo wrestler. Asia Pac J Sport Soc Sci. 2013;2(3):187–97. https://doi.org/10.1080/21640599.2013.853479.

18. Berglund L, Sundgot-Borgen J, Berglund B. Adipositas athletica: a group of neglected conditions associated with medical risks. Scand J Med Sci Sports. 2011;21(5)
19. Jonnalagadda SS, Skinner R, Moore L. Overweight athlete: fact or fiction? Curr Sports Med Rep. 2004;3(4):198–205. https://doi.org/10.1249/00149619-200408000-00005.
20. Swann C, Moran A, Piggott D. Defining elite athletes: issues in the study of expert performance in sport psychology. Psychol Sport Exerc. 2015;16:3–14. https://doi.org/10.1016/j.psychsport.2014.07.004.
21. Hoshi A, Inaba Y. Risk factors for mortality and mortality rate of sumo wrestlers. Nihon Eiseigaku Zasshi. 1995;50(3):730–6. https://doi.org/10.1265/jjh.50.730.
22. Nishizawa T, Akaoka I, Nishida Y, Kawaguchi Y, Hayashi E. Some factors related to obesity in the Japanese sumo wrestler. Am J Clin Nutr. 1976;29(10):1167–74. https://doi.org/10.1093/ajcn/29.10.1167.
23. Silva AM, Nunes CL, Matias CN, Jesus F, Francisco R, Cardoso M, Santos I, Carraca EV, Silva MN, Sardinha LB, Martins P, Minderico CS. Champ4life study protocol: a one-year randomized controlled trial of a lifestyle intervention for inactive former elite athletes with overweight/obesity. Nutrients. 2020;12(2). https://doi.org/10.3390/nu12020286.
24. Sudi K, Ottl K, Payerl D, Baumgartl P, Tauschmann K, Muller W. Anorexia athletica. Nutrition. 2004;20(7-8):657–61. https://doi.org/10.1016/j.nut.2004.04.019.
25. Tappauf M, Scheer PJ, Trabi T, Dunitz-Scheer M. Anorexia athletica – Sportanorexie. Wenn Sport krank is(s)t. Monatsschrift Kinderheilkunde. 2007;155(6):558–9. https://doi.org/10.1007/s00112-007-1523-8.
26. Smith NJ. Excessive weight loss and food aversion in athletes simulating anorexia nervosa. Pediatrics. 1980;66(1):139–42.
27. Beals KA, Manore MM. The prevalence and consequences of subclinical eating disorders in female athletes. Int J Sport Nutr. 1994;4(2):175–95. https://doi.org/10.1123/ijsn.4.2.175.
28. Sundgot-Borgen J. Risk and trigger factors for the development of eating disorders in female elite athletes. Med Sci Sports Exerc. 1994;26(4):414–9.
29. Garner D, Olmstead M, Polivy J. Development and validation of a multidimensional eating disorder inventory for anorexia nervosa and bulimia. Int J Eat Disord. 1983;1:15–34.
30. American Psychiatric Association. Diagnostic and statistical manual of mental disorders. DSM-III-R (3rd edition revised). Washington, DC: American Psychiatric Association; 1987.
31. Davison KK, Earnest MB, Birch LL. Participation in aesthetic sports and girls' weight concerns at ages 5 and 7 years. Int J Eat Disord. 2002;31(3):312–7. https://doi.org/10.1002/eat.10043.
32. Matejek N, Weimann E, Witzel C, Molenkamp G, Schwidergall S, Bohles H. Hypoleptinaemia in patients with anorexia nervosa and in elite gymnasts with anorexia athletica. Int J Sports Med. 1999;20(7):451–6. https://doi.org/10.1055/s-1999-8834.
33. Sundgot-Borgen J. Nutrient intake of female elite athletes suffering from eating disorders. Int J Sport Nutr. 1993;3(4):431–42. https://doi.org/10.1123/ijsn.3.4.431.
34. Brown K, Yates M, Meenan M, Brown AF. Increased female athlete triad knowledge among collegiate dancers following a brief educational video intervention. J Dance Med Sci. 2020;24(4):161–7. https://doi.org/10.12678/1089-313X.24.4.161.
35. Aserlind AB, Burnweit CA. Spontaneous sternal fracture during labor in a healthy primigravida with female athlete triad: a case report. Case Rep Womens Health. 2020;27:e00213. https://doi.org/10.1016/j.crwh.2020.e00213.
36. Holtzman B, Tenforde AS, Parziale AL, Ackerman KE. Characterization of risk quantification differences using female athlete triad cumulative risk assessment and relative energy deficiency in sport clinical assessment tool. Int J Sport Nutr Exerc Metab. 2019:1–7. https://doi.org/10.1123/ijsnem.2019-0002.
37. Koltun KJ, Williams NI, De Souza MJ. Female Athlete Triad Coalition cumulative risk assessment tool: proposed alternative scoring strategies. Appl Physiol Nutr Metab. 2020:1–8. https://doi.org/10.1139/apnm-2020-0131.
38. Mountjoy M, Sundgot-Borgen J, Burke L, Carter S, Constantini N, Lebrun C, Meyer N, Sherman R, Steffen K, Budgett R, Ljungqvist A, Ackerman K. RED-S CAT. Relative

energy deficiency in sport (RED-S) clinical assessment tool (CAT). Br J Sports Med. 2015;49(7):421–3. https://doi.org/10.1136/bjsports-2015-094873.
39. Tenforde AS, Barrack MT, Nattiv A, Fredericson M. Parallels with the female athlete triad in male athletes. Sports Med. 2016;46(2):171–82. https://doi.org/10.1007/s40279-015-0411-y.
40. De Souza MJ, Koltun KJ, Williams NI. The role of energy availability in reproductive function in the female athlete triad and extension of its effects to men: an initial working model of a similar syndrome in male athletes. Sports Med. 2019;49(Suppl 2):125–37. https://doi.org/10.1007/s40279-019-01217-3.
41. Kraus E, Tenforde AS, Nattiv A, Sainani KL, Kussman A, Deakins-Roche M, Singh S, Kim BY, Barrack MT, Fredericson M. Bone stress injuries in male distance runners: higher modified Female Athlete Triad Cumulative Risk Assessment scores predict increased rates of injury. Br J Sports Med. 2019;53(4):237–42. https://doi.org/10.1136/bjsports-2018-099861.
42. Bonci CM, Bonci LJ, Granger LR, Johnson CL, Malina RM, Milne LW, Ryan RR, Vanderbunt EM. National athletic trainers' association position statement: preventing, detecting, and managing disordered eating in athletes. J Athl Train. 2008;43(1):80–108. https://doi.org/10.4085/1062-6050-43.1.80.
43. American Psychiatric Association. Diagnostic and statistical manual of mental disorders, DSM IVTR, 4th edition, text revised. Washington, DC: American Psychiatric Association; 2000.
44. Turocy PS, DePalma BF, Horswill CA, Laquale KM, Martin TJ, Perry AC, Somova MJ, Utter AC, National Athletic Trainers A. National Athletic Trainers' Association position statement: safe weight loss and maintenance practices in sport and exercise. J Athl Train. 2011;46(3):322–36. https://doi.org/10.4085/1062-6050-46.3.322.
45. Thiel A, Gottfried H, Hesse FW. Subclinical eating disorders in male athletes. A study of the low weight category in rowers and wrestlers. Acta Psychiatr Scand. 1993;88(4):259–65. https://doi.org/10.1111/j.1600-0447.1993.tb03454.x.
46. Lydecker JA, Silverman JA, Grilo CM. Disentangling associations of children's sports participation and compulsive exercise with parenting practices and child disordered eating behavior. J Adolesc Health. 2020; https://doi.org/10.1016/j.jadohealth.2020.04.028.
47. Bar RJ, Cassin SE, Dionne MM. Eating disorder prevention initiatives for athletes: a review. Eur J Sport Sci. 2016;16(3):325–35. https://doi.org/10.1080/17461391.2015.1013995.
48. Stewart TM, Pollard T, Hildebrandt T, Wesley NY, Kilpela LS, Becker CB. The Female Athlete Body project study: 18-month outcomes in eating disorder symptoms and risk factors. Int J Eat Disord. 2019;52(11):1291–300. https://doi.org/10.1002/eat.23145.
49. Dittmer N, Jacobi C, Voderholzer UJJED. Compulsive exercise in eating disorders: proposal for a definition and a clinical assessment. 2018;6(1):42. https://doi.org/10.1186/s40337-018-0219-x.
50. Savidaki M, Demirtoka S, Rodriguez-Jimenez RM. Re-inhabiting one's body: a pilot study on the effects of dance movement therapy on body image and alexithymia in eating disorders. J Eat Disord. 2020;8:22. https://doi.org/10.1186/s40337-020-00296-2.
51. Herbrich L, Pfeiffer E, Lehmkuhl U, Schneider N. Anorexia athletica in pre-professional ballet dancers. J Sports Sci. 2011;29(11):1115–23. https://doi.org/10.1080/02640414.2011.578147.
52. Borgen JS, Corbin CB. Eating disorders among female athletes. Phys Sportsmed. 1987;15(2):88–95. https://doi.org/10.1080/00913847.1987.11709282.
53. Wallet M. Deux cas d'anorexie hystérique. Nouvelle iconographie de la Salpêtrière. 1892:276–80.
54. Farlex Medical Dictionary. Anorexia athletica; 2009. Retrieved December 2-2020 from https://medical-dictionary.thefreedictionary.com/anorexia+athletica
55. McCutcheon R, Nolan A. Chewing and spitting out food—a neglected symptom? Int J Eat Disord. 1995;17(2):197–200. https://doi.org/10.1002/1098-108x(199503)17:2<197::aid-eat2260170214>3.0.co;2-q.
56. Aouad P, Hay P, Soh N, Touyz S. Chew and Spit (CHSP): a systematic review. J Eat Disord. 2016;4(1):23. https://doi.org/10.1186/s40337-016-0115-1.

57. De Zwaan M. Chewing and spitting out food in eating disorder. Int J Psychiatry Clin Pract. 1997;1(1):37–8. https://doi.org/10.3109/13651509709069203.
58. Guarda AS, Coughlin JW, Cummings M, Marinilli A, Haug N, Boucher M, Heinberg LJ. Chewing and spitting in eating disorders and its relationship to binge eating. Eat Behav. 2004;5(3):231–9. https://doi.org/10.1016/j.eatbeh.2004.01.001.
59. American Psychiatric Association, editor. Diagnostic and statistical manual of mental disorders, DSM-IV. 4th ed. Washington, DC: American Psychiatric Association; 1994.
60. Kovacs D, Mahon J, Palmer RL. Chewing and spitting out food among eating-disordered patients. Int J Eat Disord. 2002;32(1):112–5. https://doi.org/10.1002/eat.10073.
61. Mitchell JE, Hatsukami D, Eckert ED, Pyle RL. Characteristics of 275 patients with bulimia. Am J Psychiatry. 1985;142(4):482–5. https://doi.org/10.1176/ajp.142.4.482.
62. Durkin NE, Swanson SA, Crow SJ, Mitchell J, Peterson CB, Crosby R. Re-examination of chewing and spitting behavior: characteristics within and across eating disorder diagnoses. Eat Weight Disord. 2014;19(3):315–20. https://doi.org/10.1007/s40519-013-0090-3.
63. Song YJ, Lee JH, Jung YC. Chewing and spitting out food as a compensatory behavior in patients with eating disorders. Compr Psychiatry. 2015;62:147–51. https://doi.org/10.1016/j.comppsych.2015.07.010.
64. Makhzoumi SH, Guarda AS, Schreyer CC, Reinblatt SP, Redgrave GW, Coughlin JW. Chewing and spitting: a marker of psychopathology and behavioral severity in inpatients with an eating disorder. Eat Behav. 2015;17:59–61. https://doi.org/10.1016/j.eatbeh.2014.12.012.
65. Aouad P, Hay P, Soh N, Touyz S. Prevalence of chew and spit and its relation to other features of disordered eating in a community sample. Int J Eat Disord. 2018;51(8):968–72. https://doi.org/10.1002/eat.22873.
66. Aouad P, Hay P, Soh N, Touyz S, Mannan H, Mitchison D. Chew and spit (CHSP) in a large adolescent sample: prevalence, impact on health-related quality of life, and relation to other disordered eating features. Eat Disord. 2019:1–14. https://doi.org/10.1080/10640266.2019.1695449.
67. Aouad P, Morad A, Hay P, Soh N, Touyz S, Rhodes P. Chew and Spit (CHSP): an interpretative phenomenological analysis (IPA). Eat Behav. 2020;37:101,388. https://doi.org/10.1016/j.eatbeh.2020.101388.
68. Inoue K, Matsubara T, Matsuo K, Watanabe Y. A case of anorexia nervosa with chewing and spitting improved by treatment with selective serotonin reuptake inhibitors. Seishin Shinkeigaku Zasshi. 2015;117(5):327–32.
69. Asher R. Munchausen's syndrome. Lancet. 1951;1(6650):339–41. https://doi.org/10.1016/s0140-6736(51)92313-6.
70. Meadow R. Munchausen syndrome by proxy. The hinterland of child abuse. Lancet. 1977;2(8033):343–5. https://doi.org/10.1016/s0140-6736(77)91497-0.
71. Katz RL, Mazer C, Litt IF. Anorexia nervosa by proxy. J Pediatr. 1985;107(2):247–8.
72. Honjo S. A mother's complaints of overeating by her 25-month-old daughter: a proposal of anorexia nervosa by proxy. Int J Eat Disord. 1996;20(4):433–7. https://doi.org/10.1002/(SICI)1098-108X(199612)20:4<433::AID-EAT12>3.0.CO;2-Z.
73. Sirois F. Anorexia nervosa by proxy: an unusual case. Presse Med. 2011;40(5):547–50. https://doi.org/10.1016/j.lpm.2010.12.007.
74. van Wezel-Meijler G, Wit JM. The offspring of mothers with anorexia nervosa: a high-risk group for undernutrition and stunting? Eur J Pediatr. 1989;149(2):130–5. https://doi.org/10.1007/bf01995864.
75. Russell GF, Treasure J, Eisler I. Mothers with anorexia nervosa who underfeed their children: their recognition and management. Psychol Med. 1998;28(1):93–108.
76. Martini MG, Barona-Martinez M, Micali N. Eating disorders mothers and their children: a systematic review of the literature. Arch Womens Ment Health. 2020;23(4):449–67. https://doi.org/10.1007/s00737-020-01019-x.
77. Cuzzolaro M, Donini LM. Orthorexia nervosa by proxy? Eat Weight Disord. 2016;21(4):549–51. https://doi.org/10.1007/s40519-016-0310-8.

78. Wu MS, Rudy BM, Arnold EB, Storch EA. Phenomenology, clinical correlates, and impairment in emetophobia. J Cogn Psychother. 2015;29(4):356–68. https://doi.org/10.1891/0889-8391.29.4.356.
79. Wu MS, Selles RR, Novoa JC, Zepeda R, Guttfreund D, McBride NM, Storch EA. Examination of the phenomenology and clinical correlates of emetophobia in a sample of salvadorian youths. Child Psychiatry Hum Dev. 2017;48(3):509–16. https://doi.org/10.1007/s10578-016-0677-9.
80. Becker ES, Rinck M, Turke V, Kause P, Goodwin R, Neumer S, Margraf J. Epidemiology of specific phobia subtypes: findings from the Dresden Mental Health Study. Eur Psychiatry. 2007;22(2):69–74. https://doi.org/10.1016/j.eurpsy.2006.09.006.
81. Dosanjh S, Fleisher W, Sam D. I think I'm going to be sick: an eight-year-old boy with emetophobia and secondary food restriction. J Can Acad Child Adolesc Psychiatry. 2017;26(2):104–9.
82. Maertens C, Couturier J, Grant C, Johnson N. Fear of vomiting and low body weight in two pediatric patients: diagnostic challenges. J Can Acad Child Adolesc Psychiatry. 2017;26(1):59–61.
83. Lipsitz JD, Fyer AJ, Paterniti A, Klein DF. Emetophobia: preliminary results of an internet survey. Depress Anxiety. 2001;14(2):149–52. https://doi.org/10.1002/da.1058.
84. van Overveld M, de Jong PJ, Peters ML, van Hout WJ, Bouman TK. An internet-based study on the relation between disgust sensitivity and emetophobia. J Anxiety Disord. 2008;22(3):524–31. https://doi.org/10.1016/j.janxdis.2007.04.001.
85. Verwoerd J, van Hout WJ, de Jong PJ. Disgust- and anxiety-based emotional reasoning in non-clinical fear of vomiting. J Behav Ther Exp Psychiatry. 2016;50:83–9. https://doi.org/10.1016/j.jbtep.2015.05.009.
86. Veale D, Ellison N, Boschen MJ, Costa A, Whelan C, Muccio F, Henry K. Development of an inventory to measure specific phobia of vomiting (emetophobia). Cogn Ther Res. 2013;37(3):595–604. https://doi.org/10.1007/s10608-012-9495-y.
87. Boschen MJ, Veale D, Ellison N, Reddell T. The emetophobia questionnaire (EmetQ-13): psychometric validation of a measure of specific phobia of vomiting (emetophobia). J Anxiety Disord. 2013;27(7):670–7. https://doi.org/10.1016/j.janxdis.2013.08.004.
88. Sykes M, Boschen MJ, Conlon EG. Comorbidity in emetophobia (specific phobia of vomiting). Clin Psychol Psychother. 2016;23(4):363–7. https://doi.org/10.1002/cpp.1964.
89. Boschen MJ. Reconceptualizing emetophobia: a cognitive-behavioral formulation and research agenda. J Anxiety Disord. 2007;21(3):407–19. https://doi.org/10.1016/j.janxdis.2006.06.007.
90. Veale D, Costa A, Murphy P, Ellison N. Abnormal eating behaviour in people with a specific phobia of vomiting (emetophobia). Eur Eat Disord Rev. 2012;20(5):414–8. https://doi.org/10.1002/erv.1159.
91. Garfinkel PE, Kaplan AS, Garner DM, Darby PL. The differentiation of vomiting/weight loss as a conversion disorder from anorexia nervosa. Am J Psychiatry. 1983;140(8):1019–22. https://doi.org/10.1176/ajp.140.8.1019.
92. Manassis K, Kalman E. Anorexia resulting from fear of vomiting in four adolescent girls. Can J Psychiatry. 1990;35(6):548–50. https://doi.org/10.1177/070674379003500614.
93. Price K, Veale D, Brewin CR. Intrusive imagery in people with a specific phobia of vomiting. J Behav Ther Exp Psychiatry. 2012;43(1):672–8. https://doi.org/10.1016/j.jbtep.2011.09.007.
94. de Jongh A. Treatment of a woman with emetophobia: a trauma focused approach. Mental illness. 2012;4(1):e3. https://doi.org/10.4081/mi.2012.e3.
95. Keyes A, Deale A, Foster C, Veale D. Time intensive cognitive behavioural therapy for a specific phobia of vomiting: a single case experimental design. J Behav Ther Exp Psychiatry. 2020;66:101,523. https://doi.org/10.1016/j.jbtep.2019.101523.
96. Riddle-Walker L, Veale D, Chapman C, Ogle F, Rosko D, Najmi S, Walker LM, Maceachern P, Hicks T. Cognitive behaviour therapy for specific phobia of vomiting (Emetophobia): a

pilot randomized controlled trial. J Anxiety Disord. 2016;43:14–22. https://doi.org/10.1016/j.janxdis.2016.07.005.
97. Wijesinghe B. A vomiting phobia overcome by one session of flooding with hypnosis. J Behav Ther Exp Psychiatry. 1974;5(2):169–70. https://doi.org/10.1016/0005-7916(74)90107-4.
98. Ritow JK. Brief treatment of a vomiting phobia. Am J Clin Hypn. 1979;21(4):293–6. https://doi.org/10.1080/00029157.1979.10403986.
99. Maack DJ, Deacon BJ, Zhao M. Exposure therapy for emetophobia: a case study with three-year follow-up. J Anxiety Disord. 2013;27(5):527–34. https://doi.org/10.1016/j.janxdis.2013.07.001.
100. Simons M, Vloet TD. Emetophobia—a metacognitive therapeutic approach for an overlooked disorder. Z Kinder Jugendpsychiatr Psychother. 2018;46(1):57–66. https://doi.org/10.1024/1422-4917/a000464.
101. Boterhoven de Haan KL, Lee CW, Fassbinder E, van Es SM, Menninga S, Meewisse ML, Rijkeboer M, Kousemaker M, Arntz A. Imagery rescripting and eye movement desensitisation and reprocessing as treatment for adults with post-traumatic stress disorder from childhood trauma: randomised clinical trial. Br J Psychiatry. 2020;217(5):609–15. https://doi.org/10.1192/bjp.2020.158.
102. Nakamura M, Kitanishi K. Morita therapy for the treatment of emetophobia: a case report. Asia Pac Psychiatry. 2019;11(1):e12343. https://doi.org/10.1111/appy.12343.
103. Sugg HVR, Richards DA, Frost J. What is morita therapy? The nature, origins, and cross-cultural application of a unique Japanese psychotherapy. J Contemp Psychother. 2020;50(4):313–22. https://doi.org/10.1007/s10879-020-09464-6.
104. Faye AD, Gawande S, Tadke R, Kirpekar VC, Bhave SH. Emetophobia: a fear of vomiting. Indian J Psychiatry. 2013;55(4):390–2. https://doi.org/10.4103/0019-5545.120556.
105. Kannappan A, Middleman AB. Emetophobia: a case of nausea leading to dehydration in an adolescent female. SAGE Open Med Case Rep. 2020;8:2050313X20951335. https://doi.org/10.1177/2050313X20951335.
106. Dovey TM, Staples PA, Gibson EL, Halford JC. Food neophobia and 'picky/fussy' eating in children: a review. Appetite. 2008;50(2-3):181–93. https://doi.org/10.1016/j.appet.2007.09.009.
107. Jacobi C, Agras WS, Bryson S, Hammer LD. Behavioral validation, precursors, and concomitants of picky eating in childhood. J Am Acad Child Adolesc Psychiatry. 2003;42(1):76–84. https://doi.org/10.1097/00004583-200301000-00013.
108. Evans A, Seth JG, Smith S, Harris KK, Loyo J, Spaulding C, Van Eck M, Gottlieb N. Parental feeding practices and concerns related to child underweight, picky eating, and using food to calm differ according to ethnicity/race, acculturation, and income. Matern Child Health J. 2011;15(7):899–909. https://doi.org/10.1007/s10995-009-0526-6.
109. Shim JE, Kim J, Mathai RA, Team SKR. Associations of infant feeding practices and picky eating behaviors of preschool children. J Am Diet Assoc. 2011;111(9):1363–8. https://doi.org/10.1016/j.jada.2011.06.410.
110. Taylor CM, Wernimont SM, Northstone K, Emmett PM. Picky/fussy eating in children: review of definitions, assessment, prevalence and dietary intakes. Appetite. 2015;95:349–59. https://doi.org/10.1016/j.appet.2015.07.026.
111. Wolstenholme H, Kelly C, Hennessy M, Heary C. Childhood fussy/picky eating behaviours: a systematic review and synthesis of qualitative studies. Int J Behav Nutr Phys Act. 2020;17(1):2. https://doi.org/10.1186/s12966-019-0899-x.
112. Tharner A, Jansen PW, Kiefte-de Jong JC, Moll HA, van der Ende J, Jaddoe VW, Hofman A, Tiemeier H, Franco OH. Toward an operative diagnosis of fussy/picky eating: a latent profile approach in a population-based cohort. Int J Behav Nutr Phys Act. 2014;11(14) https://doi.org/10.1186/1479-5868-11-14.
113. Taylor CM, Emmett PM. Picky eating in children: causes and consequences. Proc Nutr Soc. 2019;78(2):161–9. https://doi.org/10.1017/S0029665118002586.
114. Cardona Cano S, Hoek HW, Bryant-Waugh R. Picky eating: the current state of research. Curr Opin Psychiatry. 2015;28(6):448–54. https://doi.org/10.1097/YCO.0000000000000194.

115. Wildes JE, Zucker NL, Marcus MD. Picky eating in adults: results of a web-based survey. Int J Eat Disord. 2012;45(4):575–82. https://doi.org/10.1002/eat.20975.
116. Ellis JM, Zickgraf HF, Galloway AT, Essayli JH, Whited MC. A functional description of adult picky eating using latent profile analysis. Int J Behav Nutr Phys Act. 2018;15(1):109. https://doi.org/10.1186/s12966-018-0743-8.
117. Kauer J, Pelchat ML, Rozin P, Zickgraf HF. Adult picky eating. Phenomenology, taste sensitivity, and psychological correlates. Appetite. 2015;90:219–28. https://doi.org/10.1016/j.appet.2015.03.001.
118. Wardle J, Guthrie CA, Sanderson S, Rapoport L. Development of the children's eating behaviour questionnaire. J Child Psychol Psychiatry. 2001;42(7):963–70. https://doi.org/10.1111/1469-7610.00792.
119. Birch LL, Fisher JO, Grimm-Thomas K, Markey CN, Sawyer R, Johnson SL. Confirmatory factor analysis of the Child Feeding Questionnaire: a measure of parental attitudes, beliefs and practices about child feeding and obesity proneness. Appetite. 2001;36(3):201–10. https://doi.org/10.1006/appe.2001.0398.
120. Silverman AH, Berlin KS, Linn C, Pederson J, Schiedermayer B, Barkmeier-Kraemer J. Psychometric properties of the infant and child feeding questionnaire. J Pediatr. 2020;223:81–86.e82. https://doi.org/10.1016/j.jpeds.2020.04.040.
121. Ellis JM, Galloway AT, Webb RM, Martz DM. Measuring adult picky eating: the development of a multidimensional self-report instrument. Psychol Assess. 2017;29(8):955–66. https://doi.org/10.1037/pas0000387.
122. Cole NC, An R, Lee SY, Donovan SM. Correlates of picky eating and food neophobia in young children: a systematic review and meta-analysis. Nutr Rev. 2017;75(7):516–32. https://doi.org/10.1093/nutrit/nux024.
123. Xue Y, Zhao A, Cai L, Yang B, Szeto IM, Ma D, Zhang Y, Wang P. Growth and development in Chinese pre-schoolers with picky eating behaviour: a cross-sectional study. PLoS One. 2015;10(4):e0123664. https://doi.org/10.1371/journal.pone.0123664.
124. Xue Y, Lee E, Ning K, Zheng Y, Ma D, Gao H, Yang B, Bai Y, Wang P, Zhang Y. Prevalence of picky eating behaviour in Chinese school-age children and associations with anthropometric parameters and intelligence quotient. A cross-sectional study. Appetite. 2015;91:248–55. https://doi.org/10.1016/j.appet.2015.04.065.
125. Mascola AJ, Bryson SW, Agras WS. Picky eating during childhood: a longitudinal study to age 11 years. Eat Behav. 2010;11(4):253–7. https://doi.org/10.1016/j.eatbeh.2010.05.006.
126. Cardona Cano S, Tiemeier H, Van Hoeken D, Tharner A, Jaddoe VW, Hofman A, Verhulst FC, Hoek HW. Trajectories of picky eating during childhood: a general population study. Int J Eat Disord. 2015;48(6):570–9. https://doi.org/10.1002/eat.22384.
127. Ekstein S, Laniado D, Glick B. Does picky eating affect weight-for-length measurements in young children? Clin Pediatr (Phila). 2010;49(3):217–20. https://doi.org/10.1177/0009922809337331.
128. Kwon KM, Shim JE, Kang M, Paik HY. Association between picky eating behaviors and nutritional status in early childhood: performance of a picky eating behavior questionnaire. Nutrients. 2017;9(5) https://doi.org/10.3390/nu9050463.
129. Berger PK, Hohman EE, Marini ME, Savage JS, Birch LL. Girls' picky eating in childhood is associated with normal weight status from ages 5 to 15 y. Am J Clin Nutr. 2016;104(6):1577–82. https://doi.org/10.3945/ajcn.116.142430.
130. Li Z, van der Horst K, Edelson-Fries LR, Yu K, You L, Zhang Y, Vinyes-Pares G, Wang P, Ma D, Yang X, Qin L, Wang J. Perceptions of food intake and weight status among parents of picky eating infants and toddlers in China: a cross-sectional study. Appetite. 2017;108:456–63. https://doi.org/10.1016/j.appet.2016.11.009.
131. Mak VS. How picky eating becomes an illness-marketing nutrient-enriched formula milk in a Chinese society. Ecol Food Nutr. 2017;56(1):81–100. https://doi.org/10.1080/03670244.2016.1261025.
132. Zohar AH, Pick S, Lev-Ari L, Bachner-Melman R. A longitudinal study of maternal feeding and children's picky eating. Appetite. 2020;154:104,804. https://doi.org/10.1016/j.appet.2020.104804.

133. Ellis JM, Galloway AT, Webb RM, Martz DM, Farrow CV. Recollections of pressure to eat during childhood, but not picky eating, predict young adult eating behavior. Appetite. 2016;97:58–63. https://doi.org/10.1016/j.appet.2015.11.020.
134. Brown CL, Vander Schaaf EB, Cohen GM, Irby MB, Skelton JA. Association of picky eating and food neophobia with weight: a systematic review. Child Obes. 2016;12(4):247–62. https://doi.org/10.1089/chi.2015.0189.
135. Kreipe RE, Palomaki A. Beyond picky eating: avoidant/restrictive food intake disorder. Curr Psychiatry Rep. 2012;14(4):421–31. https://doi.org/10.1007/s11920-012-0293-8.
136. Zickgraf HF, Franklin ME, Rozin P. Adult picky eaters with symptoms of avoidant/restrictive food intake disorder: comparable distress and comorbidity but different eating behaviors compared to those with disordered eating symptoms. J Eat Disord. 2016;4(26) https://doi.org/10.1186/s40337-016-0110-6.
137. van Praag HM. Nosologomania: a disorder of psychiatry. World J Biol Psychiatry. 2000;1(3):151–8. https://doi.org/10.3109/15622970009150584.
138. Vandereycken W. Media hype, diagnostic fad or genuine disorder? Professionals' opinions about night eating syndrome, orthorexia, muscle dysmorphia, and emetophobia. Eat Disord. 2011;19(2):145–55. https://doi.org/10.1080/10640266.2011.551634.

CAIS Syndrome and Eating and Weight Disorders

37

Emilia Manzato and Malvina Gualandi

37.1 Definition

Androgen insensitivity syndrome (AIS) represents a spectrum of defects in androgen action due to mutations in the androgen receptor gene (AR), an X-linked recessive genetic disorder.

AIS is typically characterized by evidence of feminization or undermasculinization of the external genitalia at birth, abnormal secondary sexual development in puberty and infertility in individuals with a 46 XY karyotype.

AIS was initially known as "Morris Syndrome" from the name of John McLean Morris, an American gynecologist who, for the first time, described it in 1953 as "testicular feminization" term no longer used [1].

According to the degree of androgen insensitivity, AIS is subdivided into three phenotypes:

- Complete androgen insensitivity syndrome (CAIS), with typical female external genitalia

E. Manzato (✉)
Former University of Ferrara, Eating and Weight Disorders Center "L'Albero",
Private Hospital "Salus", Ferrara, Italy
e-mail: emilia.manzato@gmail.com

M. Gualandi
Former Day Hospital of Internal Medicine and Eating Disorders,
University Hospital S. Anna, Ferrara, Italy
e-mail: malvinagualandi@virgilio.it

- Partial androgen insensitivity syndrome (PAIS) with predominantly female, predominantly male, or ambiguous external genitalia
- Mild androgen insensitivity syndrome (MAIS) with typical male external genitalia

CAIS, the most frequent manifestation of AIS [2], is characterized by a complete resistance to androgens and by a female appearance.

AR gene mutation is found in more than 95% of patients with CAIS: 70% of them have inherited mutations from mothers "carriers" of the genetic disorder, while the remaining 30% are de novo mutations [3].

37.2 CAIS Phenotype

Women with CAIS have a 46 XY karyotype, but a female phenotype, consistent with androgen resistance even if testosterone levels are within or above the male range produced by their abdominal testes [4]. Normally, in presence of a 46 XY karyotype, the sex-determining region Y (SRY) gene situated in Y chromosome will determine, in the embryo-fetal period, the development of functioning testes and absence of female internal genitalia.

Genitalia virilization physiologically occurs between the 8th and 14th week of gestation and is strictly linked to androgen action and AR function. The complete resistance to androgens in CAIS results in female external genitalia because testosterone and dihydrotestosterone, transformed by aromatase into estrogen, determine the development of female sexual characteristics.

On the contrary internal female genitalia are absent because the abdominal testes produce the antimullerian hormone (AMH), which inhibits the development of the uterus, cervix, and proximal vagina. At first observation the individuals with CAIS may present masses in the inguinal canal, subsequently identified as testes. They have primary amenorrhea and sparse or absent pubic or axillary hair. Breasts and female adiposity develop normally. Sexual identity and orientation are typically female and heterosexual.

Gonadectomy before or just after puberty is advised for CAIS individuals to eliminate the risk of testicular tumors. Estrogen replacement therapy is recommended after gonadectomy to prevent symptoms of hypoestrogenism and to maintain secondary sexual features [5].

Final height in CAIS is above normal mean female height, likely due to the action of the growth-controlling gene (GCY) located at the Y chromosome [6].

37.3 Prevalence and Incidence

CAIS is a rare condition but one of the most common causes of disorders of sex development (DSD). Its prevalence ranges from 2:100,000 to 5:100,000 [7] and from 1:20,400 to 1:99,100 [3] depending on the study. The minimal incidence reported is 1:99,000 [8].

37.4 Psychological and Sexual Aspects

Outcome studies have focused on aspects of psychosexual development, especially gender dysphoria and sexual functioning. Conflicting data on gender identity in CAIS patients are reported [9]. Gender change is very rarely described in CAIS, and there are only four cases of gender change in individuals with CAIS [10]. Therefore, gender dysphoria in CAIS is considered truly transgenderism. However, in a long-term outcome study of disorders of sex development (DSDs) including CAIS, it was noted that dissatisfaction with original gender assignment had been underestimated, thus suggesting that gender and sexual counseling should be part of the multidisciplinary service available to individuals with DSDs [5]. Sexual functioning and sexual quality of life demonstrated a less positive outcome in CAIS patients in comparison with normal women [11].

CAIS diagnosis is also reported to be associated with psychological distress, and consequently psychosocial care along with sexual counseling should be an integral part of the management to promote positive adaptation [12]. A study carried out in Sweden in a sample of women with CAIS and gonadal dysgenesis has shown that the subgroup of women with CAIS had a higher risk than controls to satisfy the criteria for a psychiatric disorder specifically for a major depressive episode and obsessive and compulsive disorders [13].

Another interesting but poorly investigated issue in the study of subjects suffering from CAIS is their vulnerability to develop body dissatisfaction (BD).

Only Wisniewski et al. assessed physical and psychosexual status in a sample of 14 subjects (median age 45) with a diagnosis of CAIS, by using a questionnaire and medical examination.

BD was evaluated through a questionnaire with three response options (mainly satisfied, somewhat dissatisfied, mainly dissatisfied) regarding the degree of satisfaction with physical appearance.

The results showed that 57% reported a low degree of BD, while 43% of the sample reported varying degrees of BD both related to physical appearance (such as inadequate body hair, looking younger than actual age, etc.) and linked to the presence of obesity [14].

37.5 The Influence of Androgens on Weight, Metabolism, and Eating Behavior: What Happens in CAIS?

Testosterone determines a permanent imprinting on developing brain areas, functionally linked to hunger and satiety control such as increased size of nuclei involved in regulation of appetite and influences neuronal circuits involved in reward mechanisms and attitudes toward food. In addition, testosterone is involved in the regulation of energy metabolism and body weight. Males have in general a prevalent orexic-orientated attitude, and their metabolism is orientated toward anabolism.

Body composition in men is substantially different from female as testosterone promotes growth of lean mass and suppresses deposition of fat [15, 16]. The impact of altered AR signaling and consequent failure of testosterone action on the development of visceral obesity, insulin resistance, and metabolic syndrome in men is very well established [17, 18].

Dati et al. (2009) investigated body composition and metabolism assessment in a sample of middle-aged patients with CAIS, both with removed and retained testes. The body fat mass had increased in comparison with both female and male controls and high values of total cholesterol and LDL cholesterol, and high values of HOMA-IR (homeostatic model assessment for insulin resistance) were detected. An enhanced rate of obesity, especially in those who had retained testes, was reported [19].

Yang Peng et al. (2018) described the case of a 22-year-old female with CAIS and diabetes.

The authors underlined the role of AR signaling in glucose homeostasis and a link between the disruption of AR signaling and increase of body fat as well as abnormal values of cholesterol (total and LDL-c) and HOMA-IR [20].

37.6 Eating Disorders in CAIS

Eating disorders (EDs) are less frequent in men. This sexual dimorphism appears, according to a wide body of literature, to be mostly related to a two-step process where the organizational effects of a prenatal exposure to maternal and fetal testosterone on brain areas are followed, in puberty, by the activational effect of testosterone. This sequence is thought to produce a protective effect against the occurrence of EDs in males [15, 16].

The androgenic protective effect does not only depend on the hormonal level but also on its receptor sensitivity [21]. Furthermore, masculinization of the brain is also due to a direct expression of SRY region of the Y chromosome which is hormone-independent. This region—involved in testis differentiation and subsequent testosterone secretion—is chiefly expressed in the testes, but, to some extent, it is also expressed in other tissues, e.g., heart, liver, and kidneys, and in certain brain regions such as the hypothalamus and frontal and temporal cortex, therefore influencing the development of male-specific neurobiology and brain function in a direct cell-autonomous manner.

This function, together with others, related, for example, to the growth-controlling region on the long arm of the Y chromosome, is present also in CAIS subjects.

Even if the lack of testosterone action determines a female phenotype, it is not possible to exclude brain masculine modifications as the role of Y chromosome in brain function is not only mediated by hormone secretion [22, 23].

According to Savic, a mixture of "male" and "female" neuronal coding in women with CAIS is observed, but specific behavioral correlates are presently uncertain [24].

The coexistence of CAIS and EDs was reported for the first time by Manzato et al. [25] who described a case of a 22-year-old patient with CAIS and ED. The history of the subject was characterized by previous overweight—BMI was 28.4 at the age of 19 (weight 90 kg, height 1.78 m). Afterward, she followed a restricted diet and practiced compulsive exercise aiming to lose weight.

Data regarding gender differences in the clinical presentation of ED are still highly controversial.

While EDs are considered primarily female disorders, a considerable proportion of ED patients are male, and, in the last 10 years, increased attention has been paid to ED male patients. Research has particularly focused on sex differences regarding the epidemiology and the symptom profile.

In their study in 2009, Striegel-Moore et al. [26] reported that males with EDs used more frequently food restriction and physical hyperactivity as compensatory behaviors rather than purging behaviors (such as self-induced vomiting and use of laxatives), more frequent in female patients.

In a recent review on ED adolescents by Timko et al. [27], few differences between sexes were reported regarding core ED symptoms, patterns of restriction, binging, vomiting, or laxative abuse, but excessive exercise as compensatory behavior was more frequently observed in males. Furthermore, male ED patients were more likely to have a history of overweight prior to ED onset.

Core ED symptoms in females are concerns about body image and drive for thinness, whereas ED males tend to show increased concern with muscularity and shape according to [28, 29].

In our clinical case, risk factors and clinical symptoms are a mixture of risk factors and symptoms typically but not exclusively related to the male sex or the female sex.

For example, a previous overweight was present (risk factor more common in ED male patients than in females), physical hyperactivity was used as compensatory behavior, whereas purging behaviors (more present in ED female patients) were not detected.

The core symptom was the desire for thinness, more typical of females with anorexia nervosa, and no concern about muscularity was present. This behavior worsened over time leading to an episode of restrictive anorexia nervosa. The patient lost 30 kg in 1 1/2 years. Later on she had binge eating episodes and the ED shifted into bulimia nervosa. In this patient self-inducing vomiting or laxative misuse had never been present. The patient reported a severe BD exclusively related to weight gain and to the desire for thinness.

37.7 Sexual Differences of the Brain

This case offers the opportunity to speculate about possible risk factors for EDs and ED clinical picture in a condition where the Y chromosome is present but testosterone is unable to carry out its function. Since EDs are generally considered sex-bound diseases, it is worth briefly remembering a controversial and sensitive question, with important social implications, about the existence of two distinct categories "male brain" or "female brain." Cahill et al. support the hypothesis that sex differences in the brain are present and are the result of a different anatomical structure and/or a functional dimension such as the function of a neurotransmitter. According to this point of view, brains fall into two classes, one typical of males and the other typical of females. The sex bias in the incidence and prevalence of neuropsychiatric disorders (i.e., eating disorders) confirms this hypothesis [30]. However, in a recent large Israeli study by Joela et al., the authors reported MRI analysis of human brain structure concerning most regions of gray and white matter, as well as measures of connectivity, and concluded that human brains are a unique "mosaic" of male and female features. According to the authors, sex differences in brain structure are present, but brains do not fall into two classes but in a "male brain-female brain" continuum [31]. Once sex brain differences had been hypothesized, the research concentrated on the biological steps able to modify the human brain in a prevalently male or prevalently female direction, i.e., the relative role of sex chromosomes and sex steroids (maternal and fetal). As above reported androgens have organizing effects on fetal brain and, during puberty, activated by hormonal cascade. This "paradigm" of sexual differentiation of the brain was coined by Phoenix et al. (1959) and has dominated the view on cerebral sex dimorphism during the last decades [32]. Recently Hammes et al. have affirmed that the concept of "male" and "female" hormones appears to be an oversimplification of a complex biological system of steroid actions where both estrogens and androgens regulate critical biological and pathological processes in both males and females [33]. Furthermore, evidence exists that SRY and/or other genes are directly (and not through testosterone action) involved in sexual dimorphism of the brain. Independent of the masculinizing effects of gonadal secretions, XY and XX brain cells have different patterns of gene expression that influence their differentiation and function without any mediation by gonadal hormones [34]. The relative influence of genes of sexual chromosomes, sex hormones, and external environment in defining sexual differences of the brain is still under debate. CAIS represents a unique model of research in this field as Savic demonstrated in her interesting research. Three biological factors were involved according to the author in the mixture of male and female MRI images found in 16 CAIS subjects compared with samples of normal males and females: testosterone effects, Y chromosome genes, and X-chromosome inactivation escapee genes [24].

37.8 Conclusions

The biological factors possibly underlying the link between CAIS and eating disorders are not clarified. Even though a mixture of "male" and "female" neuronal coding in women with CAIS is observed, specific behavioral correlates are presently uncertain.

Reported data underline the importance of a regular assessment of body composition, metabolic status, and cardiovascular risk in all patients diagnosed with CAIS, regardless of gonadal condition.

It appears to be mandatory to perform a correct diagnostic framework of overweight, BD, and eating behaviors, which are risk factors for ED onset also in CAIS subjects.

References

1. Morris JM. The syndrome of testicular feminization in male pseudohermaphrodites. Am J Obstet Gynecol. 1953;65:1192–211.
2. Hughes IA, Davies JD, Bunch TI, Pasterski V, Mastroyannopoulou K, Macdougall J. Androgen insensitivity syndrome. Lancet. 2012;380:1419–28.
3. Oakes MB, Eyvazzadeh AD, Quint E, Smith YR. Complete androgen insensitivity syndrome- A review. J Pediatr Adolesc Gynecol. 2008;21:305–10.
4. Batista RL. Androgen insensitivity syndrome: a review. Arch Endocrinol Metab. 2018;62(2):227–35.
5. Warne GL. Long-term outcome of disorders of sex development. Sex Dev. 2008;2:268–77.
6. Danilovic DL, Correa PH, Costa EM, Melo KF, Mendonca BB, Arnhold IJ. Height and bone mineral density in androgen insensitivity syndrome with mutations in the androgen receptor gene. Osteoporos Int. 2007;18(3):369–74.
7. Gottlieb B, Trifiro MA (2017) Androgen insensitivity syndrome. In: Adam MP, Ardinger HH, Pagon RA, et al., editors. GeneReviews® [Internet]. Seattle, WA (1993–2020).
8. Boehmer AL, Brinkmann O, Bruggenwirth H, van Assendelft C, Otten BJ, Verleun-Mooijman MC, Niermeijer MF, Brunner HG, Rouwe CW, Waelkens JJ, Oostdijk W, Kleijer WJ, van der Kwast TH, de Vroede MA, Drop SL. Genotype versus phenotype in families with androgen insensitivity syndrome. J Clin Endocrinol Metab. 2001;86:4151–60.
9. Brunner F, Fliegner M, Krupp K, Rall K, Brucker S, Richter-Appelt H. Gender role, gender identity and sexual orientation in CAIS ("XY-women") compared with subfertile and infertile 46, XX women. J Sex Res. 2016;53(1):109–24.
10. Bermúdez de la Vega JA, Fernández-Cancio M, Bernal S, Audí L. Complete androgen insensitivity syndrome associated with male gender identity or female precocious puberty in the same family. Sex Dev. 2015;9(2):75–9.
11. Petroli RJ, Hiort O, et al. Functional impact of novel androgen receptor mutations on the clinical manifestation of androgen insensitivity syndrome. Sex Dev. 2018;11:238–47.
12. D'Alberton F, Assante MT, Foresti M, Balsamo A, Bertelloni S, Dati E, et al. Quality of life and psychological adjustment of women living with 46,XY differences of sex development. J Sex Med. 2015;12(6):1440–9.
13. Engberg H, et al. Increased psychiatric morbidity in women with complete androgen insensitivity syndrome or complete gonadal dysgenesis. J Psychosom Res. 2017;101:122–7.
14. Wisniewski AB, et al. Complete androgen insensitivity syndrome: long-term medical, surgical, and psychosexual outcome. J Clin Endocrinol Metab. 2000;85(8):2664–9.
15. Lombardo MV, Ashwin E, Auyeung B, et al. Fetal programming effects of testosterone on the reward system and behavioral approach tendencies in humans. Biol Psychiatry. 2012;72:839–47.
16. Culbert KM, Breedlove SM, Sisk CL, et al. The emergence of sex differences in risk for disordered eating attitudes during puberty: a role for prenatal testosterone exposure. J Abnorm Psychol. 2013;122:420–32.
17. Yu IC, Lin HY, Sparks JD, Yeh S, Chang C. Androgen receptor roles in insulin resistance and obesity in males: the linkage of androgen-deprivation therapy to metabolic syndrome. Diabetes. 2014;63(10):3180–8. https://doi.org/10.2337/db13-1505.
18. Zitzmann M. Testosterone deficiency, insulin resistance and the metabolic syndrome. Nat Rev Endocrinol. 2009;5:673–81.1,2, 15–18.
19. Dati E, Baroncelli GI, Mora S, Russo G, Baldinotti F, Parrini D, Erba P, Simi P, Bertelloni S. Body composition and metabolic profile in women with complete androgen insensitivity syndrome. Sex Dev. 2009;3:188–93.
20. Yang P, Liu X, Gao J, Qu S, Zhang M. Complete androgen insensitivity syndrome in a young woman with metabolic disorder and diabetes: a case report. Medicine (Baltimore). 2018;97(33):e11353. https://doi.org/10.1097/MD.0000000000011353.

21. Morford JJ, Wu S, Mauvais-Jarvis F. The impact of androgen actions in neurons on metabolic health and disease. Mol Cell Endocrinol. 2018;465:92–102. https://doi.org/10.1016/j.mce.2017.09.001. Epub 2017 Sep 4.
22. Arnold AP, Xu J, Grisham W, Chen X, Kim YH, Minireview IY. Sex chromosomes and brain sexual differentiation. Endocrinology. 2004;145(3):1057–62. https://doi.org/10.1210/en.2003-1491.
23. Kopsida E, Stergiakouli E, Lynn PM, Wilkinson LS, Davies W. The role of the Y chromosome in brain function. Open Neuroendocrinol J (Online). 2009;2:20–30. https://doi.org/10.2174/1876528900902010020.
24. Savic I, Frisen L, Manzouri A, Nordenstrom A, Lindén Hirschberg A. Role of testosterone and Y chromosome genes for the masculinization of the human brain. Hum Brain Mapp. 2017;38(4):1801–14. https://doi.org/10.1002/hbm.23483.
25. Manzato E, Gualandi M, Roncarati E. Complete androgen insensitivity syndrome (CAIS) and eating disorders: a case report. Eat Weight Disord. 2020; https://doi.org/10.1007/s40519-020-01069-1.
26. Striegel-Moore R, et al. Gender difference in the prevalence of eating disorder symptoms. Int J Eat Disord. 2009;42:471–4.
27. Timko CA, et al. Sex differences in adolescent anorexia and bulimia nervosa: beyond the signs and symptoms. Curr Psychiatry Rep. 2020;21(1):1. https://doi.org/10.1007/s11920-019-0988-1.
28. Rizk M, et al. Physical activity in eating disorders: a systematic review. Nutrients. 2020;12:183. https://doi.org/10.3390/nu12010183.
29. Cooper M, et al. Muscle dysmorphia: a systematic and meta-analytic review of the literature to assess diagnostic validity. Int J Eat Disord. 2020;53:1583–604.
30. Cahill L. Why sex matters for neuroscience. Nature reviews. Neuroscience. 2006;7(6):477–84. https://doi.org/10.1038/nrn1909.
31. Joel D, Tavor Berman Z, et al. Sex beyond the genitalia: the human brain mosaic. Proc Natl Acad Sci U S A. 2015;112(50):15,468–73. https://doi.org/10.1073/pnas.1509654112.
32. Phoenix CH, Goy RW, Gerall AA, Young WC. Organizing action of prenatally administered testosterone propionate on the tissues mediating mating behaviour in the female guinea pig. Endocrinology. 1959;65:369–82.
33. Hammes S, Levin E. Impact of estrogens in males and androgens in females. J Clin Invest. 2019;129(5):1818–26. https://doi.org/10.1172/JCI125.
34. Dewing P, Chiang C, Sinchak K, Sim H, Fernagut P-O, Kelly S, Chesselet M-F, Micevych P, Albrecht K, Harley V, Vilain E. Direct regulation of adult brain function by the male-specific factor SRY. Curr Biol. 2006;16:415–20. https://doi.org/10.1016/j.cub.2006.01.017.

DIE SCHÖNE APOTHEKERIN